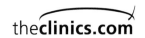

SURGICAL CLINICS
OF NORTH AMERICA

Trauma Care Today

GUEST EDITOR
Ronald V. Maier, MD

CONSULTING EDITOR
Ronald F. Martin, MD

February 2007 • Volume 87 • Number 1

SAUNDERS

An Imprint of Elsevier, Inc.
PHILADELPHIA   LONDON   TORONTO   MONTREAL   SYDNEY   TOKYO

W.B. SAUNDERS COMPANY
A Division of Elsevier Inc.

1600 John F. Kennedy Blvd., Suite 1800, Philadelphia, PA 19103-2899

http://www.theclinics.com

SURGICAL CLINICS OF NORTH AMERICA
February 2007
Editor: Catherine Bewick

Volume 87, Number 1
ISSN 0039–6109
ISBN-13: 978-1-4160-4369-0
ISBN-10: 1-4160-4369-1

Reprints. For copies of 100 or more of articles in this publication, please contact the commercial Reprints Department Elsevier Inc., 360 Park Avenue South, New York, New York 10010-1710. Tel. (212) 633-3813, Fax: (212) 462-1935, email: reprints@elsevier.com

The ideas and opinions expressed in *The Surgical Clinics of North America* do not necessarily reflect those of the Publisher. The Publisher does not assume any responsibility for any injury and/or damage to persons or property arising out of or related to any use of the material contained in this periodical. The reader is advised to check the appropriate medical literature and the product information currently provided by the manufacturer of each drug to be administered to verify the dosage, the method and duration of administration, or contraindications. It is the responsibility of the treating physician or other health care professional, relying on independent experience and knowledge of the patient, to determine drug dosages and the best treatment for the patient. Mention of any product in this issue should not be construed as endorsement by the contributors, editors, or the Publisher of the product or manufacturers' claims.

Surgical Clinics of North America (ISSN 0039–6109) is published bimonthly by Elsevier Inc., 360 Park Avenue South, New York, NY 10010-1710. Months of publication are February, April, June, August, October, and December. Business and Editorial Offices: 1600 John F. Kennedy Blvd., Suite 1800, Philadelphia, PA 19103-2899. Customer Service Office: 6277 Sea Harbor Drive, Orlando, FL 32887-4800. Periodicals postage paid at New York, NY and additional mailing offices. Subscription prices are $220.00 per year for US individuals, $347.00 per year for US institutions, $110.00 per year for US students and residents, $270.00 per year for Canadian individuals, $424.00 per year for Canadian institutions, $286.00 for international individuals, $424.00 per year for international institutions and $143.00 per year for Canadian and foreign students/residents. To receive student/resident rate, orders must be accompanied by name of affiliated institution, date of term, and the *signature* of program/residency coordinator on institution letterhead. Orders will be billed at individual rate until proof of status is received. Foreign air speed delivery is included in all *Clinics* subscription prices. All prices are subject to change without notice. POSTMASTER: Send address changes to *Surgical Clinics*, Elsevier Periodicals Customer Service, 6277 Sea Harbor Drive, Orlando, FL 32887-4800. **Customer Service: 1-800-654-2452 (US). From outside of the US, call 1-407-345-1000.**

The Surgical Clinics of North America is also published in Spanish by McGraw-Hill Interamericana Editores S.A., P.O. Box 5-237 06500 Mexico D.F. Mexico; and in Portuguese by Interlivros Edicoes Ltda., Rua Comandante Coelho 1085, CEP 21250, Rio de Janeiro, Brazil; and in Greek by Paschalidis Medical Publications, Athens Greece.

The Surgical Clinics of North America is covered in *Index Medicus, EMBASE/Excerpta Medica, Current Contents/Clinical Medicine, Current Contents/Life Sciences, Science Citation Index,* and *ISI/BIOMED*.

Printed in the United States of America.

CONSULTING EDITOR

RONALD F. MARTIN, MD, Staff Surgeon, Marshfield Clinic, Marshfield, Wisconsin; Lieutenant Colonel, Medical Corps, United States Army Reserve

GUEST EDITOR

RONALD V. MAIER, MD, FACS, Jane and Donald D. Trunkey Professor of Surgery, University of Washington; Surgeon-in-Chief, Harborview Medical Center, Seattle, Washington

CONTRIBUTORS

HASAN B. ALAM, MD, Associate Professor of Surgery, Department of Surgery; Director of Research, Division of Trauma, Emergency Surgery, and Surgical Critical Care, Massachusetts General Hospital, Boston, Massachusetts

CARLOS ARREOLA-RISA, MD, Professor and Surgeon, Department of Surgery; Director, Injury Prevention and Emergency Medicine Program, TEC de Monterrey School of Medicine, Monterrey, Mexico

ALEC C. BEEKLEY, MD, FACS, Trauma Medical Director, Staff General Surgeon, Major, United States Army Medical Corps, Madigan Army Medical Center, Tacoma, Washington

EILEEN M. BULGER, MD, Associate Professor of Surgery, Department of Surgery, University of Washington, Harborview Medical Center, Seattle, Washington

TAMMY T. CHANG, MD, PhD, Resident, Department of Surgery, University of California, San Francisco, California

RANDALL M. CHESNUT, MD, FCCM, FACS, Associate Professor of Neurosurgery and Orthopaedics, University of Washington, Harborview Medical Center, Seattle, Washington

RAUL COIMBRA, MD, PhD, Professor of Surgery and Chief, Division of Trauma, Burns and Critical Care, Department of Surgery, University of California, San Diego School of Medicine, San Diego, California

TIMOTHY C. FABIAN, MD, FACS, Harwell Wilson Alumni Professor and Chairman, Department of Surgery, University of Tennessee Health Science Center, Memphis, Tennessee

MARY E. FALLAT, MD, Professor of Surgery and Director, Division of Pediatric Surgery, Department of Surgery, University of Louisville, Louisville, Kentucky

NICOLE S. GIBRAN, MD, Professor, Department of Surgery; Director, University of Washington Burn Center, Harborview Medical Center, Seattle, Washington

J. JASON HOTH, MD, Assistant Professor, Department of General Surgery, Wake Forest University School of Medicine, Winston-Salem, North Carolina

DAVID B. HOYT, MD, FACS, John Connolly Professor of Surgery and Chairman, Department of Surgery, University of California, Irvine School of Medicine, Orange, California

MANJUL JOSHIPURA, MD, Director, Academy of Traumatology, Ahmedebad, India

GREGORY J. JURKOVICH, MD, Professor of Surgery, University of Washington, Seattle; Chief of Trauma, Harborview Medical Center, Seattle, Washington

RONALD V. MAIER, MD, FACS, Jane and Donald D. Trunkey Professor of Surgery, University of Washington; Surgeon-in-Chief, Harborview Medical Center, Seattle, Washington

KIM G. MENDELSON, MD, PhD, Pediatric Surgery Resident, Division of Pediatric Surgery, Department of Surgery, University of Louisville, Louisville, Kentucky

J. WAYNE MEREDITH, MD, Richard T. Myers Professor and Chairman, Department of General Surgery, Director of Division of Surgical Sciences, Wake Forest University School of Medicine; Chief of Surgery, Wake Forest University Baptist Medical Center, Winston-Salem, North Carolina

CHARLES MOCK, MD, PhD, Professor of Surgery, University of Washington, Seattle; and Director, Harborview Injury Prevention and Research Center, Harborview Medical Center, Seattle, Washington

TAM N. PHAM, MD, Surgical Critical Care Fellow, University of Washington Burn Center, Department of Surgery, Harborview Medical Center, Seattle, Washington

ROBERT QUANSAH, MD, PhD, Senior Lecturer, Department of Surgery, Kwame Nkrumah University of Science and Technology, Kumasi, Ghana

PETER RHEE, MD, MPH, Captain, MC, United States Navy; Professor of Surgery and Molecular Cellular Biology, Navy Trauma Training Center, University of Southern California, Los Angeles, California

WILLIAM P. SCHECTER, MD, Professor, Clinical Surgery, Department of Surgery, University of California, San Francisco, California

JAMES A. SEBESTA, MD, FACS, Chief of Bariatric Surgery, Staff General Surgeon, Major, United States Army Medical Corps, Madigan Army Medical Center, Tacoma, Washington

BENJAMIN W. STARNES, MD, FACS, Chief of Endovascular Surgery, Staff Vascular Surgeon, Lieutenant Colonel, United States Army Medical Corps, Madigan Army Medical Center, Tacoma, Washington

CONTENTS

Foreword   xi
Ronald F. Martin

Preface   xv
Ronald V. Maier

Advancing Injury Prevention and Trauma Care
in North America and Globally   1
Charles Mock, Manjul Joshipura, Robert Quansah, and
Carlos Arreola-Risa

> Injury is a major global health problem. This article reviews ways
> in which the toll from injury can be lowered through the spectrum
> of injury control, including surveillance, prevention, and trauma
> care. There is room for improvement in the application of scientifi-
> cally based, proved interventions at all points in the spectrum in all
> countries. The greatest attention is needed in low- and middle-
> income countries, however, where most of the world's people live,
> where injury rates are higher, and where few injury control activ-
> ities have yet been undertaken.

Trauma Systems   21
David B. Hoyt and Raul Coimbra

> The major goal of a trauma system is to enhance the community
> health. This occurs through a process of assessment, policy devel-
> opment, and ongoing assurance. This can be achieved by (1) iden-
> tifying risk factors in the community and creating solutions to
> decrease the incidence of injury, (2) providing optimal care during
> the acute and the late phase of injury, including rehabilitation, and
> (3) maintaining the objective to decrease overall injury-related mor-
> bidity and mortality and years of life lost. Disaster preparedness

also is an important function of trauma systems, and using an established trauma system network facilitates the care of victims of natural disasters or terrorist attacks.

Prehospital Care of the Injured: What's New   37
Eileen M. Bulger and Ronald V. Maier

Emergency medical services (EMS) play a critical role in the trauma system as the point of initial patient care and stabilization and in determining the regional flow of patients and the commitment of resources to the critically injured. Trauma surgeons and emergency physicians need to be involved in the organizational planning of EMS systems to ensure that uniform patient care protocols are developed for triage and treatment. Ongoing efforts should focus on addressing national variability in care provided after injury to ensure optimal outcome for patients in all regions. Through additional research, the best practice and optimal EMS system design will continue to be defined.

New Developments in Fluid Resuscitation   55
Hasan B. Alam and Peter Rhee

Hemorrhagic shock is the leading cause of death in civilian and military trauma. Effective hemorrhage control and optimal resuscitation are the main goals in the management of severely injured patients. This article addresses the changing trends in fluid resuscitation in regards to who, when, and how. Much of these changing trends are caused by the recognition that the current method of resuscitation with crystalloid fluids may not be optimal and may even have detrimental consequences. This article summarizes a number of studies that have evaluated the cellular toxicities of commonly used resuscitation fluids, to highlight the need for the development of new fluids.

Damage Control in Trauma: Laparotomy Wound Management
Acute to Chronic   73
Timothy C. Fabian

Damage control surgery is fundamental to operative trauma care. Prophylactic application of open abdomen techniques has led to avoidance of a great deal of the organ dysfunction associated with abdominal compartment syndrome. Surgeons are learning about management of large open abdominal wounds. There seems to be a general consensus regarding acute management of these wounds. Institutions are using staged techniques of management. Getting open wounds closed as soon as possible leads to fewer complications. The acute use of vacuum wound may provide for early secondary closure. There is less study focused on optimal definitive reconstructive techniques. Further study in all of these areas will lead to improved outcomes.

Thoracic Trauma: When and How to Intervene   95
J. Wayne Meredith and J. Jason Hoth

> Trauma is the leading cause of death in patients younger than
> 40 years of age. Thoracic injuries are common and often can be
> managed by tube thoracostomy. In many patients, however,
> the thoracic injuries must be repaired surgically in one of three time
> periods: immediate, urgent, or delayed thoracotomy. In this article,
> we describe the general approach to effectively managing thoracic
> trauma patients. We review common injuries and scenarios that
> may be encountered by the surgeon and discuss the considerations
> and variables that enter into the decision-making process for
> operative intervention.

Care of Central Nervous System Injuries   119
Randall M. Chesnut

> The primary method of improving outcome from traumatic brain
> injury is through avoiding secondary insults to the injured brain.
> Although surgery is important, most management is critical care.
> Evidence-based guidelines continue to be developed to assist in
> directing care. With modern monitoring systems, a physiologic-
> based approach is increasingly applicable, allowing focused treat-
> ment for intracranial hypertension and ischemia. It is important
> to balance and integrate the care of the injured brain into the over-
> all care of the polytrauma patient.

Lessons Learned from Modern Military Surgery   157
Alec C. Beekley, Benjamin W. Starnes, and James A. Sebesta

> The era of global terrorism and asymmetric warfare heralded by
> the September 11, 2001 attacks on the United States have blurred
> the traditional lines between civilian and military trauma. The
> lessons learned by physicians in the theaters of war, particularly
> regarding the response to mass casualties, blast and fragmentation
> injuries, and resuscitation of casualties in austere environments,
> likely resonate strongly with civilian trauma surgeons in the
> current era. The evolution of a streamlined trauma system in the
> theaters of operations, the introduction of an in-theater institution
> review board process, and dedicated personnel to collect combat
> casualty data have resulted in improved data capture and real-
> time, on-the-scene research.

Thermal and Electrical Injuries   185
Tam N. Pham and Nicole S. Gibran

> Through progress in wound management, resuscitation, intensive
> care treatment, and a coordinated rehabilitation process, modern
> burn care has been able to deliver substantial increases in survival
> and improvement in functional outcomes for burn victims. The

development of regionalized burn centers has contributed greatly to this progress. As the field of burns matures, burn centers are preparing to meet future challenges through collaborative efforts in disaster management and outcomes research.

Pediatric Injuries: Prevention to Resolution   207
Kim G. Mendelson and Mary E. Fallat

Despite improved education and prevention initiatives, trauma remains the leading cause of death in children. A variety of preventative measures have been developed to decrease the morbidity and mortality, and the financial burden on the health care system. This article discusses injury prevention strategies, issues in prehospital care, and key points of initial resuscitation. In addition, the major injury patterns are described with attention paid to the diagnosis and management of patients with multiple traumatic injuries.

Injury in the Elderly and End-of-Life Decisions   229
Tammy T. Chang and William P. Schecter

The elderly constitute the fastest growing sector of the population of the United States and geriatric trauma patients are presenting for care with increasing frequency. These patients are challenging particularly because of their vulnerability to severe injury, limited physiologic response to stress, and frequent presence of comorbid medical conditions complicating care. Many elderly trauma victims require prolonged intensive care and some fail to improve or succumb despite the best efforts because of the extent of their injuries and their underlying disease. These patients may present profound ethical challenges for trauma surgeons as the goals of care shift from salvage to end-of-life care.

Environmental Cold-Induced Injury   247
Gregory J. Jurkovich

More than 650 deaths from hypothermia occur each year in the United States. Even minor deviation from normal temperature leads to important symptoms and disability. The most significant risk factors are advanced age, mental impairment, substance abuse, and injury. This article examines the incidence of hypothermia, its detrimental effect on trauma patients, and methods of rewarming the hypothermic patient. It also looks at the controversial protective role hypothermia might play in shock, organ transplantation, cardiac arrest, and brain injury. Finally, it examines cold injuries, including frostbite, chilblain, and trench foot, and makes recommendations for their treatment.

Index   269

FORTHCOMING ISSUES

April 2007
   Breast Disorders
   Lisa Newman, *Guest Editor*

June 2007
   Inflammatory Bowel Disease
   Joseph Cullen, MD, *Guest Editor*

RECENT ISSUES

December 2006
   Critical Care for the General Surgeon
   Juan Carlos Puyana, MD, and Matthew R. Rosengart, MD, MPH,
   Guest Editors

October 2006
   Topics in Organ Transplantation for General Surgeons
   Paul Morrissey, MD, *Guest Editor*

August 2006
   **Recent Advances in the Management of Benign
   and Malignant Colorectal Diseases**
   Robin P. Boushey, MD, PhD,
   and Patricia L. Roberts, MD, *Guest Editors*

June 2006
   Surgical Response to Disaster
   Robert M. Rush, Jr, MD, *Guest Editor*

April 2006
   Current Practice in Pediatric Surgery
   Mike K. Chen, MD, *Guest Editor*

February 2006
   Evidence-Based Surgery
   Jonathan Meakins, MD and Muir Gray, MD, *Guest Editors*

The Clinics are now available online!

www.theclinics.com

SURGICAL
CLINICS OF
NORTH AMERICA

Surg Clin N Am 87 (2007) xi–xiv

Foreword

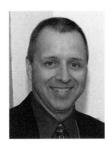

Ronald F. Martin, MD
Consulting Editor

It is said that where one stands depends upon where one sits. This is particularly true in the care of the traumatized patient. I can think of no other aspect of medical care that so well illustrates the problems of the modern meta-stable industry of health care delivery. To me the fundamental question of modern medicine in the United States is whether we are a private industry or a public utility—maybe even a fundamental right. I do not consider myself an ardent socialist or capitalist, although my participation in our profession most likely means I am a little of both. I do, however, very much consider myself a realist. And the realistic and pragmatic side of me is quite convinced that our current system of trauma care is unsustainable.

Society has an expectation that medical care for traumatic events will be available by some means. And it is expected that this situation will exist independent of society's ability to underwrite the cost of its care either privately or by third party payers. This expectation of course extends to all persons who become acutely ill but it is somewhat more dramatically displayed in the trauma population. Society has some fundamentally sound reasons to maintain this belief. Taxpayers and their elected governments provide prehospital emergency medical services, equipment, and personnel. Communities may have responders of varying levels of training and expertise; they may use full-time, part-time or volunteer personnel, and may have shared arrangements for the use of equipment. Certainly all the prehospital care services provided, independent of level of sophistication, will likely fall short without hospitals to accept the injured patients.

doi:10.1016/j.suc.2006.11.001   *surgical.theclinics.com*

Although hospitals do derive some economic support and service benefit from communities and various levels of government, the support is generally far short of the costs incurred by these institutions. There are some situations in which trauma care is profitable to the institution but there are many whereby the cost is an enormous strain on its financial survival.

The American College of Surgeons, through its commendable support of Advanced Trauma Life Support training efforts and its verified trauma center review process, has made tremendous strides in improving the care delivered to our injured fellow citizens. The American College of Surgeons, though however important, is not an elected body by the people and is not an established organ of government. Neither fellowship in the college nor participation in any of its programs is mandatory for any surgeon, let alone any trauma surgeon. And whereas voluntary acceptance and adherence to the espoused principles of the American College of Surgeons committee on trauma has improved trauma care substantially, it will unlikely carry us the rest of the distance.

Our current model of trauma care and interfacility transfer patterns by necessity requires more people to be available to handle surge capacity than one can optimally employ during more average workloads. When the percentage difference in resource requirements between peak surge and optimal efficiency is low, most systems can absorb the economic impact. As that percentage increases, the impact varies from detrimental to unsustainable. In part this is because trauma care at the physician and hospital level is reimbursed on a piecework basis whereas the readiness requirement follows a "firefighter" model. Firefighters are not paid to put out fires so much as they are compensated for their availability and willingness to put out fires. If we were to develop the practice of paying firefighters only to put fires out, we would run the risks of encouraging arson or inhibiting fire prevention, or possibly have inadequate numbers of people available to fight fires. (Let me state that by no means do I wish to suggest that firefighters would do any such thing. I have the utmost respect and admiration for their profession and use this example for the sole purpose of metaphor. Also, in many places fire and rescue responders are the prehospital trauma care support personnel —another reason to include them in this discussion). Because injury prevention and community education are part of our overall trauma project— another largely nonreimbursed effort—we find ourselves, rightfully, trying to put ourselves out of business. Ironically, we serve the public's interest to the degree to which we can keep ourselves unemployed.

The financial strains of trauma care systems coupled with the success in improvements in care of the traumatized patient have created a new— though maybe not so terribly new—problem for us as surgeons: the surgeon who feels that his operative volume and experience is suboptimal to maintain proficiency. One report suggested that many "trauma surgeons" working in level I trauma centers performed less than one laparotomy per week. This volume of operative experience was thought to be suboptimal for maintenance of technical proficiency. I agree. One solution is the development or widespread adoption of the "acute care surgery" model. There are certainly pros and cons to that approach. On the pro side it would likely yield a greater operative volume to the surgeon in question. On the con side it would not yield a higher volume of trauma-related cases. Furthermore because the science of trauma is really about the applied knowledge of the consequences of damaging levels of kinetic energy being transmitted to an unsuspecting patient, there is not necessarily a reason to believe that the acute care surgeon would have particular adeptness at managing nontraumatic acute care problems. Simply because a patient presents nonelectively does not imply what type of specialty trained physician the patient would benefit from most. It may be possible to suggest that if the modern trauma surgeon does so few laparotomies that he or she is volume-deficient for operative proficiency. Then, perhaps, we should have "abdominal surgeons" consulted for operative care of these patients as we frequently do for patients requiring the expertise of orthopedic surgeons, neurosurgeons, plastic and reconstructive surgeons, and so forth.

The modern era has also added a new wrinkle to the debate of emergency service—disaster preparedness. We have addressed this topic in some detail in our June 2006 issue of the *Surgical Clinics of North America*. Certainly the kind of surge capacity needed to manage a large-scale disaster could potentially dwarf any of the aforementioned concerns, yet the components of the dilemma are identical: resource allocation, surge capacity, and availability of expertise. Declared disasters are generally accompanied by some governmental or societal funding to help mitigate the costs of response, but the ongoing "slow disaster" that has evolved in terms of trauma and emergent care will unlikely be recognized in such terms by the public or their duly elected and appointed officials.

As I conclude this foreword I realize that its content may well irritate, if not infuriate, some of our colleagues. I would like to think that it will be read as a call to collectively address a huge societal problem rather than an attempt to fuel an already bitter "turf war." You, the reader, will have to decide how you see it. I have had the opportunity to care for traumatized patients both as attending of record and consultant, as private solo practitioner and as a member of a large group, as well as chief of surgery of a Combat Support Hospital in an active shooting war; the problems and the issues have always been similar in each of those environments: difficult systems issues, appropriate matching of skill sets to problems, distribution of finances and resources, and integration of new technology and understanding. Dr Maier and his colleagues have done an outstanding job of summarizing the scientific basis of trauma care and the concept of systems. We as general surgeons need to address these issues among ourselves and force hospital systems and government as well as third party payers to address the logistical and financial considerations previously alluded to. This topic is too important to leave unresolved. We need to definitively establish whether we are a private industry, a public utility, or a right or entitlement. Internal cost shifting and turf battles are analogous to the rearranging of deck chairs on the *Titanic*. The future of the rest of medical care may depend upon how this debate is conducted and resolved. Each of us should try our best to get it right.

Ronald F. Martin, MD
Department of Surgery
Marshfield Clinic
1000 North Oak Avenue
Marshfield, WI 54449, USA

E-mail address: martin.ronald@marshfieldclinic.org

ELSEVIER
SAUNDERS

Surg Clin N Am 87 (2007) xv–xvi

SURGICAL
CLINICS OF
NORTH AMERICA

Preface

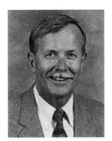

Ronald V. Maier, MD
Guest Editor

Optimal care of the injured patient continues to evolve. Seemingly well established and defined protocols and approaches to care have come under scrutiny and debate and, ultimately, driven by evidence-based data, are redefined. As in the past, many of these changes in approach to the injured patient occur in response to the knowledge gained from military conflicts. Also, it is becoming increasingly evident that "the world is flat," not only from a global economic perspective, but from a medical care initiative as well. The challenges we face in the care of the injured patient bring us all closer together. This issue of the *Surgical Clinics of North America* provides an update of knowledge in the care of the injured, and presents the latest approaches to trauma care for our global habitat. It is evident that we must continue to investigate, test, and evolve to reach the best approach to the care of the injured patient.

The current issue contains a carefully selected, broad spectrum of articles from leaders in the field, including those recently returned from military deployment, to update the surgical practitioner. Documentation continues to indicate that prevention is the most efficacious approach to lessening the impact of trauma in America. The global challenge of the injury epidemic and the importance of improvements in injury care and prevention throughout the world are increasingly recognized. The struggle for trauma system development, the threat of inadequate support, the lack of stability in infrastructure, and the challenge of maintaining the balance between inclusivity and exclusivity while optimizing standards of care, remain significant threats to advances in trauma care. The entire gamut of injury is

doi:10.1016/j.suc.2006.10.002   *surgical.theclinics.com*

addressed in this monograph, from the optimal delivery of prehospital care to the challenge of providing access to the increasing numbers of active elderly patients sustaining critical and potential life-ending injuries. New physiologic, molecular, and genomic understanding of the impact of simple maneuvers is helpful, such as in the choice of resuscitation fluid, where this understanding helps define which, when, and how much fluid to use. The concept of damage control to prevent the potential terminal sequence of events known as the "bloody triad," along with improvements in the care of specific organ injuries, including thoracic and central nervous system, and the unique physiologic concepts involved in the care of environmental injury, both thermal and cold, are presented by leaders in these fields. The unique aspects of care required by the injured child and the elderly are presented as well.

The resulting compilation is a timely and current discussion of critical issues in the care of the severely injured patient as we move into the twenty-first century. Old dictums have become challenged, new knowledge has contributed to improvements in care, and both are occurring as the access to trauma care for the critically ill is facing its greatest challenge. The improvements in care have led to an increase in survival and a decrease in long-term morbidity for the injured patient that is indeed exciting, gratifying, and encouraging, but the epidemic of death and disability from injury continues in the United States and globally. This global epidemic demands our ongoing clinical and research commitments, objective assessment, and analysis of outcomes to optimize care delivery for this critically ill patient population. We hope the reader enjoys the current updates, ongoing developments, and recurring debates in this always exciting and rewarding arena.

Ronald V. Maier, MD, FACS
Department of Surgery, University of Washington
Harborview Medical Center
325 Ninth Avenue
Box 359796
Seattle, WA 98104-2499, USA

E-mail address: ronmaier@u.washington.edu

ELSEVIER
SAUNDERS

Surg Clin N Am 87 (2007) 1–19

SURGICAL
CLINICS OF
NORTH AMERICA

Advancing Injury Prevention and Trauma Care in North America and Globally

Charles Mock, MD, PhD[a,b,*], Manjul Joshipura, MD[c],
Robert Quansah, MD, PhD[d],
Carlos Arreola-Risa, MD[e]

[a]Department of Surgery, University of Washington, Harborview Medical Center,
325 Ninth Avenue, Seattle, WA 98103, USA
[b]Harborview Injury Prevention and Research Center, Box 359960,
Harborview Medical Center, 325 Ninth Avenue, Seattle, WA 98103, USA
[c]Academy of Traumatology, A/35, Someshwara Part II, Sattelite Road, Ahmedabad, India
[d]Department of Surgery, Komfo Anokye Teaching Hospital, Kumasi, Ghana
[e]Department of Surgery, TEC de Monterrey School of Medicine, Ave. I Morones Prieto,
#3000 PTE, Monterrey, NL, CP 64710, Mexico

Historically, in all societies, infectious diseases were the leading cause of death and disability. This pattern changed in the past two centuries in high-income countries with decreases in infection as a result of improved sanitation and medical care and with consequent increases in life expectancy. Some of these gains were offset by increases by other disease, such as cancer, heart disease, and injury. In most high-income countries today injury is the leading cause of death between age 1 and 44. Similar trends are underway in today's low- and middle-income countries (LMICs) with decreases in most infectious diseases, except HIV-AIDS, and also with increases in many injury-related causes of death, especially from road traffic. Because of recent increases in use of motorized transport globally, road traffic crashes have now become a leading cause of death among young, working-aged adults in almost every country. In the age group 15 to 44 years, road traffic deaths are second only to HIV-AIDS as a cause of death [1–3].

* Corresponding author. Harborview Injury Prevention and Research Center, Box 359960, Harborview Medical Center, 325 Ninth Avenue, Seattle, WA 98103.
E-mail address: cmock@u.washington.edu (C. Mock).

0039-6109/07/$ - see front matter © 2006 Elsevier Inc. All rights reserved.
doi:10.1016/j.suc.2006.09.017   *surgical.theclinics.com*

Moreover, rates of injury-related death in LMICs today are higher than in high-income countries. Overall annual injury-related deaths in LMICs are 89 per 100,000 per year compared with 51 per 100,000 in high-income countries [3]. Despite the high burden of death and disability from injury in almost every country, policy responses have been disproportionately low. For example, in the United States, funding for trauma-related research is less than 30% of that for cancer or heart disease [4]. The lack of attention is even more pronounced in LMICs, where less than $0.6 is spent per year of life lost because of death or disability from injuries [5].

The lack of attention to injury is partly caused by the fact that populations and governments regard injury as fundamentally different from other diseases. It is believed that injuries are caused by carelessness or bad luck and that little can be done to prevent them. Much can be done, however, to lower rates of death and disability from injury by addressing the spectrum of injury control, including surveillance, prevention, and treatment. Scientifically based efforts can be applied at each point along the spectrum (Fig. 1). Such attention to the spectrum of injury control has lowered rates of injury-related death to the lowest levels recorded the past 100 years in the United States and many European counties. Obviously, injury still remains a major health problem in these countries and much remains to be done. Attention is especially needed to injury in the setting of LMICs, however, where injury rates are higher, few injury control activities have yet been undertaken, and where most of the world's people live.

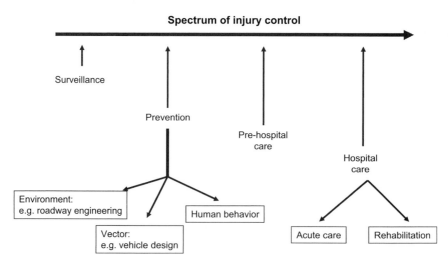

Fig. 1. Spectrum of injury control. (*From* Mock C, Quansah R, Kobusingye O, et al. Trauma care in Africa: the way forward. African Journal of Trauma 2004;2:56; with permission.)

Surveillance

Too frequently, injury control activities have been conducted without adequate assessment of their impact [6,7]. There is a need to have ongoing data regarding the extent and characteristics of the injury problem in each country. This allows better targeting of interventions and assessment of their success or failure. Most high-income countries have well-developed surveillance systems specifically for injury, such as the Fatality Analysis Reporting System [8] for automotive deaths in the United States.

Few LMICs have surveillance systems specific for injury. Most do have some system to gather information on injuries as part of their general health information systems. Data on injury usually derive from police reports and vital statistics. Several factors diminish the usefulness of such data, including lack of free availability; delays in compilation; questionable reliability of individual data elements; and underreporting. Sometimes as few as 10% of injury-related events or even injury-related deaths are recorded [9,10].

Despite these problems, several LMICs have reported sustainable improvements in injury surveillance, often by building on existing information systems [10–13]. For example, South Africa's National Non-Natural Mortality Surveillance System is built on data collated from selected mortuaries nationwide. Its data have been extensively used by both government and nongovernment organizations [14].

The World Health Organization (WHO) has made progress on promoting surveillance by published guidelines for collecting, coding, and processing injury data. These were developed to be universally applicable, but are especially useful for circumstances with limited or no electronic equipment, staff with other time demands, and limited existing expertise in injury data [15].

Prevention

All too often injury prevention is misconstrued as merely admonitions to be careful. It is a scientific field like that used to control any other health problem, however, a scientific field that (1) seeks to understand the extent and characteristics of injury through surveillance and research; (2) identifies risk factors; (3) targets these risk factors through well-developed and scientifically based prevention efforts; and (4) evaluates the results of such prevention efforts so as to know which efforts are successful and, hence, should be continued and scaled up, and which efforts are not succeeding so that they can be amended or discontinued.

Injury prevention entails actions in the overlapping spheres of environment (eg, roadway infrastructure); vector (eg, vehicle); and host (eg, human behavior). Factors contributing to high risk of injury can be modified in these locations at different points of time, including before, during, and after an event. The interactions of these factors across time in the different spheres can be conceptually visualized in Haddon's matrix (Table 1).

Table 1
Examples of the interactions of phases and factors within Haddon's matrix of injury causation and injury prevention

Phase	Human or host	Vector or vehicle	Environment: Social and physical
Pre-event	Driver intoxication experience	Condition of brakes, tires	Speed limits
			Traffic regulations
		Accessibility of moving parts in machinery in factories	Societal attitudes and laws on intoxicated driving
		Window bars at high elevations	Highway design (road curvature, intersections, road conditions)
Event	Use of safety belts	Airbags	Highway design (guard rails, breakaway poles)
		Collapsible steering column	Societal attitudes and laws regarding seatbelt use
		Side impact protection	
Postevent	Age physical conditioning	Integrity of fuel system or fire proof gasoline tanks	Trauma care systems

Adapted from Maier R, Mock CN. Injury prevention. In: Mattox K, Feliciano D, Moore E, editors. Trauma. 5th edition. New York: McGraw-Hill; 2003. p. 41–56.

Scientifically based injury prevention efforts in all the different components of Haddon's matrix have had considerable success in lowering rates of death from several injury-related causes, especially motor vehicles. Rates of motor vehicle–related death are at the lowest levels since the 1920s in the United States and most high-income countries. For example, in the United States motor vehicle–related death peaked in the 1930s at 30 deaths per 100,000 per year. They are currently at 15 deaths per 100,000 per year nationwide. Many European countries are even lower, such as Sweden at 8 deaths per 100,000 per year [4,16,17]. Such success has been achieved through many means along the spectrum of injury control. For example, surveillance systems, such as Fatality Analysis Reporting System, provide accurate and timely feedback for prevention efforts. Improvements in roadway infrastructure, such as increased use of divided highways, have decreased the rate of collisions. Improvements in the crashworthiness of vehicles as mandated by Federal Motor Vehicle Safety Standards have improved the likelihood that occupants in crashes escape major injury.

Recent developments further improving road safety in the United States have included graduated licensing and strengthened efforts to combat drunk driving, including wider adoption of blood alcohol concentration of 80 mg/dL as a per se limit for drunk driving and decreasing recidivism among intoxicated trauma patients [16].

Graduated drivers licensing

A particularly high-risk group for crashes is new teenage drivers. Rates of crashes and crash-related death are higher than for older drivers because of the younger drivers having less experience and skill coupled with more risk-taking behavior. Drivers aged 16 to 20 have an annual rate of involvement in fatal crashes of 62 per 100,000 licensed drivers, compared with 29 per 100,000 for the general public [16].

One particularly effective method to decrease the crash rate in this age group has been graduated driver licensing programs. The exact details vary between states and between countries. Several common features of these programs include new teenage drivers first obtain a learner's permit, which allows them to drive only while supervised by a licensed adult; a provisional license is next obtained, which allows new teenage drivers to drive unsupervised only under restricted conditions, such as only during certain times of day (usually not late at night), and with restrictions on the numbers and ages of passengers (eg, with only limited numbers of other adolescents). Progression from one stage to the next and to a full license only occurs after certain minimum time periods. Moreover, the potential new licensee must not have had traffic violations or at-fault crashes [18].

Graduated driver licensing programs have been shown to be effective at decreasing rates of crashes and crash-related death among new teenage drivers. For example, after institution of a graduated driver licensing system for 16-year-old drivers in North Carolina, rates of fatal crashes involving 16-year-old drivers declined by 57%, from 5 to 2 per 10,000 population per year [19].

A total of 47 states in the United States, and several other countries, have adopted graduated driver licensing. Only 21 states have achieved a rating of "good," however, according to the scale developed by the Insurance Institute for Highway Safety, which takes into account the toughness of the restrictions and the length of the period after the sixteenth birthday for which these restrictions apply. Factors in this rating include the hour at which nighttime restrictions apply, the number of adolescent passengers that are allowed, and the age at which a full license may be obtained. The other states have been rated as fair, marginal, or poor. Much work still needs to be done in terms of promoting graduated driver licensing programs [18].

Anti–drunk driving efforts

A major risk factor for motor vehicle crashes is alcohol-impaired driving. Anti–drunk driving efforts have been a cornerstone of road safety efforts in the United States and most other developed nations [20]. Such efforts have decreased the percent of alcohol involvement in fatal crashes from 50% in the 1970s down to 36% currently [3,4,21]. This is still too high. One recent development in the fight against drunk driving has been the increasing use of screening and brief intervention programs to address drunk driving recidivism. There is a high rate of recidivism among drunk drivers and among intoxicated trauma patients in general. Identification and appropriate treatment of injured persons with alcohol abuse problems is a means toward decreasing the level of alcohol-related injury from all causes. Blood alcohol screening on admission, accompanied by brief questioning, such as the Short Michigan Alcohol Screening Test, is used to identify potential problem drinkers [22–24]. Referring these patients for counseling or even engaging in very brief interventions by trained professionals in the hospital is a proved effective way of getting these patients to decrease their alcohol intake [25]. Brief interventions generally entail one or more counseling sessions, adding up to less than 1 hour. These have been shown to be effective in the context of acute injury hospitalization for all except the most severely impaired patients [22,23,25].

The effectiveness and importance of alcohol screening and brief intervention has recently led the American College of Surgeons Committee on Trauma to add a requirement that screening and brief intervention programs must be present to its list of requirements for trauma center verification for level I and II trauma centers.

Global injury prevention: recent advances

Most injury-related deaths occur in LMICs. Injury prevention efforts need to be considered globally [1–3,26]. The general injury prevention principles discussed in this article are applicable under any circumstances. Many of the specific details need to be adopted, however, to fit the circumstances of most of the world. This is because of varying injury mechanisms, resource restrictions, and cultural differences. There is a need to develop local injury prevention expertise and to develop locally applicable strategies.

After years of neglect, injury control has been gradually receiving justifiable increases in attention worldwide. Two recent landmark publications by the WHO have addressed two of the biggest injury problems: road traffic injury and violence. The *World Report on Road Traffic Injury Prevention* has raised awareness of the problem and helped to promote practical policy solutions for countries at different economic levels worldwide [17]. The *World Report on Violence and Health* has emphasized the role that the health sector can have in violence prevention, in addition to criminal justice and other sectors, which have traditionally been the foundation of violence prevention [27]. This report points out the complementary role that the health sector brings by its focus on changing behavioral, social, and environmental factors that contribute to violence. WHO also brings its focus on prevention, its scientific outlook, and its potential to coordinate multidisciplinary approaches. Readers interested in learning more about the application of injury prevention programs in LMICs are referred to these and other related [3,28,29] publications and this website (www.who.int/violence_injury_prevention/en/).

In addition to the previously noted technical considerations regarding injury prevention, broader societal issues must be dealt with. For example, land use patterns that promote large sprawling cities in turn promote car dependence. Such dependence has been supported by some governments. More compact urban planning and greater reliance on public transport are ways to decrease use of less safe transportation alternatives, such as private automobiles [30]. Similar considerations apply to almost all causes of injury, whether intentional or unintentional.

Trauma care

The past few decades have witnessed considerable improvement in the care of injured patients. Many injuries that were previously thought of as unsurvivable now have good prognosis for survival and return to active life. These achievements are caused by several factors including technologic advances, especially in intensive care. They are also caused by improved training of doctors and nurses providing trauma care. Examples of this include the growth of trauma care as a bona fide specialty within general surgery and wide promulgation of the Advanced Trauma Life Support course, which has been shown considerably to lower trauma mortality [31–33].

Another major contributor to lowering rates of trauma death has been improved organization and planning for trauma care services, which has been engendered by the growth of trauma systems. Trauma systems entail several related activities including trauma center designation and verification, improved planning for prehospital care, and the development of inter-hospital transfer agreements and protocols. Well-organized trauma systems have been consistently shown to decrease mortality among hospitalized trauma patients by 15% to 20%. They are especially effective at decreasing medically preventable death, such as death from airway obstruction or isolated intra-abdominal organ injury and other conditions that clinicians know how to treat well with existing technology. Such medically preventable deaths have been shown to decrease by over 50% with enactment of trauma systems [34,35]. In the United States, however, many areas and entire states do not have organized trauma systems [36,37]. Clearly, trauma systems need to be more widely enacted.

Improved organization and planning for trauma care services, of which trauma systems are an example, are especially needed globally. There are huge discrepancies in the outcome of trauma among countries of different economic levels. For example, mortality among patients with injury severity scores of 9 and higher increases from 35% in high-income countries, such as the United States, to 55% in middle-income countries, such as Mexico, to 63% in low-income countries, such as in Africa. Such figures include many people who are dead at the scene in all locations. The discrepancies become even more pronounced when one looks only at patients with potentially life-threatening but immanently salvageable injuries, such as those with injury scores of 15 to 24. Among such patients mortality rates have been shown to increase from 6% in high-income countries to 36% in Africa (eg, a sixfold increase in mortality). Likewise, many of the injury-related disabilities, globally, are caused by definitely treatable extremity injuries, as opposed to a higher portion of more difficult to treat neurologic-related disabilities in high-income countries [38–41]. Such extremity-related disabilities should be immanently preventable through improved orthopedic care and rehabilitation.

Much of the reason for the discrepancies in outcome between persons injured in high-income countries and those injured in LMICs is resource restrictions. There are logarithmic differences in funding available for health care, with many African countries able to afford only $10 per capita per year for health in comparison with over $5000 per capita per year for health in the United States [42]. Despite these restrictions, progress in lowering mortality rates among the injured is indeed feasible, especially through improved organization and planning for trauma care services, which has been the goal of the Essential Trauma Care (EsTC) Project.

The Essential Trauma Care Project

The EsTC Project represents an effort to set reasonable, affordable, minimum standards for trauma care services worldwide and to define the resources necessary actually to provide these services to every injured person, even in the lowest-income countries [43–46]. The basic theme of the project is that considerable improvements in trauma care and its outcome can be achieved through improved organization and planning at a very low cost. This project seeks actually to catalyze such improvements in countries worldwide.

The EsTC Project is a collaborative effort of the WHO and the International Association for Trauma Surgery and Intensive Care (IATSIC), an integrated society within the broader International Society of Surgery. A milestone of the project has been the development of the publication *Guidelines for Essential Trauma Care* [45], which is being used to catalyze improvements in trauma care globally. Outlined next are the foundations on which the EsTC Project seeks to build, the history of the development process for the *Guidelines for Essential Trauma Care*, and a summary of the progress made in implementing these guidelines in several countries.

Foundations of the Essential Trauma Care Project

The vast differences in economic resources among countries partially accounts for the previously mentioned discrepancies in trauma outcomes. There are many deficiencies in specific, critical, but low-cost trauma care resources, however, which have been documented in many LMICs. These include such items as minimal trauma care training for doctors and nurses, especially in rural areas, and deficiencies in physical resources, such as chest tubes and airway equipment, which are critically important, yet low in cost. Deficiencies in the process of care have also been documented, even when human and physical resources are more adequate [47–49].

To address such deficiencies, the EsTC Project seeks to build on two very different foundations (Fig. 2). Both have in common improvements in outcome at an affordable cost and in a sustainable fashion through improved organization and planning. One foundation is the field of international public health, which has sought to advance the concept of essential health services. These are services that are low-cost but high yield and that could be ensured to almost every member of a given population. This has included such efforts as the Expanded Program on Immunizations, the Global TB Program, the Essential Medicines Program, and on a more surgical note, the Safe Motherhood Initiative, which has sought to promulgate low-cost improvements in emergency obstetric care. All of these efforts have in common defining a core set of essential services, defining the resources necessary to ensure them, and conducting international programs to remove barriers to providing these resources [50–52]. Until recently, a similar global approach had not been used for trauma.

The other foundation to build on is the trauma system development, as described in the preceding section, which has primarily been applied in high-income countries [34,35]. The EsTC Project seeks to blend these two perspectives. In so doing it seeks to establish and promote a core set of essential trauma care services that, if widely applied, could significantly decrease the burden of preventable injury-related deaths and disabilities worldwide.

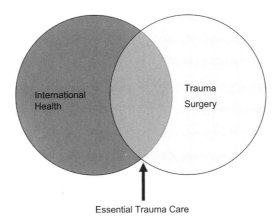

Fig. 2. Foundations of the Essential Trauma Care Project. (*From* Mock C, Joshipura M, Goosen J, et al. Overview of the Essential Trauma Care Project. World J Surg 2006;30:921; with permission.)

Development process for the Guidelines for Essential Trauma Care

In 2001, IATSIC created a Working Group for Essential Trauma Care. This Working Group made contact with the WHO, in particular the Injury and Violence Prevention Department. These two partners enlisted the aid of a network consisting of 40 persons active with providing or administering trauma care in 20 different countries, including at least one country on every continent.

In addition to long distance work, these partners and their network of collaborators held two international meetings devoted to the EsTC Project. The initial meeting in 2002 was to formulate a plan. Preliminary recommendations were developed. These were refined and expanded on by the network, followed by an extensive internal and then external review process. At the time the publication was released in 2004, another meeting was held to plan how to promulgate and institute the recommendations of the *Guidelines.* Reports from these meetings may be found on the IATISC and WHO websites: www.essentialtraumacare.org and www.who.int/violence_injury_prevention/publications/services/en/.

A major milestone of the EsTC Project has been the publication of *Guidelines for Essential Trauma Care*, a 100-page document released in June of 2004 as a collaborative publication of IATSIC, the International Society of Surgery, and the WHO. This publication may be downloaded from the previously mentioned websites. This document spells out a core set of 11 essential trauma care services, which the authors and their respective organizations believe could realistically be ensured to almost every injured person worldwide (Box 1). IATSIC has endorsed these as "The Rights of the Injured." These include such services as opening obstructed airways before hypoxia leads to death or permanent disability, stopping bleeding in a timely fashion, and correcting potentially disabling orthopedic injuries. These are services that most surgeons consider as straightforward. The reason for stating them so explicitly is that a great many injured persons in this world do not currently receive these services, and those involved in the EsTC Project believe that they can and should.

To ensure these services, the *Guidelines* delineates 260 individual items of human resources (training, skills, and sufficient staffing to ensure that someone with the skills is present when needed) and physical resources (equipment and supplies) that should be in place in institutions of varying levels worldwide. A sample of one of the tables from the *Guidelines* is shown in Table 2. The table lists individual items of human resources and physical resources that should be in place in the spectrum of health facilities globally. Such facilities range from small rural clinics, often staffed by nondoctor providers; to small rural hospitals, staffed mainly by general practitioners; to larger, specialist staffed hospitals; to tertiary care facilities. Items that are essential (E in Table 2) are those that are the most cost-effective and could realistically be provided to all injured persons treated at that level of the health

---

Box 1. Essential trauma care services: Endorsed by IATSIC as the "Rights of the Injured"

- Obstructed airways are opened and maintained before hypoxia leads to death or permanent disability.
- Impaired breathing is supported until the injured person is able to breathe adequately without assistance.
- Pneumothorax and hemothorax are promptly recognized and relieved.
- Bleeding (external or internal) is promptly stopped.
- Shock is recognized and treated with intravenous fluid replacement before irreversible consequences occur.
- The consequences of traumatic brain injury are lessened by timely decompression of space-occupying lesions and by prevention of secondary brain injury.
- Intestinal and other abdominal injuries are promptly recognized and repaired.
- Potentially disabling extremity injuries are corrected.
- Potentially unstable spinal cord injuries are recognized and managed appropriately, including early immobilization.
- The consequences to the individual of injuries that result in physical impairment are minimized by appropriate rehabilitative services.
- Medications for these services and for the minimization of pain are readily available when needed.

From Mock C, Lormand JD, Goosen J, et al. Guidelines for essential trauma care. Geneva: World Health Organization; 2004; with permission.

---

care system anywhere in the world, even in the lowest-income countries. Items that are desirable (D in Table 2) are those that increase the likelihood of successful outcome, but are higher in cost and not as universally affordable. They are more applicable to middle-income countries or to very busy trauma care facilities in any location. These resource tables are intended to be a flexible matrix to be adjusted by planners in ministries of health or administrators and clinicians in individual hospitals to fit the particular circumstances of that country or facility.

A key point for emphasis is that the essential items should not just be physically present. Essential resources and services should actually be provided to all who need them in a timely fashion, without regard of ability to pay. Having a piece of equipment does not meet essential status if the equipment is nonfunctional for long periods of time while awaiting repairs, nor if it is unused because of insufficient staffing during periods of time (eg,

Table 2
Airway management resource matrix

	Facility level[a]			
	Basic	GP	Specialist	Tertiary
Airway: knowledge & skills				
Assessment of airway compromise	E	E	E	E
Manual maneuvers (chin lift, jaw thrust, recovery position, and so forth)	E	E	E	E
Insertion of oral or nasal airway	D	E	E	E
Use of suction	D	E	E	E
Assisted ventilation using bag–valve–mask	D	E	E	E
Endotracheal intubation	D	D	E	E
Cricothyroidotomy (with or without tracheostomy)	D	D	E	E
Airway: equipment & supplies				
Oral or nasal airway	D	E	E	E
Suction device: at least manual (bulb) or foot pump	D	E	E	E
Suction device: powered, electric or pneumatic	D	D	D	D
Suction tubing	D	E	E	E
Yankauer or other stiff suction tip	D	E	E	E
Laryngoscope	D	D	E	E
Endotracheal tube	D	D	E	E
Esophageal detector device	D	D	E	E
Bag–valve–mask	D	D	E	E
Basic trauma pack	D	E	E	E
Magill forceps	D	D	E	E
Capnography	I	D	D	D
Other advanced airway equipment	I	D	D	D

Abbreviations: D, desirable; E, essential; I, irrelevant (not usually to be considered at the level in question, even with full resource availability).

[a] Basic: outpatient clinics, often staffed by nondoctors; GP: hospitals staffed by general practitioners; Specialist: hospitals staffed by specialists, usually including a general surgeon; Tertiary: tertiary care hospitals, often university hospitals, with a wide range of specialists.

From Mock C, Lormand JD, Goosen J, et al. Guidelines for essential trauma care. Geneva: World Health Organization; 2004; with permission.

nights and weekends) when most injured patients need the equipment. Having medications or other supplies in stock does not meet essential status if their use depends on a patient's insurance status or payment in advance. These stipulations do not rule out the need for billing or cost-recovery later, after essential items of care have been rendered. Cost-recovery, however, should not prevent rendering such essential care when it is needed.

The *Guidelines* cover the breadth of trauma care, including initial resuscitation, acute definitive care of injuries to specific body regions, and long-term rehabilitation. In general terms, some of the types of services that the *Guidelines* seek to promote include, for the circumstances of low-income countries, such as in Africa and South Asia, the following:

- Rural clinics (basic level) should have capabilities for rapid basic first aid, which many currently do not have. Although usually having only very basic capabilities, many of these facilities do receive considerable numbers of injured persons, either because of the clinics' locations on major roadways or because of their geographic isolation and lack of any other health facilities in their vicinity.

- Small hospitals should have capabilities for chest tube insertion and airway maintenance and certain minimum blood transfusion capabilities, which many do not have.
- Specialists and tertiary care facilities should have capabilities for advanced airway management, including endotracheal intubation, on an emergency basis, which many do not have. These larger hospitals should also have trauma-related quality improvement or medical audit programs in place, which few currently have.

Similar recommendations pertain to middle-income settings, such as Latin America, but desirable items figure more prominently.

Finally, the *Guidelines* provide more general recommendations on ways to implement the resource recommendations. These include (1) training programs; (2) performance improvement strategies; (3) trauma team organization; (4) hospital inspection programs, such as with trauma center verification; and (5) political interactions among stakeholders.

The *Guidelines* is intended to be part planning guide for ministries of health or individual facilities and part advocacy document to be used by whoever wishes to push for actual improvements in trauma care. The legitimacy of this document for such advocacy is increased by the fact that it was created by the three bodies in the world that have the most credibility to do so (IATSIC, the International Society of Surgery, and WHO) and by the fact the *Guidelines* was created with the review and other input of persons directly involved with trauma care from many countries, including at least one on every continent, and with the input of many other trauma-related specialty organizations [44–46].

Progress on the ground

The value of the *Guidelines for Essential Trauma Care* lies in its actually promoting improvements of the care of the injured on the ground in individual countries. There has already been progress in this regard. The *Guidelines* have already been put to use in several countries. In four of these countries, it has been the basis for needs assessments (situation analysis) of trauma care capabilities [53–56]. These needs assessments have helped to identify priorities for low-cost improvements. They have identified several deficiencies in human and physical resources that could be remedied primarily by greater attention to detail in planning and administering trauma care services. In all of these countries, the *Guidelines* have shown their usefulness in providing an internationally applicable, standardized template or yardstick for countries to use to assess the trauma care capabilities of their facilities and their trauma systems.

Likewise, the *Guidelines* have already been used by ministry of health planners and have received considerable political endorsement in several countries. This publication and the overall EsTC Project have stimulated several important stakeholder meetings in all of the countries mentioned. These meetings brought together ministry of health planners, WHO country offices, representatives of many professional societies that deal with trauma, nongovernment organizations, and others. At these meetings, priorities from the needs assessments were identified, the resource templates were adjusted for local circumstances, and implementation plans were developed. Most participants felt that these meetings constituted the highest governmental attention to trauma care ever in those countries [44]. High points of these developments are summarized next.

India

The guidelines have been endorsed by the Academy of Traumatology (India). India became one of the first early innovators to use the *Guidelines*, even while it was in its draft stages. In 2003, a meeting was held of stakeholders in trauma care in Gujarat State, at which time the resource template was adjusted for the Indian circumstances, in which there are five, rather than four, levels. This meeting stimulated a needs assessment of trauma care capabilities in that state. This meeting also stimulated an expanded, nationwide meeting in 2005 entitled "First National Consultation Meeting on Trauma System Development in India," which expanded the EsTC concept to a nationwide scale and also incorporated planning for prehospital services [44,57]. Reports from these meetings are available at www.essentialtraumacare.org. The *Guidelines* have also been used in the development of legislation relating to trauma system development in Gujarat State.

Ghana

The *Guidelines* have been endorsed by the Ghana Medical Association. A nationwide needs assessment based on the EsTC criteria was conducted, highlighting priorities for low-cost improvements [56]. A stakeholder conference in June, 2005, brought together trauma care professionals; ministry of health planners; WHO personnel; several members of Parliament, including representatives of the two main political parties; and members of the Committees on Health and on Transportation. At this meeting the EsTC criteria were adapted for the Ghanaian circumstances. This meeting also addressed heavily emphasized implementation methods. Supplemental ways in which to provide adequate funding to promote trauma system development were proposed, including the development of a "trauma fund" subsidized from sources such as a portion of the tax on gasoline. The meeting concluded with the development of a document "Recommendations for a National Policy on Strengthening the Care of Injured Persons in Ghana," coauthored by the Ministry of Health and the WHO Country office, which has been provided to Ghana's Parliament. Especially notable is that, as a result of this meeting, strengthening trauma care is part of the WHO country office's plan of technical collaboration with the Ministry of Health. This is an important step in getting trauma care better institutionalized in health policy [44,58,59].

Mexico

The *Guidelines* have been endorsed by the Mexican Association for the Medicine and Surgery of Trauma. A nationally representative, three-state needs assessment was conducted using the *Guidelines* as basis [53]. A stakeholder conference was conducted in 2004 to adapt the *Guidelines* to Mexican circumstances. This was sponsored by the national Ministry of Health and WHO. Stakeholders included presidents or representatives of most national professional societies that deal with trauma and critical care, and ministry of health planners. The *Guidelines* have been used by the National Ministry of Health in its latest modifications of "normas" or standards for prehospital and emergency medical services for the country. The activities in Mexico have created interest in the EsTC Project among other countries in Latin America, including Ecuador and Columbia [44].

Vietnam

One of the best examples of use of the *Guidelines* in individual countries comes from Vietnam. A needs assessment of trauma care capabilities using the *Guidelines* as a template was conducted in the Hanoi area in 2002, while the *Guidelines* were still in draft form. This demonstrated several low-cost, but highly important, deficiencies in human and physical resources in trauma care facilities. There were moderate deficiencies, especially in airway management, in the larger hospitals in that city, and more extensive deficiencies in capabilities in the commune health stations and smaller hospitals serving the nearby rural areas. Drawing attention to these deficiencies increased attention to the administration and organization of trauma care, which in turn resulted in improvements in capabilities when the survey was repeated the following year. These improvements occurred with no additional budget having been allotted to trauma care by the health department [55]. The *Guidelines* has been translated into Vietnamese and republished locally [44]. A non-government organization, Counterpart International, has also been active in promoting the recommendations of the *Guidelines* in its own work with health system development. These activities and the experiences from Hanoi have helped to stimulate and have been part of increasing attention to trauma care nationwide, both locally in individual provinces and in national Ministry of Health planning.

Sri Lanka

As with some of the other countries mentioned previously, the EsTC project catalyzed a nationwide trauma care stakeholder meeting in 2005 [44].

This meeting was sponsored by College of Surgeons of Sri Lanka and Sri Lanka Medical Association and involved the ministry of health and the WHO country office, nongovernment organizations, and others. This meeting expanded the EsTC concept to integrate disaster preparedness in light of that country's involvement with the tsunami in December 2004. This process has helped to increase support for other ongoing efforts to improve trauma care, such as the development of a Trauma System Development Committee.

Next steps in the Essential Trauma Care Project

The most important next steps to further the EsTC Project globally include advancing the adaptation and implementation of the EsTC resource criteria in institutions in individual countries. Such on-the-ground work is the foundation of the project. In so doing, there is a role to link with other international efforts, such as those to improve emergency care services in general. Likewise, there is increased collaboration between those involved in the EsTC Project and related efforts to improve prehospital trauma care. The latter has been stimulated by a related WHO publication, *Prehospital Trauma Care Systems* [60].

Global uptake of the EsTC recommendations can be promoted by increased political will, both in individual countries and among international organizations. For this reason, several of the partners involved in the EsTC project have drawn up a draft resolution for consideration by the World Health Assembly. This is the governing board of the WHO and consists of every minister of health in all United Nations member states. World Health Assembly resolutions form the basis for much of what the WHO does and are also very influential in setting the agenda of national ministries of health, donors, and other international organizations. The draft World Health Assembly resolution calls on governments to implement the recommendations of the *Guidelines for Essential Trauma Care* and the *Prehospital Trauma Care Systems* as part of their national health policy [57].

Summary

Injury is a major global health problem. Increased attention to this problem is desperately needed. Much can be done to lower the rates of injury-related death and disability by addressing the spectrum of injury control, including surveillance, prevention, and trauma care. There is room for improvement in the application of scientifically based, proved interventions at all points in this spectrum in all countries in the world. Especially notable is the fact that there are many effective interventions for road safety that are only partially applied globally. Likewise, improved organization and planning for trauma care services needs to be better applied in most countries. The Essential Trauma Care Project has defined the minimum standards for trauma care services, as applicable to countries at all economic levels. These standards are already proving useful at improving trauma care services in several countries and need to be more widely used. For all aspects of injury control, much remains to be done in high-income countries. Even greater attention is needed in low- and middle-income countries, however, where most of the world's people live, where injury rates are higher, and where few injury control activities have yet been undertaken. Finally, injury, as with other diseases, must be viewed within the context of broader societal issues. In all countries, people in lower socioeconomic groups are most at risk for injury and often have the least access to quality trauma care [3,26,61,62]. Surgeons and those from other professions who confront injury must develop skills in advocacy and politics and must be prepared to take on difficult issues of equity and human rights.

References

[1] Krug E. Injury: a leading cause of the global burden of disease (WHO/HSC/PVI/99.11). Geneva: World Health Organization; 1999.
[2] Krug EG, Sharma GK, Lozano R. The global burden of injuries. Am J Public Health 2000; 90:523–6.
[3] Mock C, Quansah R, Krishnan R, et al. Strengthening the prevention and care of injuries worldwide. Lancet 2004;363:2172–9.
[4] Baker SP, O'Neill B, Ginsburg MJ, et al. The injury fact book. 2nd edition. New York: Oxford University Press; 1992.
[5] Michaud C, Murray CJ. External assistance to the health sector in developing countries. Bull World Health Organ 1994;72:639–51.
[6] Maier R, Mock CN. Injury prevention. In: Mattox K, Feliciano D, Moore E, editors. Trauma. 4th edition. New York: McGraw-Hill; 1999. p. 41–55.
[7] O'Neill B, Mohan D. Reducing motor vehicle crash deaths and injuries in newly motorising countries. BMJ 2002;324:1142–5.
[8] Fatality Analysis Reporting System. Available at: www-fars.nhtsa.dot.gov. Accessed January 3, 2004.
[9] Salifu M, Mock CN. Pedestrian injuries in Kumasi: results of an epidemiologic survey. The Ghana Engineer 1998;18:23–7.
[10] London J, Mock CN, Abantanga FA, et al. Using mortuary statistics in the development of an injury surveillance system in Ghana. Bull World Health Organ 2002;80:357–64.
[11] Kobusingye OC, Lett RR. Hospital based trauma registries in Uganda. J Trauma 2000;48: 498–502.
[12] Ghaffar A, Hyder AA, Mastoor MI, et al. Injuries in Pakistan: directions for future health policy. Health Policy Plan 1999;14:11–7.
[13] Rahman F, Andersson R, Svanstrom L. Potential of using existing injury information for injury surveillance at the local level in developing countries. Public Health 2000;114: 133–6.
[14] The Injury and Violence Surveillance Consortium and Participating Forensic Pathologists. The South African National Non-Natural Mortality Surveillance System. Africa Safecom Newsletter 2000;1:1, 5.
[15] Holder Y, Peden M, Krug E, et al. Injury surveillance guidelines. Geneva: World Health Organization; 2001.

[16] National Highway Traffic Safety Administration. Traffic safety facts 2004. Washington: National Center for Statistics and Analysis, US Department of Transportation; 2005.

[17] Peden M, Scurfield R, Sleet D, et al. World report on road traffic injury prevention. Geneva: World Health Organization; 2004.

[18] Insurance Institute for Highway Safety. Graduated licensing: a blueprint for North America. Available at: www.iihs.org/laws/state_laws/pdf/blueprint.pdf. Accessed November 1, 2006.

[19] Foss R, Feaganes J, Rodgman E. Initial effects of graduated driver licensing on 16-year-old driver crashes in North Carolina. JAMA 2001;286:1588–92.

[20] DeJong W, Hingson R. Strategies to reduce driving under the influence of alcohol. Annu Rev Public Health 1998;19:359–78.

[21] Voas RB, Wells J, Lestina D, et al. Drinking and driving in the United States: the 1996 National Roadside Survey. Accid Anal Prev 1998;30:267–75.

[22] Dunn CW, Donovan DM, Gentilello LM. Practical guidelines for performing alcohol interventions in trauma centers. J Trauma 1997;42:299–304.

[23] Gentilello LM, Donovan DM, Dunn CW, et al. Alcohol interventions in trauma centers. JAMA 1995;274:1043–8.

[24] Rivara FP, Grossman DC, Cummings P. Injury prevention: first of two parts. N Engl J Med 1997;337:543–8.

[25] Gentilello L, Rivara F, Donovan D, et al. Alcohol interventions in a trauma center as a means of reducing the risk of injury recurrence. Ann Surg 1999;230:473–80.

[26] Nantulya V, Reich M. The neglected epidemic: road traffic injuries in developing countries. BMJ 2002;324:1139–41.

[27] Krug E, Dahlberg L, Mercy J, et al. World report on violence and health. Geneva: World Health Organization; 2002.

[28] Barss P, Smith G, Baker S, et al. Injury prevention: an international perspective. New York: Oxford University Press; 1998.

[29] Berger LR, Mohan D. Injury control: a global view. Delhi: Oxford University Press; 1996.

[30] Newman P, Kenworthy J. Sustainability and cities: overcoming automobile dependence. Washington: Island Press; 1999.

[31] Ali J, Adams R, Butler AK, et al. Trauma outcome improves following the advanced trauma life support program in a developing country. J Trauma 1993;34:890–8.

[32] American College of Surgeons. Advanced trauma life support: student course manual. 7th edition. Chicago: American College of Surgeons; 2004.

[33] Mock CN, Jurkovich GJ. Trauma system development in the United States. Trauma Q 1999; 14:197–210.

[34] Jurkovich G, Mock C. A systematic review of trauma system effectiveness based on registry comparisons. J Trauma 1999;47:S46–55.

[35] Mann N, Mullins R, MacKenzie E, et al. A systematic review of published evidence regarding trauma system effectiveness. J Trauma 1999;47:S25–33.

[36] Bazzoli GJ. Community-based trauma system development: key barriers and facilitating factors. J Trauma 1999;47:S22–4.

[37] Bazzoli GJ, Madura K, Cooper GG, et al. Progress in the development of trauma systems in the United States: results of a national survey. JAMA 1995;273:395–401.

[38] MacKenzie EJ, Siegel JH, Shapiro S, et al. Functional recovery and medical costs of trauma: an analysis by type and severity of injury. J Trauma 1988;28:281–97.

[39] Mock C, Boland E, Acheampong F, et al. Long-term injury related disability in Ghana. Disabil Rehabil 2003;25:732–41.

[40] Mock CN, Adzotor KE, Conklin E, et al. Trauma outcomes in the rural developing world: comparison with an urban level I trauma center. J Trauma 1993;35:518–23.

[41] Mock CN, Jurkovich GJ, nii-Amon-Kotei D, et al. Trauma mortality patterns in three nations at different economic levels: implications for global trauma system development. J Trauma 1998;44:804–14.

[42] World Health Organization. Available at: www.who.int/countries/en/. Accessed July 18, 2006.
[43] Mock C, Joshipura M, Goosen J. Global strengthening of care of the injured. Bull World Health Organ 2004;82:241.
[44] Mock C, Joshipura M, Goosen J, et al. Overview of the Essential Trauma Care Project. World J Surg 2006;30:919–29.
[45] Mock C, Lormand JD, Goosen J, et al. Guidelines for essential trauma care. Geneva: World Health Organization; 2004.
[46] Mock C, Joshipura M, Goosen J, et al. Strengthening trauma systems globally: the Essential Trauma Care Project. J Trauma 2005;59:1243–6.
[47] London JA, Mock CN, Quansah RE, et al. Priorities for improving hospital based trauma care in an African city. J Trauma 2001;51:747–53.
[48] Mock C, Arreola-Risa C, Quansah R. Strengthening care for injured persons in less developed countries: a case study of Ghana and Mexico. Inj Control Saf Promot 2003;10: 45–51.
[49] Quansah RE, Mock CN. Trauma care in Ghana. Trauma Q 1999;14:283–94.
[50] Maher D. Clinical audit in a developing country. Trop Med Int Health 1996;1:409–13.
[51] Pio A, Luelmo F, Kumaresan J, et al. National tuberculosis programme review: experience over the period 1990–95. Bull World Health Organ 1997;75:569–81.
[52] Rosenfield A. The history of the Safe Motherhood Initiative. Int J Gynaecol Obstet 1997;59: S7–9.
[53] Arreola-Risa C, Mock C, Vega Rivera F, et al. Evaluating trauma care capabilities in Mexico with the World Health Organization's Guidelines for Essential Trauma Care. Pan American Journal of Public Health 2006;19:94–103.
[54] Mock C, Nguyen S, Quansah R, et al. Evaluation of trauma care capabilities in four countries using the WHO-IATSIC Guidelines for Essential Trauma Care. World J Surg 2006;30: 946–56.
[55] Nguyen S, Mock C. Improvements in trauma care capabilities in Vietnam through use of the WHO-IATSIC Guidelines for Essential Trauma Care. Inj Control Saf Promot 2006;13: 125–7.
[56] Quansah R, Mock C, Abantanga F. Status of trauma care in Ghana. Ghana Med J 2004;38: 149–52.
[57] Joshipura M. Guidelines for essential trauma care: Progress in India. World J Surg 2006;30: 930–3.
[58] Quansah R. Essential trauma care in Ghana: Adaptation and implementation on the tough political road. World J Surg 2006;30:934–9.
[59] Anonymous. Strengthening care for injury victims: Recommendations for a National policy. From Consultation Meeting held 17–18 June, 2005, Akosombo. Kumasi, Ghana: University Printing Press; 2006.
[60] Sasser S, Varghese M, Kellermann A, et al. Prehospital trauma care systems. Geneva: World Health Organization; 2005.
[61] Roberts I. Cause specific social class mortality differentials for child injury and poisoning in England and Wales. J Epidemiol Community Health 1997;51:334–5.
[62] Maier R, Mock CN. Injury prevention. In: Mattox K, Feliciano D, Moore E, editors. Trauma. 5th edition. New York: McGraw-Hill; 2003. p. 41–56.

SURGICAL
CLINICS OF
NORTH AMERICA

Surg Clin N Am 87 (2007) 21–35

Trauma Systems

David B. Hoyt, MD[a],*, Raul Coimbra, MD, PhD[b]

[a]*Department of Surgery, University of California, Irvine School of Medicine, City Tower, 333 City Boulevard West, #700, Orange, CA 92868, USA*
[b]*Division of Trauma, Burns and Critical Care, Department of Surgery, University of California, San Diego School of Medicine, San Diego, CA, USA*

Definition of trauma system

A trauma system is an organized approach to patients who are acutely injured. It should occur in a defined geographic area and provide optimal care that is integrated with the local or regional emergency medical service (EMS) system.

The major goal of a trauma system is to enhance the community health. This occurs through a process of assessment, policy development, and ongoing assurance (Fig. 1). This can be achieved by (1) identifying risk factors in the community and creating solutions to decrease the incidence of injury, (2) providing optimal care during the acute and the late phase of injury, including rehabilitation, and (3) maintaining the objective to decrease overall injury-related morbidity and mortality and years of life lost. Disaster preparedness also is an important function of trauma systems, and using an established trauma system network facilitates the care of victims of natural disasters or terrorist attacks.

Regionalization is an important goal of a trauma system as it promotes the efficient use of health care facilities and the rational use of equipment and resources. Trauma care within a trauma system is multidisciplinary and is provided along a continuum that includes all phases of care.

Important historical events in trauma systems development

In 1966, the National Academy of Sciences and the National Research Council published a landmark white paper—"Accidental Death and

* Corresponding author. Department of Surgery, University of California, Irvine, City Tower, 333 City Boulevard West, #700, Orange, CA 92868.
E-mail address: dhoyt@uci.edu (D.B. Hoyt).

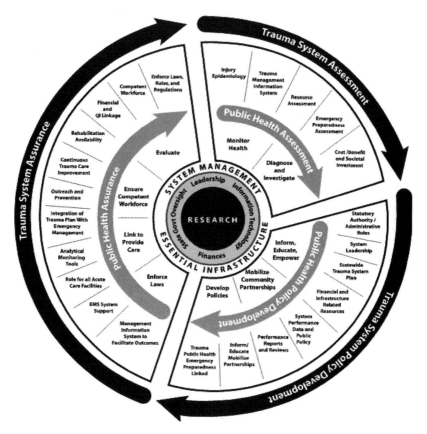

Fig. 1. The public health approach to trauma system development. (*From* the United States De-partment of Health and Human Services Health Resources and Services Administration. Model trauma system planning and evaluation. Available at http://www.hrsa.gov/trauma/model.htm. Accessed August 1, 2006.)

Disability: The Neglected Disease of Modern Society" [2]. This was fol-lowed by the Airlie Conference on Emergency Medical Services, in 1969, where the need to develop EMS was addressed [3].

The American College of Surgeons Committee on Trauma (ACSCOT) developed the guideline "Optimal Hospital Resources for the Care of the Se-riously Injured" in 1976 [4]. This document was the first to set out specific criteria for the categorization of hospitals as trauma centers. This document is revised periodically, is recognized nationally and internationally as the standard for hospitals aspiring to be trauma centers, and established a stan-dard for evaluation of care. It recently was translated into Chinese and will help develop trauma systems in the Pacific Rim. The current version, "Re-sources for Optimal Care of the Injured Patient," published in 2006, estab-lishes criteria for prehospital and trauma care personnel and establishes the importance of ongoing quality assessment [5]. The ACSCOT also developed an advanced trauma life support (ATLS) course in 1980, which has contributed to the uniformity of initial care and the development of a common language for all care providers. It has been taken by more than 450,000 physicians throughout the world [6].

In 1985, the National Research Council and the Institute of Medicine published "Injury in America: A Continuing Health Care Problem." This document concludes that despite considerable funding used to develop trauma systems, little progress had been made toward reducing the burden of injury [7]. This document also reinforces the necessity of investments in epidemiologic research and injury prevention. After the publication of this document, the Centers for Disease Control and Prevention (CDC) was chosen as the site for an injury research center to coordinate efforts at the national level in injury control, injury prevention, and all other aspects of trauma care. The CDC has established a national inquiry research agenda and compliments other previous efforts by the National Institutes of Health [8,9].

In 1987, the ACSCOT instituted the Verification/Consultation Program, which provided further opportunities and incentives for trauma system development and a trauma centers' designation. The ACSCOT published a document, entitled "Consultation for Trauma Systems," with the objective of providing guidelines for trauma system evaluation and enhancement [10]. In 1987, the American College of Emergency Physicians published "Guidelines for Trauma Care Systems" [11]. This document focused on the continuum of trauma care and identified essential criteria for trauma care systems.

In 1988, the National Highway Traffic Safety Administration (NHTSA) established the Statewide EMS Technical Assessment Program and the Development of Trauma Systems Course, important tools for assessing the effectiveness of trauma systems components and for system development. NHTSA also developed standards for quality EMS, including trauma care [12]. The standard required that the trauma care system be integrated fully into a state's EMS system and have specific legislation. The trauma care component must include designated trauma centers, transfer and triage guidelines, trauma registries, and initiatives in public education and injury prevention.

In 1990, the Trauma Systems Planning and Development Act created the Division of Trauma and EMS within the Health Resources and Services Administration (HRSA) to improve EMS and trauma care. The program lost funding between 1995 and 2000 and many states that were in the process of developing trauma systems lost momentum [13]. Two initiatives from this legislation were noteworthy: (1) planning grants for statewide trauma system development that were provided to states on a competitive basis and (2) the Model Trauma Care System Plan, which was published as a consensus document [14]. The Model Trauma Care System Plan established a nonpolitical framework for measuring progress in trauma system development and set the standard for the promulgation of systems of trauma care. The program was funded again in fiscal year 2001—but lost funding in 2006.

New legislation is being written to further this effort. The newest document is comprehensive and has tools for successful assessment, policy development, and assurance [1]. With appropriate federal funding this approach will be successful.

Trauma systems development

The criteria for a statewide EMS and trauma systems have been determined and are identified in Box 1. The first step is to establish legal authority for the development of a system. This usually requires legislation at a state or local level that provides public agency authority. Determining the need for such a system has been done in communities by reviewing the outcome of trauma cases in the region. Such reviews have focused on preventable deaths, and surgeons' role is critical in leadership and commitment to establish a better standard of care. The designated agency in combination with local trauma surgeons and other medical personnel develop criteria for a trauma system, determine which facilities are designated trauma centers, and establish a trauma registry, a fundamental component of a quality assurance (QA) program.

Trauma system components

Recent data demonstrate that only 50% of states in the United States have statewide trauma systems [15,16]. The essential elements are access to care, prehospital care, hospital care, and rehabilitation. In addition, prevention, disaster medical planning, patient education, research, and rational financial planning are essential. Prehospital communications, a transport system, trained personnel, and qualified trauma care personnel for all phases of care are of utmost importance for a system's success.

External peer review is used to verify specific hospital's capabilities. The verification process can be accomplished through the ACSCOT or by inviting experts in the field of trauma as outside reviewers. QI is a vital component of

---

Box 1. Criteria for statewide trauma care system

Legislative authority for designation
Formal designation process
American College of Surgeons standards or equivalent
Use of nonbiased survey teams (out of town)
Population- or volume-based trauma center designation
Triage criteria that requires direct transport to trauma center
Quality improvement (QI) systems
Full geographic coverage

the system. It provides constant evaluation of a system's performance, needs, and outcomes.

The Model Trauma Care System Plan formalized the concept of the "inclusive system" with trauma centers identified by their ability to provide definitive care to those injured most critically [14]. Only 15% of all trauma patients benefit from the resources of a level I or II trauma center. Recent data suggest, however, that many patients who are severely injured are not taken to trauma centers [17]. It is expected in an inclusive system to encourage participation and to enhance capabilities of the smaller hospitals, while maintaining appropriate triage of those injured most severely to level I or II trauma centers. Surgical leadership is of fundamental importance and trauma systems cannot develop without the commitment of the surgeons of a hospital or community.

Public information, education, and injury prevention

Death after trauma occurs in a trimodel distribution and effective trauma programs also must focus on injury prevention as potentially the most important aspect of trauma system development. More than half of deaths occur within minutes of injury even in established trauma systems and never are able to be addressed by acute care [18]. A trauma system also must focus on injury prevention based on local injury data. Identification of risk factors and high-risk groups and development of strategies to alter personal behavior through education and legislation have the greatest impact on trauma in the community. Efforts to increase awareness of the public and instruct the public about how the system operates are important, as trauma generally is not perceived as an important public health problem. A recent Harris Poll, conducted by the American Trauma Society, shows that most citizens value the importance of a trauma system as the same importance as fire and police services [19].

Human resources

A quality trauma system provides quality education to its providers. This includes all personnel along the trauma care continuum: physicians, nurses, emergency medical technicians (EMTs), and many others who have an impact on patients or patients' families. Recently, adequate physician resources have become a challenge for trauma surgeons and surgical specialists. Interest in care of injured patients continues to decline and access to care for injured patients is becoming a major problem in many parts of the country [20]. The development of the acute care surgeon model (providing care not only for the acutely injured but also for all patients requiring acute surgical intervention) may help address increasing trauma surgeon shortages [21].

Prehospital

Trauma care before hospital arrival has a direct effect on survival and a system must ensure prompt access and dispatch of qualified personnel, appropriate care at the scene, and safe and rapid transport of patients to the closest and most appropriate facility. Effective prehospital care requires coordination between various public safety agencies and hospitals to maximize efficiency, minimize duplication of services, and provide care at a reasonable cost. Training is the most important aspect of a successful prehospital program and the prehospital trauma life support (PHTLS) has standardized this effort in line with ATLS training [22].

Communication system

A reliable communications system is essential for providing optimal trauma care. Many urban centers use modern electronic technology to establish emergency notification systems. Universal access to emergency telephone numbers (eg, 9-1-1), trained dispatch personnel who can dependably match EMS expertise with the patient's needs, and the capability of EMS personnel at trauma incidents to communicate with prehospital dispatch, with trauma hospitals, and with other units are essential components. Maintenance of the system, particularly during disasters, remains a major, evolving, unresolved challenge.

Medical direction

Medical direction provides oversight for care provided while granting freedom of action and limitations to EMTs who must perform independently in the field. Medical directors are responsible for the design and implementation of field treatment guidelines, their timely revision, and their quality control. Ongoing field audit of care is mandatory to demonstrate that prehospital practices are not harmful to patients [23].

Triage and transport

The word triage derives from the French word, meaning "to sort." It involves the initial evaluation of patients and the determination of priorities and levels of medical care necessary for victims. The purpose of triage is to be selective, so that limited medical resources are allocated to patients who receive the most benefit. Proper triage should ensure that patients who are seriously injured be taken to a facility capable of treating their types of injuries—a trauma center. Patients who have lesser severity of injuries may be transported safely to other closest and appropriate medical facilities for care. Because of the complexities of patient evaluation and injury determination, however, the perfect triage system has yet to be developed.

The primary goal of an effective triage system is to identify which patients are seriously injured and in need of immediate surgical or medical care. Many triage methods can be used and often they rely on physiologic, anatomic, and mechanism of injury information to assist in the triage decision. The ACSCOT triage system uses a combination of anatomic and physiologic criteria [5]. In addition, a concise prehospital radio report enables the receiving medical personnel to anticipate emergent equipment and personnel needs. The few minutes of preparation before a patient's arrival may make the difference in patient survival.

The goal of identifying major trauma victims may be easy to conceptualize but difficult to quantify. Prompt recognition of those patients who are at immediate risk for life (eg, loss of airway or hemorrhagic shock) or loss of a limb (ischemia) or who need immediate operative or life-saving interventions is not difficult. Patients who have a less clear threat to life are challenging to triage so as not to overburden the system. Retrospectively, the Injury Severity Score (ISS) provides a means for a trauma system to triage major trauma victims as those who have an ISS of greater than 15, a commonly accepted level [24]. Another less used definition of major trauma is provided by the Major Trauma Outcome Study, which defines trauma patients as all patients who died resulting from their injuries or were admitted to the hospital [25].

After a traumatic event, the effectiveness of a triage system should be analyzed based on expected performance standards. One of the accepted performance markers is undertriage and overtriage rates. Undertriage is defined as a triage decision that classifies patients as not needing a higher level of care (eg, trauma center), when in fact they do. Undertriage (false-negative triage) is a medical problem that may result in an adverse patient outcome. Generally, undertriage rates should be less than 5%, but recent data suggest that patients who are severely injured still frequently are triaged to no-trauma centers [17]. Overtriage is a decision that classifies patients incorrectly as needing a trauma center, although retrospective analysis suggests that such care was not justified. Overtriage has been claimed to result potentially in overuse and consumption of finite, expensive resources. In most moderate volume centers, however, overtriage rates, even as high as 50%, result in only 1 to 3 additional patients per day to a trauma center [26]. This problem becomes magnified in high-volume, overloaded trauma centers.

Trauma center facilities and leadership

Level I trauma centers

Level I trauma centers are tertiary care hospitals that demonstrate a leadership role in system development, optimal trauma care, QI, education, and research. They are regional resources for the provision of the most sophisticated trauma care, managing large numbers of patients who are severely injured through immediate 24-hour availability of an attending trauma surgeon. Level I trauma centers address public education and prevention issues and provide education for all levels of trauma care providers. They lead research efforts to advance care, which may extend from prehospital clinical trials to rehabilitation.

Level II trauma centers

Level II trauma centers also provide definitive care to those who are injured and may be the principal trauma provider in a community. Their approach to trauma is comprehensive and an attending trauma surgeon's availability is equivalent to a Level I trauma center in the early care of patients. Graduate education and research are not required.

Level III trauma centers

Level III trauma centers generally are large community hospitals that serve a community that lacks level I or II facilities. Commitment is required to assess, resuscitate, and, when necessary, provide definitive operative therapy. When capabilities for definitive care are exceeded, transfer agreements and protocols are essential for level III trauma centers. Education for health care personnel may be part of a level III center's role, as the hospital may be the only designated trauma center in a community.

Level IV trauma centers

Level IV trauma centers usually are hospitals located in rural areas and are expected to provide initial evaluation of patients who are acutely injured, with transfer to a higher level of care anticipated. Transfer agreements and protocols must be in place, because most of these hospitals have no definitive surgical capabilities on a regular basis.

Acute care facilities within the system

Many general hospitals exist within a trauma care system, at which patients who are injured less severely may arrive. The system should provide for interfacility transfer of patients if major trauma patients are mistriaged to one of these hospitals.

Specialty trauma centers

Specialty facilities concentrate expertise in a specific discipline and serve as a regional resource for patients who have specialty focus. Examples include pediatric trauma, burn, spinal cord injuries, and hand (replantation) trauma. These facilities provide a valuable resource to the community and region and should be included in the needs assessment when designing a system.

Rehabilitation

Rehabilitation is as important as prehospital and hospital care. It often is the longest and most difficult phase of the trauma care continuum for patients and families. Few patients in the United States have access to truly optimal rehabilitation programs because of lack of an adequate national commitment and financially supported infrastructure. Rehabilitation can be provided by a designated program within a trauma center or by agreement with a freestanding rehabilitation center.

System evaluation

A trauma system has to monitor its performance over time and determine areas where improvement is needed. This principle is in the public's best interest, as patients generally are taken (regardless of individual wishes) to designated trauma centers and, therefore, public trust in the quality of care is essential. Reliable data collection and analysis through a system-wide trauma registry are critical. Compatibility between data collection during different phases of care is important to determine the effects of certain interventions in any phase on long-term outcome accurately. System evaluation instruments are needed to identify where a system falls short operationally to allow for improvements in system design.

The implementation of trauma care systems coupled with trauma registry databases, injury severity indices, and measurable outcome indicators has led to many improvements in systems. Systems also can be evaluated during trauma center verification to see if individual trauma centers are identifying their problems and responding correctly.

Trauma system quality improvement

A system-wide QI program's most important role is to monitor the quality of trauma care from incident through rehabilitation and create solutions to correct identified problems. The purpose of QI is to provide care in a planned sequence, to measure compliance with defined standards of care, and to reduce variability and cost while maintaining quality. A comprehensive downloadable guide to this process is detailed on the American College of Surgeons Web site [27].

Errors occur resulting from the complexity of trauma care and because of the involvement of many providers. It is important to make a distinction between process complexity and human errors when developing a QI program in trauma [28–30]. A peer process must be established to review individual problems [31]. The process must be documented accurately, corrective action instituted and applied uniformly across the system, and results reassessed. These principles apply to system-wide QA/QI and to the process within the hospital. Corrective action is taken through changes in existing policies or

protocols, through education targeted at the problem, or, occasionally, by restriction of privileges. A successful trauma system monitors the performance
of the EMS agency and prehospital operations, individual trauma hospitals,
and, importantly, care in nondesignated hospitals. The prehospital audit process should include timeliness of arrival, timeliness of transport, application of
prehospital procedures, and treatments and outcomes.

Standards of care are defined in relation to the availability of resources
and personnel, timeliness of physician response, diagnosis, and therapy.
Guidelines or protocols then are developed and audit filters are established
to monitor the guidelines. Tracking complications and process errors allows
trends to be monitored over time [32]. Death reviews should be conducted in
an attempt to determine preventability. Adoption of guidelines reduces variability and, consequently, fewer errors are made [33].

The trauma registry provides objective data to support continuous QI.
The registry should be designed to collect and calculate response times, admission diagnoses, diagnostic and therapeutic procedures, discharge diagnoses, complications, costs, and functional recovery. Trauma coordinators are
of utmost importance in making the QI process effective. They assure timely
recognition of problems, use of the registry to document problems, and that
problems are resolved.

Standardized definition of errors and preventable death

The development of trauma systems led to a significant reduction in the
number of preventable deaths after injury. It now is accepted commonly
that a preventable death rate of less than 1% to 2% is ideal in a trauma
system. According to the ACSCOT "Resources for Optimal Care of the
Injured Patient: 2006" document, an event is defined as nonpreventable
when it is a sequela of a procedure, disease, or injury for which reasonable
and appropriate preventable steps had been observed and taken. A potentially preventable event or complication is a sequela of a procedure, disease,
or injury that has the potential to be prevented or substantially ameliorated.
A preventable event or complication is an expected or unexpected sequela of
a procedure, disease, or injury that could have been prevented or substantially ameliorated [5].

A preventable death usually includes an injury or combination of injuries
considered survivable. Patients in this category generally are stable or, if unstable, respond adequately to treatment. If the evaluation or treatment is
suspect in any way, and the calculated probability of survival is greater
than 50%, then it would be classified as preventable. The causes of preventable deaths in trauma centers are different from those occurring at nontrauma hospitals. In nontrauma hospitals, preventable deaths occur
because the severity or multiplicity of injuries is not appreciated fully, leading to delays in diagnosis, lack of adequate monitoring, and delays to definitive therapy. In trauma hospitals, the causes of preventable death include

errors in judgment or errors in technique. In trauma centers, the diagnostic modalities used and potential for correct diagnosis normally are adequate.

These definitions are useful to monitor trauma systems performance and to compare different trauma systems. Once the preventable death rate reaches a plateau after trauma system implementation, system performance should focus on tracking provider-related complications. This approach has been proved adequate for identifying problems and implementing solutions [28].

Analysis of trauma system performance

Different study designs are used to evaluate trauma system effectiveness. The most common scientific approaches include panel-review preventable death studies, trauma registry performance comparisons, and population-based studies.

The data on trauma system effectiveness published in the literature are difficult to interpret because of great variability in study design, type of analysis, and definition of outcome variables. In an attempt to review the existing evidence on the effectiveness of trauma systems, the Oregon Health Sciences University, with support from the NHTSA and the National Center for Injury Prevention and Control of the CDC, organized the "Academic Symposium to Evaluate Evidence Regarding the Efficacy of Trauma Systems," also known as the Skamania conference [34].

Trauma care providers, policy makers, administrators, and researchers reviewed and discussed the available literature in an attempt to determine the impact of trauma systems on quality of patient care. The available literature on trauma system effectiveness until recently did not contain class I (prospective randomized controlled) trials or class II (well-designed, prospective, or retrospective controlled cohort or case-controlled) studies. There were several class III (panel studies, case series, or registry-based) studies reviewed and discussed during the symposium.

According to Mann and colleagues [35], who reviewed the published literature in preparation for the Skamania symposium, it is appropriate to conclude that the implementation of trauma systems decreases hospital mortality of patients who are severely injured. Independent of the methodology (panel review, registry based, or population based) used, a decrease in mortality of 15% to 20% is shown with the implementation of trauma systems [36–38]. A subsequent study using a rigid case-controlled methodology shows mortality reduction during system maturity of 8% to 10% [39].

A recent study investigated whether or not mortality is lower in inclusive systems compared with exclusive systems. The study concludes that patients who are severely injured are more likely to survive in states with the most inclusive trauma system, independent of the triage system in place. A possible explanation to these findings includes better initial care in referring hospitals [40].

A recent landmark study using prospectively collected data comparing mortality in trauma centers to nontrauma centers shows a 25% mortality reduction for patients under age 55 when treated in a trauma center [41].

Trauma systems report card

Despite the experience acquired on trauma system development in the United States during the past 3 decades, trauma systems still face many problems and challenges. A recent national inventory of trauma centers shows significant growth in the number of trauma centers during the last 10 years. This, however, is challenged by great variability in the number

---

Box 2. Current problems of trauma systems

Urban
Financial challenges
Uncompensated care
Closure of trauma centers
Source of funding for indigent care
Overdesignations of trauma center
Ineffective triage

Rural
Sparse population
Long distances
Difficult patient access
Weather conditions
Delays in notification
Treatment delays resulting from interfacility transfer needs
Lack of medical oversight

Pediatric
Lack of integration into the system
Inadequate education

Elderly
Increased costs
Increased morbidity and mortality
Inadequate prevention

Funding requirements
National level: national trauma system development
State/local level: to finance the EMS system
Research/prevention/avoidance of duplication

---

of trauma centers per million population throughout the United States. And, much of the United States remains uncovered by an organized trauma system [42]. When considering also the variability in triage effectiveness, the successful implementation of a countrywide trauma system remains a major challenge and needs continuous ongoing attention.

The financial challenge linked to the problem of uncompensated care has led to the closure of several trauma centers and the collapse of some trauma systems. Alternative and stable sources for funding indigent care have to be part of an agenda for legislative action in support of trauma systems. Box 2 lists the actual problems faced by regionalized trauma systems as documented by a strengths, weaknesses, opportunities, and threats analysis conducted by the HRSA in 2003 [16,19].

Despite the realization that trauma systems reduce morbidity and mortality, there remain several barriers to full implementation. The recent Model Trauma System Plan is well conceived and provides the strategic plan needed [1]. It is imagined that trauma systems, when implemented fully, will enhance community health through an organized system of injury prevention, acute care, and rehabilitation that is integrated fully into the public health system of a community. In addition to addressing the daily demands of trauma, they will form the basis for disaster preparedness and possess the distinct ability to identify risk factors and early interventions to prevent injuries in a community while integrating a delivery of optimal resources for patients who ultimately need acute trauma care.

The availability of federal dollars to assist in the development of trauma systems remains essential. Trauma systems need to be built that do not over-designate trauma centers and master resources yet meet the needs of all components of trauma patients. The biggest challenge is the implementation of what already is known how to do. Politicians need to be educated and the will of the public developed. Surgeons need to be relied on to provide leadership for this crucial effort.

References

[1] US Department of Health and Human Services. Health Resources and Services Administration, Trauma-EMS Systems Program. Model trauma system planning and evaluation; trauma systems collaborating with public health for improved injury outcomes. 2006. Available at: www.HRSA.gov/trauma/model.htm. Accessed August 1, 2006.

[2] Accidental death and disability: the neglected disease of modern society. Washington, DC: National Academy of Sciences; 1966.

[3] Emergency medical services: recommendations for an approach to an urgent national problem. In: Airlie Conference on Emergency Medical Services, Warrenton, Virginia, May 5–6, 1969. Chicago: American College of Surgeons; 1969.

[4] Committee on Trauma, American College of Surgeons. Optimal hospital resources for care of the seriously injured. Bull Am Coll Surg 1976;61:15–22.

[5] American College of Surgeons Committee on Trauma. Resources for optimal care of the injured patient: 2006. Chicago: American College of Surgeons; 2006.

[6] American College of Surgeons Committee on Trauma. Advanced trauma life support course: instructor manual. Chicago: American College of Surgeons; 2004.

[7] National Research Council. Injury in America: a continuing health care problem. Washington, DC: National Academy Press; 1985.

[8] National Center for Injury Prevention and Control. CDC injury research agenda. Atlanta: Centers for Disease Control and Prevention; 2002.

[9] A report of the Task Force on Trauma Research. Bethesda (MD): National Institutes of Health; 1994.

[10] Committee on Trauma, American College of Surgeons. Consultation for trauma systems. Chicago: American College of Surgeons; 1998.

[11] American College of Emergency Physicians. Guidelines for trauma care systems. Ann Emerg Med 1987;16:459.

[12] Development of trauma systems (DOT). Washington, DC: National Highway Traffic Safety Administration; 1988.

[13] Bass R, Gainer P, Carlini A. Update on trauma system development in the US. J Trauma 1999;47:S15–21.

[14] Model trauma care system plan. Rockville (MD): Department of Health and Human Services, Health Resources and Services Administration; 1992.

[15] California statewide trauma system plan. Sacramento (CA): Emergency Medical Services; 2005.

[16] US Department of Health & Human Services. A 2002 national assessment of state trauma system development, emergency medical services resources, and disaster readiness for mass casualty events. Washington (DC): HRSA; 2003

[17] Nathens A, Jurkovich G, MacKenzie E, et al. A resource-based assessment of trauma care in the United States. Trauma 2004;56:173–8.

[18] Potenza B, Hoyt D, Coimbra R, et al. Trauma Research and Education Foundation. The epidemiology of serious and fatal injury in San Diego County over an 11-year period. J Trauma 2004;56:68–75.

[19] American Trauma Society. Harris poll. Available at: www.amtrauma.org. Accessed August 1, 2006.

[20] Growing A. Crisis in patient access to emergency surgical care. Chicago: American College of Surgeons, Division of Advocacy and Health Policy; 2006.

[21] Moore E, Maier R, Hoyt D, et al. Acute care surgery: eraritjaritjaka. J Am Coll Surg 2006; 202:655–67.

[22] Pre-Hospital Trauma Life Support. Basic and advanced prehospital trauma life support. St. Louis (MO): Mosby; 1999.

[23] Davis D, Peay J, Sise M, et al. The impact of prehospital endotracheal intubation on outcome in moderate to severe traumatic brain injury. J Trauma 2005;58:933–9.

[24] Baker S, O'Neill B, Hadden W, et al. The injury severity score: a method for describing patients with multiple injuries and evaluating emergency care. J Trauma 1974;14:187.

[25] Champion H, Copes W, Sacco W, et al. The Major Trauma Outcome Study: establishing national norms for trauma care. J Trauma 1990;30:1356.

[26] County of San Diego Health and Human Services Agency Division of Emergency Medical Services. San Diego County trauma system report San Diego County; July 1, 2003 to June 30, 2004.

[27] Available at: http://www.facs.org/dept/trauma/handbook.html. Accessed August 1, 2006.

[28] Hoyt D, Hollingsworth-Fridlund P, Winchell R, et al. An analysis of recurrent process errors leading to provider-related complications of an organized trauma services; directions for care improvement. J Trauma 1994;36(3):377–84.

[29] Davis J, Hoyt D, McArdle M, et al. The significance of critical care errors in causing preventable death in trauma patients in a trauma system. J Trauma 1991;31:813–23.

[30] Davis J, Hoyt D, McArdle M, et al. An analysis of errors causing morbidity and mortality in a trauma system: a guide for quality improvement. J Trauma 1992;32:660–72.

[31] Shackford S, Hollingsworth-Fridlund P, Cooper G, et al. The effect of regionalization upon the quality of trauma care as assessed by concurrent audit before and after institution of a trauma system: a preliminary report. J Trauma 1986;26:812–20.

[32] Hoyt D, Coimbra R, Potenza B, et al. A twelve-year analysis of disease and provider complications on an organized level 1 trauma services: as good as it gets? J Trauma 2003;54: 26–36.

[33] Gruen R, Jurkovich G, McIntyre L, et al. patterns of errors contributing to trauma mortality: lessons learned from 2594 deaths. Ann Surg, submitted for publication.

[34] The Skamania Conference proceedings. J Trauma 1999;47(Suppl).

[35] Mann N, Mullins R, Mackenzie E, et al. Systematic review of published evidence regarding trauma system effectiveness. J Trauma 1999;47:S25–33.

[36] Mackenzie E. Review of evidence regarding trauma system effectiveness resulting from panel studies. J Trauma 1999;47(Suppl):S42–3.

[37] Jurkovich G, Mock C. Systematic review of trauma system effectiveness based on registry comparisons. J Trauma 1999;47(Suppl):S46–55.

[38] Mullins R, Mann N. Population-based research assessing the effectiveness of trauma systems. J Trauma 1999;47(Suppl):S59–66.

[39] Nathens A, Jurkovich G, Cummings P, et al. The effect of organized systems of trauma on motor vehicle crash mortality. JAMA 2000;283:1990–4.

[40] Utter G, Maier R, Rivara F, et al. Inclusive trauma systems: do they improve triage or outcomes of the severely injured? J Trauma 2006;60:529–37.

[41] MacKenzie E, Rivara F, Jurkovich G, et al. A national evaluation of the effect of trauma-center care on mortality. N Engl J Med 2006;354:366–78.

[42] MacKenzie E, Hoyt D, Sacra J, et al. National inventory of hospital trauma centers. JAMA 2003;289:1515–22.

ELSEVIER
SAUNDERS

SURGICAL
CLINICS OF
NORTH AMERICA

Surg Clin N Am 87 (2007) 37–53

Prehospital Care of the Injured: What's New

Eileen M. Bulger, MD*, Ronald V. Maier, MD

Department of Surgery, University of Washington, Harborview Medical Center, Box 359796, 325 9th Avenue, Seattle, WA 98104, USA

Prehospital care of patients who are injured can trace its roots to the care provided to those wounded in action in military conflicts. Over time, the commitment of military physicians has led to improvements in care of injured soldiers that subsequently have translated into the civilian environment. The advent of modern civilian prehospital trauma care is attributed to JD "Deke" Farrington and Sam Banks, who developed the first trauma course for ambulance personnel in 1962 [1]. During the 1970s, advanced prehospital care for cardiac emergencies was established, which led to the development of structured emergency medical services (EMS) supported by the EMS Systems Act passed in 1973. During the 1980s and 1990s, although advanced prehospital care proved beneficial for management of medical emergencies, especially after cardiac arrest, there was considerable debate about its usefulness in managing patients who were injured. Several physicians raised concern that the delay in transport for field interventions was detrimental to patients in hemorrhagic shock, as it delayed the time to operative control of the hemorrhage. This was supported by several studies suggesting that outcome for trauma patients managed by advanced life support (ALS) was not better, and in some cases worse, than those managed by basic life support alone [2–8]. Other reports, however, suggest benefit from ALS care for patients who are severely injured [9–12]. In addition, several recent studies call into question the specific procedures performed by paramedics in this setting.

A primary limitation to research in prehospital settings has been the significant variability that exists in the EMS systems and care delivered across the United States, making it difficult to generalize the results of these studies. The recently published Institute of Medicine report, "Emergency

---

* Corresponding author.
E-mail address: ebulger@u.washington.edu (E.M. Bulger).

0039-6109/07/$ - see front matter
doi:10.1016/j.suc.2006.09.009
surgical.theclinics.com

Medical Services at the Crossroads," highlights this variability, including the lack of national standards for training and patient care [13]. This report describes the fragmented responsibility for EMS systems that currently exists at the federal level and indicates the need to address regionalization of care. Survival to hospital discharge after cardiac arrest is reported to range from 3% to 45% across regions of the country [14–17]. Although this has been used as a benchmark to evaluate EMS system performance, little attention has been paid to how the variability in care provided has an impact on outcome after traumatic injury. The authors recently evaluated the prehospital care provided to patients who were injured in the 15 metropolitan regions in the United States that were involved in the National Study on the Costs and Outcomes of Trauma [18]. These data confirmed the significant variability in the care provided, which persisted even when patients were stratified based on injury severity. For example, the rate of prehospital endotracheal intubation (ETI) ranged from 5% to 48% among these regions, and intubation success rates varied from 33% to 100%.

This review seeks to summarize the current literature regarding the prehospital care of patients who are injured, recognizing that further research is necessary in most areas to develop clear standards of care. The initial evaluation and management of patients who are injured involves assessment and management of airway, breathing, circulation, and disability or the potential for neurologic injury. Based on this approach, the prehospital care surrounding each of these issues is reviewed and then field triage issues and the integration of prehospital providers into the overall trauma system are discussed. The ultimate goal of any EMS or trauma system is to get the right patient to the right place at the right time ultimately to optimize their outcome.

Airway management

There is perhaps no greater area of controversy in prehospital care than optimal management of the airway. It is clear from hospital-based studies that failure to manage the airway properly is a leading cause of preventable death after injury [19–21]. There are several clinical scenarios that require the need for urgent airway intervention. These include impending airway obstruction resulting from severe upper airway burns, expanding neck hematoma, direct trauma to the upper airway, inability to protect the airway because of altered level of consciousness or severe traumatic brain injury (TBI), and severe respiratory compromise with the need for assisted ventilation. Few would argue that these patients require early intubation; however, many would debate whether or not this is accomplished best in a prehospital setting or on arrival to an emergency department (ED).

Several studies report that the primary reason for failed prehospital intubation is muscle trismus or clenched jaw [22–24]. This factor is eliminated if paramedics are allowed to use neuromuscular blocking agents (NMBA) to facilitate intubation. The introduction of neuromuscular blockade to prehospital settings also is associated with higher rates of success at achieving ETI [25,26]. Prehospital intubation success rates are reported as high as 98% in systems using this approach [27]. Concern has been raised, however, that given the large number of ALS providers in many communities, the opportunity for individual paramedics to perform a rapid sequence intubation (RSI) using neuromuscular blockade is less than one per year and that this is insufficient exposure for individuals to maintain the skills necessary for this complex procedure [28]. In addition, if NMBA are given and patients cannot be intubated, a rescue airway procedure needs to be available, such as Combitube (Kendall-Sheridan Corporation, Argyle, New York) [29] or cricothyrotomy, and the training and skills maintenance for these procedures may be even more difficult. Some investigators suggest that there is overuse of surgical airway procedures in prehospital settings [30,31]; however, in a system using NMBA, the cricothyrotomy rate was only 1% of all intubation attempts [25]. In summary, it seems that ETI facilitated by neuromuscular blockade can be performed safely in prehospital settings, with improved success at achieving appropriate endotracheal tube placement and reduction in the need for surgical airway access. The question remains, however, whether or not prehospital ETI improves outcome for patients who are severely injured.

To address this issue, recent studies have focused specifically on patients who have severe TBI. Several studies demonstrate that hypoxia worsens outcome after severe TBI and this patient population usually requires early intubation for airway protection because of severe depression in the level of consciousness [32]. As a result, these patients are among those expected to derive the greatest benefit from prehospital ETI. An initial retrospective study of patients who had severe TBI in the San Diego area demonstrated decreased mortality for patients undergoing prehospital intubation versus those who did not, with the greatest improvement in those who had the most severe injuries (57% versus 36% mortality) [33]. This led to a prospective study in which paramedics were trained to perform RSI, and patients who had a prehospital Glasgow Coma Scale (GCS) score less than 8 were enrolled and compared with matched historical nonintubated controls [34]. This study was stopped early because of higher mortality in the patients who had RSI (33% versus 24% mortality). This analysis was limited by the requirement to match patients based on their head Abbreviated Injury Scale score rather than prehospital GCS score, as these data were not available for the historical controls. Regardless, these results led to the suspension of prehospital RSI in this region. In addition, subsequent analysis of these data suggests that the increased mortality may not be the result of the intubation itself but rather of inadvertent hyperventilation, which was common in these patients [35,36]. Hyperventilation leads to hypocapnea, which may result in cerebral vasoconstriction and, thus, reduced cerebral blood flow after brain injury. A recent analysis of the aeromedical transport system in San Diego demonstrated improved outcome for intubated TBI patients, which was associated with the continuous use of end-tidal CO_2 monitoring to avoid hyperventilation [37]. Thus, ETI may facilitate inadvertent hyperventilation, which may impair outcome (see ventilation discussion below).

Another study that has questioned the role of prehospital intubation in children was a prospective, randomized, controlled trial conducted by Gausche and colleagues [38]. This study randomized pediatric patients to bag-valve-mask ventilation versus ETI without the use of neuromuscular blockade and found no difference in mortality, neurologic outcome, or aspiration rates between the groups. This led them to conclude that prehospital ETI was not beneficial. This study was limited by the inexperience of the providers who were not performing pediatric intubations before the start of the trial and received only a 6-hour manikin training module before the start of the study. The intubation success rate in the trial was only 57% with a 14% rate of tube dislodgement and a 2% esophageal intubation rate. This study also highlights the difficulty with skills maintenance, as there were 416 intubations over the study period for 2584 paramedics. This equates to one intubation for every six paramedics over the course of the study. Similarly, data from the San Diego RSI trial suggest that individual paramedics participate in an RSI procedure an average of only once every 2 years.

Three other retrospective studies have specifically addressed prehospital RSI after severe TBI. Bochicchio and coworkers compared outcome for patients intubated in the field versus those intubated in the ED and identified a higher mortality for those intubated in the field (odds ratio [OR] 2.1; 95% CI, 0.9–5.0). Domier and colleagues evaluated outcome before and after institution of an RSI program for patients who had GCS scores 3 to 8 [39]. Survival to hospital discharge improved after beginning the RSI program but outcomes also were improved for the group without prehospital ETI for the same time period. Finally, the authors reported an analysis of 2012 intubated patients who had severe TBI treated at their institution over a 5-year period and, after adjustment for injury severity, found that those undergoing prehospital RSI had a reduced odds of mortality (OR 0.61; 95% CI, 0.41–0.97) and improved adjusted OR of "good" neurologic outcome (OR 1.7; 95% CI, 1.2–2.6) compared with those intubated without the use of NMBA [40]. All these studies suffer from the limitation that patients who undergo prehospital intubation are likely to be more severely injured than those who do not. Thus, there may be a confounding variable that cannot be accounted for in a retrospective analysis. The Brain Trauma Foundation recently convened a panel of experts in this field, which included all of the investigators in these studies. This panel concluded that the available literature addressing prehospital RSI after severe TBI is inconclusive and emphasized the importance of future studies that appropriately account for the impact of airway- and nonairway-related factors on outcome after TBI [40a]. In addition, this group emphasized the importance of adequate system infrastructure to support a prehospital RSI program, including strong medical direction and oversight, protocol development, cognitive and technical training that includes a focus on appropriate patient ventilation, appropriate prehospital triage, a skills maintenance program, and a performance improvement program. These sentiments are echoed by the position paper on prehospital RSI published by the National Association of EMS Physicians [41].

Ventilation

As indicated in the discussion of prehospital intubation, appropriate ventilation of patients has emerged as a critical factor that may have impact on outcome. Hyperventilation may be detrimental for patients who have severe TBI and those in hypovolemic shock. Previous studies have shown that hyperventilation leads to hypocapnea, which results in cerebral vasoconstriction [42–44]. This impairs cerebral blood flow and could contribute to secondary brain injury. Furthermore, for patients who have severe hypovolemia, excessive ventilation can raise the intrathoracic pressure and, thus, impair venous return further, contributing to cardiovascular collapse [45].

Hyperventilation is common in prehospital settings and seems to be facilitated by ETI. In the San Diego RSI study, 50% of patients were hypocapneic on arrival to the ED ($Pco_2 < 33$ mm Hg) [34,35]. Recent studies demonstrate an association between end-tidal CO_2 levels less than 30 mm Hg and increased mortality after TBI [46,47]. Recent work by Davis and colleagues suggests that the use of continuous end-tidal CO_2 monitoring in prehospital settings may help avoid inadvertent hyperventilation [48]. Further study is warranted to determine the optimal use of this technology, including the appropriate target range for the EMS providers. The reliability of end-tidal CO_2 in low flow states, such as severe hypovolemia, remains to be determined. In addition to avoiding hyperventilation, hypoventilation in patients who have severe chest injury may be just as detrimental. In the authors' institution, mortality for TBI patients who arrive hypercapneic ($Pco_2 > 45$ mm Hg) exceeds 50% (Eileen Bulger, MD, unpublished data, 2006).

In summary, there is growing recognition that how patients are ventilated early after injury may have an impact on outcome. Further study is needed to determine the optimal monitoring approach to avoid hyper- or hypoventilation after injury. Ventilation using a standard Ambu bag is difficult to regulate, especially in often chaotic, prehospital environments. Future studies will evaluate technologic aids, including end-tidal CO_2 monitoring; the use of transport ventilators; the use of a SMART BAG (O-Two Medical Technologies), which resists excessive ventilation; and the addition of timing lights to prompt a more regulated ventilatory rate.

Management of circulation

The basic tenets of circulatory management after injury are control of hemorrhage and resuscitation with intravenous fluids. In prehospital settings, control of hemorrhage is focused primarily on application of pressure to control external bleeding and rapid transport to a trauma center to address internal hemorrhage. There are several new products introduced to the marketplace to aid in the control of external hemorrhage. These dressings are impregnated with substances to promote coagulation including: microporous polysaccharide hemospheres (TraumaDEX), mineral zeolite (QuikClot), poly-N-acetylglucosamine (HemCon), and microporous hydrogel-forming polyacrylamide (BioHemostat). Although these dressings show promise in animal models and several have been piloted by the United States military, they have yet to prove superior to direct pressure for control of external bleeding in patients who are injured [49]. The QuikClot product also is hampered by the initial induction of an exothermic reaction, which can result in burns to an ungloved rescuer. Further studies are ongoing, with fibrin-impregnated bandages that may prove useful in the future. For now, direct pressure and rapid transport are the mainstays of therapy in civilian settings.

The second area of focus for prehospital resuscitation is the administration of intravenous fluids. One study questions the advantages of intravenous fluids for patients who have penetrating torso trauma and a short transport time to the hospital [50]. In this study, patients were randomized to no fluid before surgery versus conventional resuscitation. These investigators report better outcome in the no fluid group. The theory is that patients who have isolated vascular trauma may form a temporary clot over the injury site, which may be dislodged by excessive fluid resuscitation, leading to increased blood pressure, leading to increased bleeding. Concern is raised, however, about generalizing these results to all trauma patients. The majority of traumatic injury in the United States is a result of blunt trauma, commonly with associated TBI. Prehospital hypotension after severe TBI is associated with increased mortality; thus, the principles of limited fluid resuscitation may not be applicable in this circumstance [32,51]. In addition, patients transported from rural areas may not tolerate a prolonged period of hypoperfusion. Thus, administration of intravenous fluid remains an important component of prehospital care after injury. One approach that is advocated is a controlled fluid resuscitation strategy, which targets fluid administration to a blood pressure threshold [52]. Further study is warranted to determine the appropriate prehospital resuscitation targets for patients who have multisystem injury.

Intravenous access usually is achieved in adults by using upper extremity peripheral veins. There has been a recent renewed interest in intraosseous access for adults for whom peripheral intravenous access cannot be achieved. Tibial intraosseous access has been used for children under age

6 for many years. A recent consensus conference on the resuscitation of combat casualties recommends the use of sternal intraosseous access for the resuscitation of injured soldiers because of the simplicity of insertion in a battlefield environment [53]. This has contributed to the development of several new sternal intraosseous devices marketed to the EMS community. A report of the early experience with one of these devices from an EMS system in Canada demonstrates an 84% success rate with placement and reasonable flow rates [54]. There are complications reported, however, and, given the limited data available, these devices should be used only in patients who have a critical need for access for whom intravenous access cannot be established.

Once intravenous access is obtained for trauma patients, the next question is what the best fluid is to give. Current standard of care involves resuscitation with either lactated Ringer's solution or normal saline. Although these fluids have been in use for more than 30 years, there remain problems with this approach. High volumes of normal saline can lead to the development of a hyperchloremic metabolic acidosis. In addition, several studies suggest that lactated Ringer's solution may induce a proinflammtory response in patients that could exacerbate the development of inflammatory organ injury [55–57]. Two promising alternatives for prehospital resuscitation of traumatic hemorrhagic shock currently are in clinical trials. These are hypertonic resuscitation with either 7.5% saline with or without 6% Dextran 70 and polymerized hemoglobin blood substitutes.

Hypertonic resuscitation is not a new concept. Initial studies were conducted in the 1980s after a series of animal studies that suggested that resuscitation with a small volume of 7.5% saline improved outcome in models of hemorrhagic shock [58,59]. There were eight clinical trials published in the late 1980s and early 1990s of resuscitation with hypertonic saline/dextran (HSD). Six were prehospital based and two were ED based [60–68]. All the prehospital trials suggested a survival advantage but were underpowered and many were stopped prematurely for logistic reasons. These initial trials focused primarily on the hemodynamic effects of this resuscitation strategy. Subsequently, a large number of laboratory studies demonstrated that hypertonicity has profound effects on the inflammatory response with transient suppression of neutrophil and monocyte function while enhancing T-cell function [69–74]. Studies in animal models of acute respiratory distress syndrome (ARDS) subsequently demonstrated significant attenuation of lung injury after resuscitation with hypertonic saline [75,76]. In addition, during this time, frame hypertonicity also was being evaluated as an effective means to control intracranial pressure after severe TBI [77–79].

After these initial studies, there were four meta-analyses conducted by Wade and coworkers [80–83]. The first was a traditional meta-analysis of all the trials using HSD or HTS published as of 1997. The conclusion from this article was that HSD offers a survival benefit for the treatment of traumatic hypotension, although there was no benefit from HTS alone. These investigators acknowledged the limitations of including studies with significant differences in design and went on to perform two individual patient cohort analyses. The first, which included 1395 patients from previous trials, demonstrated an improvement in overall survival to discharge in the HSD group (OR 1.47; 95% CI, 1.04–2.08). Furthermore, patients who required blood transfusion or immediate surgical intervention for bleeding showed an even greater survival benefit from HSD. The second analysis focused on 223 patients who had hypotension and TBI. This article concludes that HSD treatment in these patients resulted in a twofold increase in survival compared with conventional resuscitation. Finally, in 2003, a meta-analysis was conducted for the subgroup of patients who had penetrating torso trauma and demonstrated improved survival for patients in the HSD group (82.5% versus 75.5%). This improvement was even more notable among those requiring immediate surgery.

Despite the suggestion of benefit in these early trials and regulatory approval for use of HSD in Europe, United States Food and Drug Administration approval has not been achieved. This may be the result in large part of the lack of a driving corporate sponsor to fund a large multicenter trial. Two additional trials recently have been completed. Cooper and coworkers conducted a prehospital trial of 7.5% saline without dextran as the initial resuscitation fluid for patients who were hypotensive (systolic blood pressure [SBP] < 100 mm Hg) and who had severe TBI (GCS < 8 in the field) [84]. This study enrolled 229 patients and demonstrated no difference in neurologic outcome 6 months after injury based on the extended Glasgow outcome score. As this trial was confined to patients who had prehospital hypotension, the hospital mortality was 50%, thus limiting the number of patients available for follow-up and limiting the power of the trial. Although not statistically significant, there was a trend toward improved 6-month survival in the hypertonic group (OR 1.17; 95% CI, 0.9–1.5). Of the patients who survived to an ED, the long-term survival was 67% for those receiving hypertonic saline versus 55% for the controls (OR 1.72; 95% CI, 0.95–3.1, $P = .07$). The authors also recently completed a trial of HSD versus lactated Ringer's solution as the initial resuscitation fluid for blunt trauma patients in hypovolemic shock (SBP < 90 mm Hg) with a primary endpoint of 28-day ARDS-free survival [85]. This trial enrolled 209 patients with a planned enrollment of 400 patients but was stopped early for futility with no significant difference in outcome between the groups. In reviewing this data, the authors identified a suggestion of benefit among those at highest risk for ARDS based on the need for massive transfusion (> 10 U packed red blood cells in the first 24 hours after injury). The authors believe the finding of futility was the result of enrollment of too many patients who were not in severe shock, with 44% of patients not requiring any blood in the first 24 hours.

Based on the results of these studies, the Resuscitation Outcomes Consortium, which is supported by the National Institutes of Health, is launching a multicenter trial of hypertonic resuscitation, which seeks to evaluate the impact on outcome for patients who have hypovolemic shock and/or severe TBI. This trial will randomize patients to receive HSD, 7.5% saline without dextran, or normal saline as their initial resuscitation fluid in prehospital settings. The primary outcome for patients in hypovolemic shock will be 28-day survival and for TBI, 6-month neurologic outcome. The entry criteria for the hypovolemic shock cohort has been modified based on the experience in the Seattle trial to SBP less than 70 mm Hg or SBP 70 to 90 mm Hg with heart rate greater than 108 beats per minute. The power calculations suggest an anticipated enrollment of 3726 patients in the hypovolemic shock cohort and 2122 patients in the TBI cohort. This study is now enrolling patients and should provide a definitive answer regarding the future use of this resuscitation strategy for trauma patients.

The second promising line of research for prehospital resuscitation is the use of the hemoglobin-based blood substitute oxygen carriers. These products have the advantage of oxygen-carrying capacity and improved oxygen delivery, which cannot be accomplished with other crystalloid or colloid solutions. In addition, they are shown to result in less stimulation of the inflammatory response than is found after conventional blood transfusion [86,87]. There are three primary products under investigation. These include Polyheme and Hemolink, which are human forms of polymerized hemoglobin, and Hemopure, which is a bovine-based hemoglobin solution [88]. Polyheme was piloted in an initial hospital-based study where it was found to have a good safety profile, and patients had improved survival compared with historical controls [89]. Polyheme currently is being studied in a phase III randomized prehospital trial in the United States and the results of this trial should clarify the role of this treatment strategy further.

In summary, the current standard of care for fluid resuscitation of patients who are injured in prehospital settings is the intravenous administration of crystalloid solutions. The results of ongoing clinical trials are awaited to further define the use of hypertonic solutions and hemoglobin-based oxygen carriers.

Disability: spinal injury

The standard prehospital approach to patients who have a mechanism of injury that may result in spinal injury is to maintain alignment with spinal immobilization devices. These techniques are taught at the basic EMT level. Spinal immobilization criteria were incorporated into EMS training in the 1970s, and in 1988, a report from the Northwestern University Spinal Cord Injury Center noted a progressive decline in the proportion of patients presenting with neurologic deficit from 70% in 1972 to 33% in 1986 [90]. They attributed this improvement to adoption of immobilization protocols by EMS. Widely accepted guidelines suggest that the criteria for spinal immobilization should include any mechanism of injury suggesting violent or sudden forces to the spine regardless of the absence of other signs and symptoms; injury patterns that suggest violent forces have acted on the spine; or the presence of any signs or symptoms of spinal injury [91].

Some investigators question the liberal use of spinal immobilization, suggesting that there are some adverse effects of prehospital immobilization, including increased risk for aspiration, airway compromise, delay in transport, and patient discomfort [92]. One retrospective study has compared outcome between patients treated at the University of New Mexico, where spinal immobilization was common, versus the University of Kuala Lumpur, where no prehospital immobilization occurred [93]. These investigators suggest a higher rate of neurologic injury among the patients treated at the University of New Mexico and conclude that there is a 98% probability that immobilization is harmful or of no value. This study has several limitations, including vast differences in the mechanism of injury between the patient groups and a small sample size. It does highlight, however, the lack of clinical data supporting current practice. Some investigators have reported on the use of selective prehospital spinal immobilization using defined protocols [92,94,95]. One report suggests that the use of a prehospital spine assessment protocol resulted in an EMS decision not to immobilize 40% of the patients who previously would have been immobilized [96]. These studies are limited, however, and the number of spinal cord injuries in the population meeting criteria for immobilization is so small that large numbers of patients need to be enrolled to determine the true impact on outcome. In this study, for example, there were only seven spine fractures among 2220 patient encounters. It is estimated that 20% of spinal cord injury patients die before reaching the hospital and 25% of spinal cord damage may occur or worsen after an initial event [96]. Based on these statistics, and the lack of randomized controlled trial data to guide therapy, it seems that the most conservative approach, which includes liberal spinal immobilization, is warranted.

Prehospital trauma triage

The EMS system plays a critical role in the trauma system, as prehospital providers are responsible for determining which patients warrant transport to a trauma center, which may involve bypassing closer hospital without a trauma designation. A recent national study demonstrates that patients cared for at designated trauma centers have improved outcome compared with those treated at nondesignated centers [97]. Furthermore, the viability of the trauma system is dependent on appropriate triage, as undertriage can lead to impaired patient outcome and overtriage can lead to an excessive burden on regional trauma centers and, thus, impair availability to care for patients who are injured most severely. Several groups have sought to develop prehospital trauma triage criteria, which are based on a combination of physiologic indicators and mechanism of injury along with special considerations for high-risk populations, such as children and the elderly. Recent studies have focused on the reliability of prehospital vital signs and GCS score to predict the need for a lifesaving intervention. Two reports by Holcomb and colleagues suggest that for adults, prehospital SBP less than 90 mm Hg, GCS motor score less than 6, and radial pulse character are predictors for the need of a lifesaving intervention [98,99]. A recent study suggests that reduced heart rate variability also may be a useful marker of decreased survival, but this was not superior to the GCS score and requires sophisticated monitoring [100]. Another recent report suggests that automated blood pressure measurements are not reliable in prehospital settings, so criteria should be based on manual assessment [101].

The Centers for Disease Control recently sponsored a multidisciplinary committee to review the evidence and recommend national standards for prehospital trauma triage (Jerry Jurkovich, MD, personal communication, 2006). This algorithm will be published in the upcoming revision of the "Resources for the Optimal Care of the Injured Patient," published by the American College of Surgeons Committee on Trauma. This triage scheme involves a 4-step evaluation process beginning with assessment of impaired vital signs and GCS score, followed by evaluation for critical injury patterns, then assessment of high-energy impact mechanism, and, finally, the assessment of special patient considerations, including the extremes of age, pregnancy, anticoagulation, burns, and end-stage renal disease. This algorithm should serve as a springboard for each region to evaluate their local trauma triage guidelines, to ensure that they are evidenced based, and to address local transport challenges.

In addition to transport guidelines, another area of controversy surrounds which patients can be pronounced dead in the field, thereby avoiding excess use of resources and increased risks to providers because of transport of nonsalvageable patients. The American College of Surgeons Committee on Trauma and the National Association for EMS Physicians recently published consensus guidelines for withholding or terminating resuscitation after prehospital traumatic cardiopulmonary arrest [102]. In summary, these guidelines suggest that for patients who have blunt trauma, resuscitation may be withheld if patients are found apneic, pulseless, and without organized electrical activity on EMS arrival. For penetrating trauma, additional signs of life, such as pupillary responses and spontaneous movement, should be assessed and, if absent, resuscitation may be withheld. In addition, termination of resuscitation may be considered after 15 minutes of unsuccessful efforts or if the transport time to a trauma center is more than 15 minutes. The latter guidelines based on the 15-minute time limit were challenged by recent data from the authors' institution [103], where 184 patients who had prehospital traumatic arrest were reviewed, of whom 138 were transported to the hospital. Among these were 14 survivors (10.1%). Among the survivors, 21% had an EMS cardiopulmonary resuscitation time greater than 15 minutes and 93% exceeded the recommended 15-minute transport time. Further study is warrant to continue to refine these guidelines.

Summary

In summary, EMS plays a critical role in the trauma system not only as the point of initial patient care and stabilization but also for determining the regional flow of patients and the commitment of resources to the critically injured. Trauma surgeons and emergency physicians need to be involved in the organizational planning of the EMS system to ensure that uniform patient care protocols are developed for triage and treatment of patients who are injured. Ongoing efforts should focus on addressing the national variability in care provided after injury to ensure optimal outcome for patients in all regions. The Institute of Medicine report on EMS makes several recommendations in this regard, including the development of evidence-based protocols for the treatment, triage, and transport of patients; a common scope of practice for EMS personnel with state licensing reciprocity; national certification as a prerequisite for state licensure and local credentialing; state requirements for national accreditation of paramedic education programs; creation of subspecialty certification in EMS to enhance training of medical directors; and the development of evidence-based indicators of emergency care system performance. Finally, it is only through additional research that the best practice and optimal EMS system design will continued to be defined.

References

[1] Salomone JP, Frame SB. Prehospital care. In: Moore EE, Feliciano DV, Mattox KL, editors. Trauma. New York: McGraw-Hill; 2004. p. 105–25.
[2] Cayten CG, Murphy JG, Stahl WM. Basic life support versus advanced life support for injured patients with an injury severity score of 10 or more. J Trauma 1993;35:460–6 [discussion: 466–7].
[3] Cornwell EE 3rd, Belzberg H, Hennigan K, et al. Emergency medical services (EMS) vs non-EMS transport of critically injured patients: a prospective evaluation. Arch Surg 2000;135:315–9.
[4] Demetriades D, Chan L, Cornwell E, et al. Paramedic vs private transportation of trauma patients. Effect on outcome. Arch Surg 1996;131:133–8.
[5] Eckstein M, Chan L, Schneir A, et al. Effect of prehospital advanced life support on outcomes of major trauma patients. J Trauma 2000;48:643–8.
[6] Liberman M, Mulder D, Sampalis J. Advanced or basic life support for trauma: meta-analysis and critical review of the literature. J Trauma 2000;49:584–99.
[7] Liberman M, Mulder D, Lavoie A, et al. Multicenter Canadian study of prehospital trauma care. Ann Surg 2003;237:153–60.
[8] Sampalis JS, Lavoie A, Williams JI, et al. Impact of on-site care, prehospital time, and level of in-hospital care on survival in severely injured patients. J Trauma 1993;34:252–61.

[9] Hu SC, Kao WF. Outcomes in severely ill patients transported without prehospital ALS. Am J Emerg Med 1996;14:86–8.

[10] Messick WJ, Rutledge R, Meyer AA. The association of advanced life support training and decreased per capita trauma death rates: an analysis of 12,417 trauma deaths. J Trauma 1992;33:850–5.

[11] Quintans-Rodriquez A, Turegano-Fuentes F, Hernandez-Granados P, et al. Survival after prehospital advanced life support in severe trauma. Eur J Emerg Med 1995;2:224–6.

[12] Sanson G, Di Bartolomeo S, Nardi G, et al. Road traffic accidents with vehicular entrapment: incidence of major injuries and need for advanced life support. Eur J Emerg Med 1999;6:285–91.

[13] Emergency medical services at the crossroads. Washington, DC: Institute of Medicine of the National Academies; 2006.

[14] Davis R. Many lives are lost across USA because emergency services fail. USA Today. July 28, 2003:1A, 6A–7A.

[15] Cobb LA. Variability in resuscitation rates for out-of-hospital cardiac arrest. Arch Intern Med 1993;153:1165–6.

[16] Fredriksson M, Herlitz J, Nichol G. Variation in outcome in studies of out-of-hospital cardiac arrest: a review of studies conforming to the Utstein guidelines. Am J Emerg Med 2003;21:276–81.

[17] Rea TD, Eisenberg MS, Sinibaldi G, et al. Incidence of EMS-treated out-of-hospital cardiac arrest in the United States. Resuscitation 2004;63:17–24.

[18] Bulger EM, Nathens AB, Rivara FP, et al. National variability in out of hospital treatment after traumatic injury. Ann Emerg Med. Available at: www.ncbi.nih.gov/entrez/query.fcgi? Electronic publication 1097-6760, September 13, 2006.

[19] Esposito TJ, Sanddal ND, Dean JM, et al. Analysis of preventable pediatric trauma deaths and inappropriate trauma care in Montana. J Trauma 1999;47:243–51 [discussion: 251–3].

[20] Esposito TJ, Sanddal ND, Hansen JD, et al. Analysis of preventable trauma deaths and inappropriate trauma care in a rural state. J Trauma 1995;39:955–62.

[21] Rivara FP, Maier RV, Mueller BA, et al. Evaluation of potentially preventable deaths among pedestrian and bicyclist fatalities. JAMA 1989;261:566–70.

[22] Wang HE, Kupas DF, Paris PM, et al. Multivariate predictors of failed prehospital endotracheal intubation. Acad Emerg Med 2003;10:717–24.

[23] Doran JV, Tortella BJ, Drivet WJ, et al. Factors influencing successful intubation in the prehospital setting. Prehospital Disaster Med 1995;10:259–64.

[24] Krisanda TJ, Eitel DR, Hess D, et al. An analysis of invasive airway management in a suburban emergency medical services system. Prehospital Disaster Med 1992;7:121–6.

[25] Davis DP, Ochs M, Hoyt DB, et al. Paramedic-administered neuromuscular blockade improves prehospital intubation success in severely head-injured patients. J Trauma 2003;55: 713–9.

[26] Syverud SA, Borron SW, Storer DL, et al. Prehospital use of neuromuscular blocking agents in a helicopter ambulance program. Ann Emerg Med 1988;17:236–42.

[27] Bulger EM, Copass MK, Maier RV, et al. An analysis of advanced prehospital airway management. J Emerg Med 2002;23:183–9.

[28] Wang HE, Kupas DF, Hostler D, et al. Procedural experience with out-of-hospital endotracheal intubation. Crit Care Med 2005;33:1718–21.

[29] Davis DP, Valentine C, Ochs M, et al. The Combitube as a salvage airway device for paramedic rapid sequence intubation. Ann Emerg Med 2003;42:697–704.

[30] Fortune JB, Judkins DG, Scanzaroli D, et al. Efficacy of prehospital surgical cricothyrotomy in trauma patients. J Trauma 1997;42:832–6 [discussion: 837–8].

[31] Gerich TG, Schmidt U, Hubrich V, et al. Prehospital airway management in the acutely injured patient: the role of surgical cricothyrotomy revisited. J Trauma 1998; 45:312–4.

[32] Chesnut RM, Marshall LF, Klauber MR, et al. The role of secondary brain injury in deter-mining outcome from severe head injury. J Trauma 1993;34:216–22.

[33] Winchell RJ, Hoyt DB. Endotracheal intubation in the field improves survival in patients with severe head injury. Trauma Research and Education Foundation of San Diego. Arch Surg 1997;132:592–7.

[34] Davis DP, Hoyt DB, Ochs M, et al. The effect of paramedic rapid sequence intubation on outcome in patients with severe traumatic brain injury. J Trauma 2003;54:444–53.

[35] Davis DP, Heister R, Poste JC, et al. Ventilation patterns in patients with severe traumatic brain injury following paramedic rapid sequence intubation. Neurocrit Care 2005;2: 165–71.

[36] Davis DP, Stern J, Sise MJ, et al. A follow-up analysis of factors associated with head-injury mortality after paramedic rapid sequence intubation. J Trauma 2005;59:486–90.

[37] Poste JC, Davis DP, Ochs M, et al. Air medical transport of severely head-injured patients undergoing paramedic rapid sequence intubation. Air Med J 2004;23:36–40.

[38] Gausche M, Lewis RJ, Stratton SJ, et al. Effect of out-of-hospital pediatric endotracheal intubation on survival and neurological outcome: a controlled clinical trial [comments] [published erratum appears in JAMA 2000;283:3204]. JAMA 2000;283:783–90.

[39] Domeier RM, Frederiksen SM, Chudnofsky CF, et al. The effect of paramedic rapid se-quence intubation on outcome in trauma patients [abstract]. Prehosp Emerg Care 2005; 9:114–5.

[40] Bulger EM, Copass MK, Sabath DR, et al. The use of neuromuscular blocking agents to facilitate prehospital intubation does not impair outcome after traumatic brain injury. J Trauma 2005;58:718–23 [discussion: 723–4].

[40a] Davis D, Fakhry S, Wang H, et al. Paramedic rapid sequence intubation for severe trau-matic brain injury: Perspectives from an expert panel. Prehospital Emergency Care. In press 2006.

[41] Wang HE, Davis DP, O'Connor RE, et al. Drug-assisted intubation in the prehospital set-ting (resource document to NAEMSP Position Statement). Prehosp Emerg Care 2006;10: 261–71.

[42] Hemphill JC 3rd, Knudson MM, Derugin N, et al. Carbon dioxide reactivity and pres-sure autoregulation of brain tissue oxygen. Neurosurgery 2001;48:377–83 [discussion: 383–4].

[43] Coles JP, Minhas PS, Fryer TD, et al. Effect of hyperventilation on cerebral blood flow in traumatic head injury: clinical relevance and monitoring correlates. Crit Care Med 2002;30: 1950–9.

[44] Imberti R, Bellinzona G, Langer M. Cerebral tissue PO2 and SjvO2 changes during moderate hyperventilation in d severe traumatic brain injury. J Neurosurg 2002;96: 97–102.

[45] Manley GT, Hemphill JC, Morabito D, et al. Cerebral oxygenation during hemorrhagic shock: perils of hyperventilation and the therapeutic potential of hypoventilation. J Trauma 2000;48:1025–32 [discussion: 1032–3].

[46] Davis DP, Idris AH, Sise MJ, et al. Early ventilation and outcome in patients with moderate to severe traumatic brain injury. Crit Care Med 2006;34:1202–8.

[47] Davis DP, Dunford JV, Poste JC, et al. The impact of hypoxia and hyperventilation on out-come after paramedic rapid sequence intubation of severely head-injured patients. J Trauma 2004;57:1–8 [discussion: 8–10].

[48] Davis DP, Dunford JV, Ochs M, et al. The use of quantitative end-tidal capnometry to avoid inadvertent severe hyperventilation in patients with head injury after paramedic rapid sequence intubation. J Trauma 2004;56:808–14.

[49] Neuffer MC, McDivitt J, Rose D, et al. Hemostatic dressings for the first responder: a review. Mil Med 2004;169:716–20.

[50] Bickell WH, Wall MJ Jr, Pepe PE, et al. Immediate versus delayed fluid resuscitation for hypotensive patients with penetrating torso injuries. N Engl J Med 1994;331:1105–9.

[51] Chesnut RM, Marshall SB, Piek J, et al. Early and late systemic hypotension as a frequent and fundamental source of cerebral ischemia following severe brain injury in the Traumatic Coma Data Bank. Acta Neurochir Suppl (Wien) 1993;59:121–5.

[52] Burris D, Rhee P, Kaufmann C, et al. Controlled resuscitation for uncontrolled hemorrhagic shock. J Trauma 1999;46:216–23.

[53] Champion HR. Combat fluid resuscitation: introduction and overview of conferences. J Trauma 2003;54(5 Suppl):S7–12.

[54] Susak L, Macnab AJ, Christenson J, et al. Early report on emergency sternal intraosseous infusion in adults. Prehosp Disast Med 2000;15:s51.

[55] Rhee P, Burris D, Kaufmann C, et al. Lactated Ringer's solution resuscitation causes neutrophil activation after hemorrhagic shock. J Trauma 1998;44:313–9.

[56] Rhee P, Wang D, Ruff P, et al. Human neutrophil activation and increased adhesion by various resuscitation fluids. Crit Care Med 2000;28:74–8.

[57] Rizoli SB. Crystalloids and colloids in trauma resuscitation: a brief overview of the current debate. J Trauma 2003;54(5 Suppl):S82–8.

[58] Rowe GG, McKenna DH, Corliss RJ, et al. Hemodynamic effects of hypertonic sodium chloride. J Appl Physiol 1972;32:182–4.

[59] Velasco IT, Pontieri V, Rocha e Silva M Jr, et al. Hyperosmotic NaCl and severe hemorrhagic shock. Am J Physiol 1980;239:H664–73.

[60] Holcroft JW, Vassar MJ, Perry CA, et al. Use of a 7.5% NaCl/6% Dextran 70 solution in the resuscitation of injured patients in the emergency room. Prog Clin Biol Res 1989;299: 331–8.

[61] Holcroft JW, Vassar MJ, Turner JE, et al. 3% NaCl and 7.5% NaCl/dextran 70 in the resuscitation of severely injured patients. Ann Surg 1987;206:279–88.

[62] Vassar MJ, Fischer RP, O'Brien PE, et al. A multicenter trial for resuscitation of injured patients with 7.5% sodium chloride. The effect of added dextran 70. The Multicenter Group for the Study of Hypertonic Saline in Trauma Patients. Arch Surg 1993;128:1003–11 [discussion: 1011–3].

[63] Vassar MJ, Perry CA, Gannaway WL, et al. 7.5% sodium chloride/dextran for resuscitation of trauma patients undergoing helicopter transport. Arch Surg 1991;126: 1065–72.

[64] Vassar MJ, Perry CA, Holcroft JW. Prehospital resuscitation of hypotensive trauma patients with 7.5% NaCl versus 7.5% NaCl with added dextran: a controlled trial. J Trauma 1993;34:622–32 [discussion: 632–3].

[65] Younes RN, Aun F, Accioly CQ, et al. Hypertonic solutions in the treatment of hypovolemic shock: a prospective, randomized study in patients admitted to the emergency room. Surgery 1992;111:380–5.

[66] Mattox KL, Maningas PA, Moore EE, et al. Prehospital hypertonic saline/dextran infusion for post-traumatic hypotension. The U.S.A. Multicenter Trial. Ann Surg 1991; 213:482–91.

[67] Maningas PA, Mattox KL, Pepe PE, et al. Hypertonic saline-dextran solutions for the prehospital management of traumatic hypotension. Am J Surg 1989;157:528–33 [discussion: 533–4].

[68] Younes RN, Aun F, Ching CT, et al. Prognostic factors to predict outcome following the administration of hypertonic/hyperoncotic solution in hypovolemic patients. Shock 1997;7: 79–83.

[69] Cuschieri J, Gourlay D, Garcia I, et al. Hypertonic preconditioning inhibits macrophage responsiveness to endotoxin. J Immunol 2002;168:1389–96.

[70] Rizoli SB, Kapus A, Parodo J, et al. Hypertonic immunomodulation is reversible and accompanied by changes in CD11b expression. J Surg Res 1999;83:130–5.

[71] Rizoli SB, Kapus A, Parodo J, et al. Hypertonicity prevents lipopolysaccharide-stimulated CD11b/CD18 expression in human neutrophils in vitro: role for p38 inhibition. J Trauma 1999;46:794–8 [discussion: 798–9].

[72] Rizoli SB, Rotstein OD, Parodo J, et al. Hypertonic inhibition of exocytosis in neutrophils: central role for osmotic actin skeleton remodeling. Am J Physiol Cell Physiol 2000;279: C619–33.

[73] Junger WG, Coimbra R, Liu FC, et al. Hypertonic saline resuscitation: a tool to modulate immune function in trauma patients? Shock 1997;8:235–41.

[74] Junger WG, Liu FC, Loomis WH, et al. Hypertonic saline enhances cellular immune function. Circ Shock 1994;42:190–6.

[75] Angle N, Hoyt DB, Coimbra R, et al. Hypertonic saline resuscitation diminishes lung injury by suppressing neutrophil activation after hemorrhagic shock. Shock 1998;9:164–70.

[76] Rizoli SB, Kapus A, Fan J, et al. Immunomodulatory effects of hypertonic resuscitation on the development of lung inflammation following hemorrhagic shock. J Immunol 1998;161: 6288–96.

[77] Hartl R, Ghajar J, Hochleuthner H, et al. Hypertonic/hyperoncotic saline reliably reduces ICP in severely head- injured patients with intracranial hypertension. Acta Neurochir Suppl (Wien) 1997;70:126–9.

[78] Hartl R, Medary MB, Ruge M, et al. Hypertonic/hyperoncotic saline attenuates microcirculatory disturbances after traumatic brain injury. J Trauma 1997;42(5 Suppl): S41–7.

[79] Schmoker JD, Zhuang J, Shackford SR. Hypertonic fluid resuscitation improves cerebral oxygen delivery and reduces intracranial pressure after hemorrhagic shock. J Trauma 1991;31:1607–13.

[80] Wade C, Grady J, Kramer G. Efficacy of hypertonic saline dextran (HSD) in patients with traumatic hypotension: meta-analysis of individual patient data. Acta Anaesthesiol Scand Suppl 1997;110:77–9.

[81] Wade CE, Grady JJ, Kramer GC. Efficacy of hypertonic saline dextran fluid resuscitation for patients with hypotension from penetrating trauma. J Trauma 2003;54(5 Suppl): S144–8.

[82] Wade CE, Grady JJ, Kramer GC, et al. Individual patient cohort analysis of the efficacy of hypertonic saline/dextran in patients with traumatic brain injury and hypotension. J Trauma 1997;42(5 Suppl):S61–5.

[83] Wade CE, Kramer GC, Grady JJ, et al. Efficacy of hypertonic 7.5% saline and 6% dextran-70 in treating trauma: a meta-analysis of controlled clinical studies. Surgery 1997;122: 609–16.

[84] Cooper DJ, Myles PS, McDermott FT, et al. Prehospital hypertonic saline resuscitation of patients with hypotension and severe traumatic brain injury: a randomized controlled trial. JAMA 2004;291:1350–7.

[85] Bulger EM, Jurkovich GJ, Nathens AB, et al. Hypertonic resuscitation of hypovolemic shock after blunt trauma: a randomized controlled trial. Arch Surg in press 2006.

[86] Johnson JL, Moore EE, Gonzalez RJ, et al. Alteration of the postinjury hyperinflammatory response by means of resuscitation with a red cell substitute. J Trauma 2003;54:133–9 [discussion: 139–40].

[87] Johnson JL, Moore EE, Offner PJ, et al. Resuscitation with a blood substitute abrogates pathologic postinjury neutrophil cytotoxic function. J Trauma 2001;50:449–55 [discussion: 456].

[88] Greenburg AG, Kim HW. Hemoglobin-based oxygen carriers. Crit Care 2004;8(Suppl 2): S61–4.

[89] Gould SA, Moore EE, Hoyt DB, et al. The life-sustaining capacity of human polymerized hemoglobin when red cells might be unavailable. J Am Coll Surg 2002;195:445–52 [discussion: 452–5].

[90] Meyer PR. Annual progress report of the Midwest Regional Spinal Cord Injury Care System; Northwestern University McGaw Medical Center. Chicago: Northwestern Memorial Hospital, Rehabilitation Institute of Chicago; 1988.

[91] Butman AM, Schelble DT, Vomacka RW. The relevance of the occult cervical spine controversy and mechanism of injury to prehospital protocols: a review of the issues and literature. Prehospital Disaster Med 1996;11:228–33.
[92] Brouhard R. To immobilize or not immobilize: that is the question. Emerg Med Serv 2006; 35:81–2, 84–6.
[93] Hauswald M, Ong G, Tandberg D, et al. Out-of-hospital spinal immobilization: its effect on neurologic injury. Acad Emerg Med 1998;5:214–9.
[94] Domeier RM, Swor RA, Evans RW, et al. Multicenter prospective validation of prehospital clinical spinal clearance criteria. J Trauma 2002;53:744–50.
[95] Burton JH, Harmon NR, Dunn MG, et al. EMS provider findings and interventions with a statewide EMS spine-assessment protocol. Prehosp Emerg Care 2005;9:303–9.
[96] Bernhard M, Gries A, Kremer P, et al. Spinal cord injury (SCI)—prehospital management. Resuscitation 2005;66:127–39.
[97] MacKenzie EJ, Rivara FP, Jurkovich GJ, et al. A national evaluation of the effect of trauma-center care on mortality. N Engl J Med 2006;354:366–78.
[98] Holcomb JB, Salinas J, McManus JM, et al. Manual vital signs reliably predict need for life-saving interventions in trauma patients. J Trauma 2005;59:821–8 [discussion: 828–9].
[99] Holcomb JB, Niles SE, Miller CC, et al. Prehospital physiologic data and lifesaving interventions in trauma patients. Mil Med 2005;170:7–13.
[100] Cooke WH, Salinas J, Convertino VA, et al. Heart rate variability and its association with mortality in prehospital trauma patients. J Trauma 2006;60:363–70 [discussion: 370].
[101] Davis JW, Davis IC, Bennink LD, et al. Are automated blood pressure measurements accurate in trauma patients? J Trauma 2003;55:860–3.
[102] Hopson LR, Hirsh E, Delgado J, et al. Guidelines for withholding or termination of resuscitation in prehospital traumatic cardiopulmonary arrest: joint position statement of the National Association of EMS Physicians and the American College of Surgeons Committee on Trauma. J Am Coll Surg 2003;196:106–12.
[103] Pickens JJ, Copass MK, Bulger EM. Trauma patients receiving CPR: predictors of survival. J Trauma 2005;58:951–8.

ELSEVIER
SAUNDERS

Surg Clin N Am 87 (2007) 55–72

SURGICAL
CLINICS OF
NORTH AMERICA

New Developments in Fluid Resuscitation

Hasan B. Alam, MD[a,b], Peter Rhee, MD, MPH[c,*]

[a]Department of Surgery, Massachusetts General Hospital, 55 Fruit Street, WHT 1,
Boston, MA 02114, USA
[b]Division of Trauma, Emergency Surgery, and Surgical Critical Care,
Massachusetts General Hospital, 55 Fruit Street, WHT 1, Boston, MA 02114, USA
[c]Navy Trauma Training Center, University of Southern California, LACMC, Room 6336,
1200 North State Street, Los Angeles, CA 90033, USA

Hemorrhage control and resuscitation are the top priorities in trauma care. Exsanguination is the leading cause of possibly preventable death in civilian [1,2] and military trauma [3]. The optimal resuscitative strategy, however, remains controversial: who, when, and how are questions that have yet to be answered fully in regards to fluid resuscitation.

Evolution of fluid use in trauma

During the Vietnam War era, aggressive crystalloid resuscitation became popular because of seminal research by Shires, Moyer, Moss, and others [4–7]. Their work suggested that infusion of large-volume isotonic crystalloids improved survival, and resuscitation fluids were needed not only to replace the intravascular volume loss, but also to replenish interstitial deficits. These investigators recommended fluid replacement equal to three times the volume of blood loss (and as high as 8:1 for severe shock). Reflecting the technology and knowledge available at that time, the focus of research was on physiology, and investigators concentrated primarily on the restoration of intravascular and interstitial fluid deficits. As a result emphasis was placed on establishing intravenous access in all trauma patients to initiate early resuscitation. The Advanced Trauma Life Support course, which has been instrumental in standardizing trauma care, recommends that for patients in shock, 2 L of crystalloids be infused followed by packed red blood cell transfusions. This recommendation has been

The opinions and assertions contained herein are the private ones of the authors and are not to be construed as official or reflecting the views of the Department of Defense at large.
* Corresponding author.
E-mail address: prhee@nshs-sd.med.navy.mil (P. Rhee).

surgical.theclinics.com

extrapolated and it is now common that all trauma patients (not just patients in shock) are infused with two or more liters of lactated Ringer's (LR) solution.

In addition, Shoemaker and coworkers [8] suggested that there was an oxygen debt that needed to be repaid, and popularized aggressive resuscitation in the intensive care setting. This oxygen debt to the tissues was repaid by "maximizing or supernormalizing" cardiac output [9] with volume loading, blood transfusion, and inotropic drugs. This was continued until cardiac output no longer improved, or when oxygen consumption became independent of oxygen delivery. Numerous subsequent studies have shown, however, that this approach does not improve outcome [10–15]. On the other hand, aggressive fluid resuscitation may contribute to such conditions as abdominal compartment syndrome [16–18].

If early use of fluids is beneficial, there should be some data to support this practice. Isotonic fluids were used widely during the Vietnam conflict as the fluid of choice in massive resuscitations, but the mortality rates failed to improve compared with previous conflicts (Table 1). The only real change in outcome was noted between the first and second World Wars, and this was attributed to the widespread use of antibiotics. Coincidentally, "shock lung" or "Da Nang lung," which is now commonly referred to as acute respiratory distress syndrome [19], was first described during this period. The Navy Field Hospital in Da Nang, Vietnam, described this as a common finding in severely injured patients who were aggressively resuscitated. Current research suggests that it is caused by aberrant immune activation and immune-mediated organ injury. This condition is thought to be a part of a spectrum that can progress to multiple organ dysfunction syndrome. Since the 1990s these conditions have become main causes of death in trauma patients [1,20,21], and have been extensively investigated.

Prehospital fluids

Although it was once widely believed that early aggressive fluid resuscitation is beneficial, many are questioning this approach because clinical and

Table 1
Mortality rates of military conflicts

	KIA%	DOW%
US Civil War	16	13
Russo-Japanese War	20	9
WW I	19.6	8.1
WW II	19.8	3
Korean War	19.5	2.4
Vietnam War	20.2	3.5

Abbreviations: DOW, died of wounds refers to casualties that died after reaching a facility with a physician; KIA, killed in action refers to casualties that died before arriving at a medical facility with a physician.

basic science literature fails to provide conclusive evidence supporting this theory [22–29]. It is interesting that as early as 1918, Cannon and coworkers [30] stated "inaccessible or uncontrolled sources of blood loss should not be treated with intravenous fluids until the time of surgical control." The most controversial study proving this in humans was published in the *New England Journal of Medicine* in 1994 [24]. In that study, hypotensive patients with penetrating injury to the torso were randomized to routine fluid resuscitation, or resuscitation that was delayed until bleeding had been surgically controlled. The results of this study demonstrated a survival advantage in the delayed resuscitation group (70% versus 62%, $P = .04$). This study has generated a vigorous debate, and its findings have been extensively scrutinized for faults. Despite all the controversy, the most impressive finding remains the fact that delaying fluid resuscitation did not increase mortality in these patients. The issue of timing and volume of fluid resuscitation in bleeding patients has also been addressed by The Cochrane Database of Systematic Reviews. Only six randomized clinical trails met the inclusion criteria, and a careful review failed to provide any evidence in support of (or against) early or large-volume intravenous fluid administration in uncontrolled hemorrhage [30a]. Theoretically, fluid resuscitation in uncontrolled hemorrhage exacerbates bleeding because of the disruption of early soft thrombus, coagulopathy, and hemodilution [31–34]. A systematic review of 52 animal trials concluded that fluid resuscitation seemed to decrease the risk of death in models of severe hemorrhage (relative risk [RR] = 0.48), but increased the risk of death in those with less severe hemorrhage (RR = 1.86) [35]. Furthermore, hypotensive resuscitation, whenever tested, reduced the risk of death (RR = 0.37).

Trauma as an immune disease

Experts in the field tend to agree that serious traumatic and thermal injuries lead to immune dysfunction and subsequent cellular damage [20]. According to this concept, trauma patients who survive the early postinjury period may develop a spectrum of conditions, such as systemic inflammatory response syndrome, acute lung injury, acute respiratory distress syndrome, and multiple organ dysfunction syndrome. Most seriously injured patients survive the initial systemic inflammatory response syndrome response (without developing early multiple organ dysfunction syndrome), however, and manifest a compensatory anti-inflammatory response syndrome with suppressed immunity and significant risk of developing an infection. The resultant infection can then lead to late multiple organ dysfunction syndrome and death. A number of approaches have been tried, albeit unsuccessfully, to correct this posttraumatic immune dysfunction [36–38].

Fluids causing inflammation: changing paradigm

It is now recognized that resuscitation fluids are not completely innocuous, and they may actually potentate the cellular injury caused by hemorrhagic shock. This concept of "resuscitation injury" has steadily gained attention in recent years. A report by the Institute of Medicine (IOM) in 1999 described in detail the wide spectrum of adverse consequences that can follow resuscitative efforts [39]. Most of the adverse findings were cytotoxic effects of various fluids. The IOM report acknowledged that the D-isomer found in LR solution as a racemic mixture along with the L-isomer was not optimal and recommended that efforts be made to eliminate the D-isomer of lactate. Since that report, a number of studies have provided evidence to support the new paradigm that cellular injury is influenced not only by shock, but also by resuscitation strategies. The IOM report also recommended the replacement of lactate with other substances, such as ketone bodies. Today, with the availability of advanced cellular research techniques, one can study the effect of resuscitation fluids on the biologic systems in much greater detail. These findings now have practical implications. Although some of the modified Ringer's solutions (ketone and pyruvate based) remain experimental, LR is commercially available in the conventional racemic formulation or as a pure L-isomer solution, with markedly different properties. It is not clearly known whether the attenuation of cellular injury markers seen in the preclinical studies will translate into a measurable improvement in clinical outcome in trauma patients. Once activated, neutrophils bind to complimentary adhesion molecules (selectins, β_2 integrins) on the endothelium before transmigration into the tissues. It has been demonstrated that these adhesion molecules are up-regulated following resuscitation with racemic LR in a rodent model of hemorrhagic shock [40,41]. Furthermore, in these studies LR resuscitation was associated with histologic evidence of acute lung injury, whereas none of these adverse findings were noted following resuscitation with fresh whole blood.

Effect of resuscitation fluids on cellular regulation and functions

There is now accumulating evidence that most cellular functions are influenced by infusion of resuscitation fluids. There are a number of key variables that govern the response: (1) fluid composition, (2) fluid tonicity, (3) duration of exposure, (4) type of cells that are exposed, (5) presence or absence of infection or inflammation, (6) presence or absence of second hit, and (7) timing of fluid administration. Although cellular responses during the postresuscitation period involve almost all cell types through multiple interconnected cascades, for ease of presentation, findings from selected studies have been summarized under discrete categories.

Effects of resuscitation strategies on neutrophil excitation and immune activation in vivo

Neutrophil-mediated tissue injury has been identified as a key mechanism of postresuscitation organ damage [42]. In a swine model of hemorrhagic shock, it has been shown that resuscitation with racemic LR solution (equal amounts of D and L isomers of lactate) or mere infusion of racemic LR (without hemorrhage) caused an increase in neutrophil oxidative burst [43]. In a similar model, neutrophil excitation was influenced by the dose and rate of racemic LR administration, and resuscitation with artificial colloids (dextran and Hespan) had an even more pronounced effect on neutrophil excitation [44]. No significant neutrophil excitation was seen, however, in animals that were resuscitated with hypertonic saline (HTS) or fresh whole blood.

Impact of resuscitation fluids on human white blood cells (ex vivo)

Similar to the animal data, exposure of human blood to isotonic crystalloids and artificial colloids has been shown to cause an increase in oxidative burst, and the expression of adhesion molecules on the neutrophils in a dose-dependent fashion [45]. Interestingly, in that study natural colloids (albumin) did not excite the neutrophils, and exposure to HTS actually suppressed neutrophil functions. This suppressive effect of HTS on neutrophil functions may be through the modulation of chemoattractant receptor signaling pathways [46]. When HTS is combined with dextran, the suppressive properties of HTS overcome the stimulatory properties of dextran [47]. Response of cells to LR solution depends on its composition. Although conventional LR containing racemic lactate (D- and L-isomer) is proinflammatory, substitution of racemic lactate with L-isomer of lactate, or ketone bodies (β-hydroxybutyrate), can attenuate neutrophil activation and alter the expression of leukocyte genes known to be involved in inflammation, cell migration, and apoptosis [48]. Using customized cDNA microarrays, it has been shown that isotonic and hypertonic fluids do not differ in their effect on the cytokine genes in human leukocytes [49], but hypertonicity decreases the expression of immune activation associated genes [50]. Furthermore, the composition and tonicity of the resuscitation fluids can also have a dramatic influence on the life span of circulating cells [51].

Differential effects of resuscitation fluids on markers of cellular injury in various organs

Injured cells undergo death by two distinct mechanisms: apoptosis and necrosis. Apoptosis, although more controlled, requires energy. In the absence of energy the cells may undergo death by the poorly controlled process of necrosis. Although balanced apoptosis is essential for homeostasis and in the recovery from certain disease processes [52–55], a marked increase in apoptosis can be a marker of cellular injury and organ dysfunction [56,57]. Using apoptosis as a marker of diffuse cellular injury, it has been shown that resuscitation with racemic LR results in increased apoptosis in intestinal mucosa, smooth muscle, liver [58], and lung [59] in rodents. Pulmonary and hepatic apoptosis is markedly reduced if lactate in the solution is substituted with β-hydroxybutyrate (ketone Ringer's) or sodium pyruvate (pyruvate Ringer's) [60–62]. Designer fluids containing other formulations of pyruvate (eg, ethylpyruvate) are also superior to conventional solutions [63]. In a recent study Shires and coworkers [64] have confirmed that fluids differ dramatically in their capacity to induce tissue apoptosis, and that modified Ringer's solutions (ketone and bicarbonate Ringer's) cause significantly less apoptosis compared with the racemic LR. These findings, noted in small animal models (rodents), have also been validated in a clinically relevant model of hemorrhage in swine, where resuscitation with conventional LR solution increased apoptotic cell death in liver and lung [65]. This was easily prevented by simple elimination of D-lactate from the Ringer's solution. The modified Ringer's solutions exert their protective effects through posttranslational modifications of key regulatory proteins [66], and by selective acetylation of histones (with subsequent alterations in gene transcription) [67]. The impact of resuscitation strategies can also be seen in well-protected sites, such as the brain, where the physiologic state of the central nervous system cells can be altered by changing the composition of resuscitation fluids (across the blood-brain barrier) [68]. Furthermore, resuscitation influences not only the regulation and functions of cells but also the integrity of the surrounding extracellular matrix [69].

Effect on gene regulation: integrated approach to data analysis

Similar to the circulating cells, regulation of gene expression in the tissues is also influenced by resuscitation strategies. The authors have discovered that approximately 7% of genes in rats are altered following shock and resuscitation. In each organ studied, the gene expression profile was dependent on the fluid used for resuscitation [70]. Although transcriptional profiling is now a well-established technique, its application to systematic studying of various biologic phenomena is still limited because of problems with high-volume data analysis and interpretation. Interpretation of these large datasets in the context of accumulated knowledge on human functional networks could yield biologically meaningful information. Using this integrated approach to data analysis, a comprehensive database has now been published, which further confirms that cellular mechanisms at the level of gene regulation are profoundly influenced by shock, and by the choice of resuscitation strategy [71].

Pharmacologic resuscitation

Although resuscitation restores tissue perfusion, it does not have any specific anti-inflammatory or prosurvival properties. To improve the outcome, investigators have added various protective agents to the resuscitation regimen with good results [72–75]. An even more exciting approach is to improve survival through specific pharmacologic agents without any fluid resuscitation, that can alter gene transcription (epigenetic code) to create a prosurvival phenotype. A brief description of the underlying mechanisms may help to clarify this concept. The key regulatory site of gene transcription (and subsequent downstream pathways) is located at the level of chromatin, a 1:1 complex of DNA and proteins, predominantly composed of histone proteins. Various regulatory signals can affect gene transcription by influencing the activity of histones, most notably through acetylation. The two enzymes that govern the process of acetylation are histone acetyl transferase [76], and histone deaceylase [77,78]. Modulation of the histone code is one of the most upstream cellular events, which simultaneously regulates a subset of genes that are coordinately expressed to produce specific downstream effects. The authors have previously shown that hemorrhagic shock is associated with an imbalance in histone acetyl transferase/histone deaceylase ratio, an altered acetylation pattern of histones, and a decrease in gene transcription potential [67]. In that experiment, resuscitation reversed the shock-induced suppression of gene transcription in a fluid-specific fashion (ie, each resuscitation fluid had a distinctive pattern of histone acetylation [histone code]). Interestingly, brief administration of histone deaceylase inhibitors in this model, during 45 minutes of resuscitation, was even more effective in reversing the shock-induced imbalance, and increasing acetylation of histones. The follow-up experiments have now established that directly targeting the histones with histone deaceylase inhibitors, such as valproic acid (300 mg/kg) and suberoylanilide hydroxamic acid, can rapidly correct shock-induced alterations and improve survival in preclinical models of hemorrhage [79]. Impressively, this survival advantage was achieved without administration of any resuscitation fluids. The effect of hemorrhage and resuscitation on histone acetylation is almost identical in rodents and swine [80], and theoretically administration of histone deaceylase inhibitors should improve survival in large animal models in a similar fashion (under investigation). This raises the possibility that cell survival, and ultimately organism survival, can be improved through direct modulation of gene transcription in the setting of lethal hemorrhage. This exciting approach is currently being tested and refined under the Defense Advanced Research Programs Agency "Surviving Blood Loss" program.

Hypertonic saline and the clinical experience

The use of HTS for resuscitation from hemorrhage was first described in 1980, when Velasco and coworkers [81] and DeFelippe and coworkers [82] reported in separate studies that hypersomotic sodium chloride rapidly expands plasma volume after major blood loss. Because of its ability to mobilize interstitial fluids into the vascular space, 250 mL of 7.5% saline can achieve results comparable with resuscitation with 2 to 3 L of 0.9% saline. Since the original reports, HTS has been used in a variety of circumstances and thousands of papers have appeared in the literature, including eight double-blinded randomized trials evaluating HTS or HTS with dextran for prehospital or emergency department treatment of traumatic hypotension. Improved rates of survival with HTS were reported with HTS in seven of eight trials, although statistically significant improvement in overall survival was seen in only one trial. A meta-analysis for the evaluation of HTS with dextran as the initial treatment for hypovolemic shock reviewed the original records from six trials (and 604 subjects) [83]. Overall survival rates were better with HTS with dextran resuscitation as compared with conventional resuscitation. HTS with dextran resuscitation was particularly effective for the subgroup of patients that had sustained head injury with a discharge survival rate of 38%, as compared with a rate of 27% for the control group receiving saline. In the clinical literature, there has been a remarkable absence of deleterious effects with HTS administration in more than 1000 trauma and surgical patients. No increase in the incidence of hypernatremic seizure, increased bleeding or blood transfusion requirement, coagulopathies, renal failure, cardiac arrhythmias, or central pontine myelinolysis has been attributed to hypertonic resuscitation in trauma patients. These clinical trials had used HTS as a volume expander, but a more advantageous effect of HTS administration may be the attenuation of immune-mediated cellular injury. A number of preclinical studies have demonstrated that HTS has the potential to modulate the posttrauma immune response, with an overall attenuation of immune-mediated cellular injury [84,85]. The salutary properties of HTS are primarily exerted through its effects on neutrophil-endothelial interactions. For example, in addition to decreasing neutrophil excitation [43–45], HTS resuscitation decreases inflammation [86], neutrophil-endothelial binding [87], lung damage [88], and bowel injury [89]. A number of elegant studies have further elucidated the subcellular pathways that are influenced by exposure to HTS [90–93]. The recently established Resuscitation Outcome Consortium [94], funded by the National Institutes of Health and the US Department of Defense, has started two multicenter trials of hypertonic resuscitation in two populations of trauma patients to be conducted simultaneously. Study 1 determines the impact of hypertonic resuscitation on survival for blunt or penetrating trauma patients in hypovolemic shock, whereas study 2 evaluates its impact on long-term (6 month) neurologic outcome after severe traumatic brain injury. Both studies are three-arm, randomized, blinded intervention trials comparing HTS with dextran (7.5% saline, 6% dextran 70), HTS alone (7.5% saline), and normal saline as the initial resuscitation fluid administered to these patients in the prehospital setting. In addition to the primary end points, comprehensive data about the immunologic consequences of hypertonic resuscitation are also being collected. It is hoped that these studies would provide the conclusive evidence that is needed to get Food and Drug Administration (FDA) approval for the routine use of HTS in the treatment of trauma patients.

Fluid resuscitation for combat casualties: consensus conferences

Control of hemorrhage and judicious resuscitation are critical elements of early battlefield care. The optimal strategy for both of these goals is highly controversial, because of a general lack of category I-II clinical evidence. In addition to clinical benefits, the military must also take into account the logistical aspects of the approach (weight, volume, storage requirements, and so forth). The Office of Naval Research and the United States Army Medical Research and Material Command have supported the basic research in this field for many years. Primarily as a result of leadership and funding by the Office of Naval Research, three significant consensus conferences were held where data on fluid resuscitation were analyzed by experts, and recommendations made to improve clinical practice and to guide future research. The first meeting was under the supervision of the IOM in 1998. The IOM report concluded that the current resuscitation strategies were inadequate, potentially harmful, and needed radical changes. It identified numerous areas of future research, and recommended that combat casualties should be resuscitated with 250 mL bolus of 7.5% saline [39]. Unfortunately, the FDA has not yet approved this fluid for clinical use. In the follow-up meeting (June 2001, Uniformed Services University) a number of clinical recommendations were made including who should (and should not) be resuscitated; end point of resuscitation; and the optimal fluid [95]. Because the choice was deliberately limited to FDA-approved agents (available in the United States), hetastarch (hydroxy ethyl starch, 500 mL) was narrowly recommended as the fluid of choice for use in the battlefield. In the third meeting (October 2001, Toronto, Canada) the scope was widened to include fluids that were available in other NATO countries (even if not available in the United States) [96]. At this meeting a combination fluid (7.5% saline and 6% dextran [HTS with dextran]) was recommended as the initial fluid of choice [97]. At all of these meetings experts agreed that aggressive resuscitation is deleterious, an ideal fluid is yet not available, and low-volume resuscitation (hypertonic, colloid, or combination) is the most suitable choice for military needs. Proceedings of the last two meetings have been published as a special supplement of the *Journal of Trauma* (May 2003), including the recommendations for the initial fluid resuscitation of combat casualties [98].

The glaring absence of good clinical evidence has prompted collaboration between the National Institutes of Health and the United States Department of Defense to establish a consortium of clinical centers for conducting resuscitation research. It is hoped that this consortium will provide the much-needed clinical data to validate and confirm the promising basic science findings.

Changes in the military practice

The consensus conferences described here systematically evaluated all the available data and made strong recommendations that have catalyzed a noticeable paradigm shift. For example, the United States Army and Navy have authorized the use of low-volume resuscitation for combat casualty care and other NATO forces have developed similar protocols. The US Military's Committee on Tactical Combat Casualty Care is a standing committee comprised of members from the Army, Air Force, Navy, and Marines. This committee currently advocates the use of "permissive hypotension," which is to administer low-volume resuscitation to keep the casualty alive with a palpable pulse or consciousness but not to restore the blood pressure to normal until definitive control of hemorrhage. Early aggressive fluid resuscitation, in the absence of hemorrhage control, is no longer recommended. As a result, resuscitation in the combat zones is more selective (fluids given only when needed); is low volume; and aims for practical end points (eg, palpable pulse). Colloid fluids (eg, Hespan and Hextand) are replacing conventional crystalloids for early resuscitation, minimizing the logistical burden. Also, early hemorrhage control is being prioritized over aggressive fluid resuscitation. The resuscitation strategies that are being used by the US military in Iraq and Afghanistan already reflect the changing trends. It is too early to determine the direct impact of these new hemorrhage control and resuscitation strategies on combat casualty outcomes. It is very encouraging to note, however, that for the first time since the Crimean war the killed in action rate has markedly dropped below the historic 20% to around 10% to 14% [99,100].

Summary on current and future resuscitation fluids

Isotonic crystalloids

Significant immune activation and induction of cellular injury are seen with these fluids, especially racemic LR solution. It is known that a very large number of trauma patients receive LR and do well clinically. The patients who develop late complications of increased inflammatory response, however, are usually the ones who also have undergone severe hemorrhagic shock and massive fluid resuscitation. LR may be safe in small doses that the body can obviously tolerate, but not in larger amounts given over short periods following hemorrhagic shock and trauma. Modifications of LR, such as elimination of D-lactate, can decrease these adverse effects, and complete substitution of lactate with other monocarboxytates (eg, ketone bodies or pyruvate) seems to be beneficial.

Hypertonic crystalloids

As compared with LR, HTS causes suppression of neutrophil oxidative burst activity, decreases neutrophil-endothelial adhesions, and attenuates immune-mediated cellular injury. Because of its logistic advantages (smaller volume) and immunologic benefits, HTS with or without a colloid seems to be the ideal fluid today for military application. A manufacturer has to obtain FDA approval, however, for its use as a volume expander in the United States. Although addition of dextran to HTS tends to prolong the volume expansion response, the authors believe that it might be easier to obtain FDA approval for a simple solution (HTS) than a combination solution (HTS and dextran). Studies scheduled to be performed under the National Institutes of Health–sponsored Resuscitation Outcome Consortium are expected to provide the conclusive evidence.

Artificial colloids

Dextran and Hespan cause significant neutrophil activation. Combination of dextran with HTS, however, blunts this response. When given in combination, colloids add the theoretical advantage of prolonging the hemodynamic response of HTS resuscitation.

Plasma

Plasma has a favorable effect, because it does not seem to activate neutrophils and numerous other pathways of cellular injury. Plasma is also a very effective volume expander. It has all the well-recognized problems, however, that are associated with storage, transport, and infusion of blood products. Autologous freeze-dried plasma is a promising alternative that can be reconstituted in a hyperoncotic, hypertonic fashion when needed. This is currently a focus of active investigations under the Department of Defense funded research programs.

Fresh whole blood

Fresh whole blood is by far the best and most effective fluid for resuscitation of hemorrhagic shock in animal models. Fresh whole blood is, however, not clinically available. Even if available, logistics of storage and transport make it an unrealistic option. One exception is the use of the "walking blood bank" by the military, where fresh whole blood is used in emergency situations. There is currently tremendous interest in investigating whether early use of whole blood (or components combined to create whole blood) benefits the severely traumatized [101].

Artificial blood

All the artificial blood products tested to date have failed to live up to expectations. There are now reasons, however, for developing and testing fluids that actually mimic the constituents of what humans bleed, which is whole blood. This starts with the recognition that currently available fluids are not optimal. There is currently an ongoing multi-institutional phase III trial testing a human hemoglobin–based solution. If this type of product is deemed to be safe and beneficial, perhaps a combination product that combines freeze dried plasma along with oxygen-carrying hemoglobin may be of benefit.

Pharmacologic resuscitation

Administering specific agents to protect against ischemia-reperfusion injury and therapies that can induce a prosurvival phenotype (through up-regulation of selected genes) are attractive concepts. These are likely to be the next frontier in resuscitation research. In the future, severely traumatized patients may be treated with "designer fluids" supplemented with a cocktail of agents specifically chosen to augment the intrinsic survival pathways.

Who, when, and how?

The answers are simple but these questions are often never asked. In trauma, fluid resuscitation is only needed in patients who have lost blood. It is clear that not all the trauma patients need fluid resuscitation. For bleeding patients intravenous access is critical but should not be synonymous with fluid infusion. In the absence of traumatic brain injury, "permissive hypotension" with systolic pressures greater than 80 mm Hg, consciousness, or palpable pulse are reasonable goals until hemorrhage has been controlled. Rather than resuscitating the patient before definitive hemorrhage control, emphasis should be on controlling hemorrhage and using fluids only to keep the patient alive during the process. It can be argued that the initial fluid of choice among commercially available fluids in the United States should be 5% HTS because it is commercially available. Two 250-mL boluses are safe and offer many potential advantages. This should be followed by infusion of L-isomer LR (Baxter, Deerfield, Illinois) if further volume expansion is needed. For the hypotensive bleeding patient, initiation of blood transfusion should be early, and blood component therapy should be initiated immediately without waiting for the development of coagulopathy. Thawed fresh frozen plasma should be given in a 1:1 ratio to packed red blood cells. For the military, fresh whole blood from the walking blood bank should be obtained immediately for early use.

This aggressive approach is already being practiced at some centers with excellent results. For example, at the Los Angeles County Medical Center, six units of thawed fresh frozen plasma and platelets are given when six units of packed red blood cells are transfused (Fig. 1). For patients with thoracic hemorrhage, strong emphasis is placed on auto transfusion of blood collected from the chest tube. In the intensive care unit, blood pressure, urine output, and clinical judgment are used to guide the fluid resuscitation. As long as the serum lactate or base excess are trending toward normal, gentle resuscitation is preferred with an aim to correct acidosis over approximately

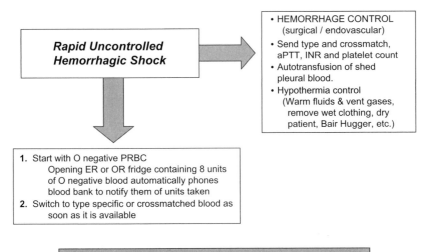

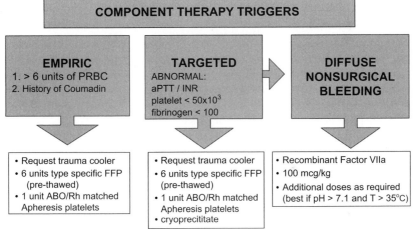

Fig. 1. LAC-USC trauma transfusion protocol. aPTT, activated partial thromboplastin time; FFP, fresh frozen plasma; INR, international normalized ratio; PRBC, packed red blood cells.

24 hours. The rate of acute respiratory distress syndrome in the authors' intensive care unit has decreased from the national average of 24% to 9% in severely injured trauma patients requiring intensive care admission [102]. Although the exact causes for this dramatic reduction cannot be specifically pinpointed, it coincides with a documented reduction in the volume of fluids used for resuscitation.

Summary

An ideal fluid for the resuscitation of trauma victims should be safe; efficacious; cheap; easy to store and transport (especially important for the military); have the capacity to carry oxygen and nutrients to the cells; and protect the cells from resuscitation injury. Unfortunately, such a fluid is not available today. Because of the emerging data on fluid cytotoxicity, clinicians should consider resuscitation fluids as drugs, with well-defined indications and contraindication, safe dosages, and side effects. A logical approach is to prevent the onset of immune dysfunction, rather than try to control multiple interconnected cascades once they have been activated. Patient's response to trauma is influenced by a number of variables (comorbid problems, severity of injuries, degree of shock, delay in definitive care, and so forth). As compared with most of the other variables that cannot be altered, resuscitative strategy is entirely under clinicians' control. They choose the nature of the fluids, rate of administration, timing, and the end points of resuscitation. They also may decide not to resuscitate in selected patients.

References

[1] Sauaia A, Moore FA, Moore EE, et al. Epidemiology of trauma deaths: a reassessment. J Trauma 1995;38:185–93.
[2] Acosta JA, Yang JC, Winchell RJ, et al. Lethal injuries and time to death in a level I trauma center. J Am Coll Surg 1998;186:528–33.
[3] Wound Data and Munitions Effectiveness Team. The WDMET Study. Bethesda: Uniformed Services University of the Health Sciences; 1970.
[4] Shires GT, Carrico CJ, Baxter CR, et al. Principles in treatment of severely injured patients. Adv Surg 1970;4:255–324.
[5] Shires GT, Coln D, Carrico J, et al. Fluid therapy in hemorrhagic shock. Arch Surg 1964; 88:688–93.
[6] Dillon J, Lunch LJ, Myers R, et al. A bioassay of treatment of hemorrhagic shock. Arch Surg 1966;93:537–55.
[7] Cervera AL, Moss G. Progressive hypovolemia leading to shock after continuous hemorrhage and 3:1 crystalloid replacement. Am J Surg 1975;129:670–4.
[8] Shoemaker WC, Appel PL, Kram HB, et al. Prospective trial of supranormal values of survivors as therapeutic goals in high-risk surgical patients. Chest 1988;94:1176–86.
[9] Bishop MH, Shoemaker WC, Appel PL, et al. Prospective, randomized trial of survivor values of cardiac index, oxygen delivery, and oxygen consumption as resuscitation endpoints in severe trauma. J Trauma 1995;38:780–7.
[10] Lobo SM, Lobo FR, Polachini CA, et al. Prospective, randomized trial comparing fluids and dobutamine optimization of oxygen delivery in high-risk surgical patients. Crit Care 2006;10:R72.
[11] McKinley BA, Kozar RA, Cocanour CS, et al. Normal versus supranormal oxygen delivery goals in shock resuscitation: the response is the same. J Trauma 2002;53:825–32.
[12] Velmahos GC, Demetriades D, Shoemaker WC, et al. Endpoints of resuscitation of critically injured patients: normal or supranormal? A prospective randomized trial. Ann Surg 2000;232:409–18.
[13] Marr AB, Moore FA, Sailors RM, et al. Preload optimization using "starling curve" generation during shock resuscitation: can it be done? Shock 2004;21:300–5.
[14] Yu M, Levy MM, Smith P, et al. Effect of maximizing oxygen delivery on morbidity and mortality rates in critically ill patients: a prospective, randomized, controlled study. Crit Care Med 1993;21:830–8.
[15] Durham RM, Neunaber K, Mazuski JE, et al. The use of oxygen consumption and delivery as endpoints for resuscitation in critically ill patients. J Trauma 1996;41:32–9.

[16] Kirkpatrick AW, Balogh Z, Ball CG, et al. The secondary abdominal compartment syndrome: iatrogenic or unavoidable? J Am Coll Surg 2006;202:668–79.
[17] Balogh Z, McKinley BA, Cocanour CS, et al. Supranormal trauma resuscitation causes more cases of abdominal compartment syndrome. Arch Surg 2003;138:637–42.
[18] Puritt BA. Protection from excessive resuscitation: pushing the pendulum back. J Trauma 2000;49:567–8.
[19] Ashbaugh DG, Bigelow DB, Petty TL, et al. Acute respiratory distress in adults. Lancet 1967;12:319–23.
[20] Mannick JA, Rodrick ML, Lederer JA. The immune response to injury. J Am Coll Surg 2001;193:237–44.
[21] Jarrar D, Chaudry IH, Wang P. Organ dysfunction following hemorrhage and sepsis: mechanisms and therapeutic approaches. Int J Mol Med 1999;4:575–83.
[22] Aprahamian C, Thompson BM, Towne JB, et al. The effect of a paramedic system on mortality of major open intra-abdominal vascular trauma. J Trauma 1983;23:687–90.
[23] Kaweski SM, Sise MJ, Virgilio RW. The effect of prehospital fluids on survival in trauma patients. J Trauma 1990;30:1215–8.
[24] Bickel WH, Wall MJ, Pepe PE, et al. Immediate versus delayed fluid resuscitation for hypotensive patients with penetrating torso injuries. N Engl J Med 1994;331:1105–9.
[25] Turner J, Nicholl J, Webber L, et al. A randomized controlled trial of prehospital intravenous fluid replacement therapy in serious trauma. Health Technol Assess 2000;4:1–57.
[26] Kwan I, Bunn F, Roberts I. WHO Pre-Hospital Trauma Care Steering Committee: timing and volume of fluid administration for patients with bleeding following trauma. Cochrane Database Syst Rev 2001;1:CD003345.
[27] Greaves MW, Hussein SH. Fluid resuscitation in pre-hospital trauma care: a consensus view. J R Coll Surg Edinb 2002;47:451–7.
[28] Dula DJ, Wood GC, Rejmer AR, et al. Use of prehospital fluids in hypotensive blunt trauma patients. Prehosp Emerg Care 2002;6:417–20.
[29] Dutton RP, Mackenzie CF, Scalea TM. Hypotensive resuscitation during active hemorrhage: impact on in-hospital mortality. J Trauma 2002;52:1141–6.
[30] Cannon WB, Faser J, Collew EM. The preventive treatment of wound shock. JAMA 1918;47:618.
[30a] Kwan I, Bunn F, Roberts I. WHO Pre-hospital trauma care steering committee: Timing and volume of fluid administration for patients with bleeding following trauma. Cochrane Database Syst Rev 2003;(3):CD002245.
[31] Stern SA, Dronen SC, Birrer P, et al. Effect of blood pressure on hemorrhage volume and survival in a near-fatal hemorrhage model incorporating a vascular injury. Ann Emerg Med 1993;22:155–63.
[32] Selby JB, Mathis JE, Berry CF, et al. Effects of isotonic saline solution resuscitation on blood coagulation in uncontrolled hemorrhage. Surgery 1996;119:528–33.
[33] Sondeen JL, Coppes VG, Holcomb JB. Blood pressure at which rebleeding occurs after resuscitation in swine with aortic injury. J Trauma 2003;54:S100–7.
[34] Rotondo MF, Schwab CW, McGonigal MD, et al. Damage control: an approach for improved survival in exsanguinating penetrating abdominal trauma. J Trauma 1993;35:375–83.
[35] Mapstone J, Roberts I, Evans P. Fluid resuscitation strategies: a systematic review of animal trials. J Trauma 2003;55:571–89.
[36] Demetriades D, Smith JS, Jacobson LE, et al. Bactericidal/permeability-increasing protein (rBPI21) in patients with hemorrhage due to trauma: results of a multicenter phase II clinical trial. rBPI21 Acute Hemorrhagic Trauma Study Group. J Trauma 1999;46:667–76.
[37] Rhee P, Morris J, Durham R, et al. Recombinant humanized monoclonal antibody against CD18 in traumatic hemorrhagic shock: results of a phase II clinical trial. J Trauma 2000;49:611–20.

[38] Seekamp A, van Griensven M, Dhondt E, et al. The effect of anti-L-selectin (aselizumab) in multiple traumatized patients: results of a phase II clinical trial. Crit Care Med 2004;32: 2021–8.

[39] Committee on Fluid Resuscitation for Combat Casualties. Fluid resuscitation: state of the science for treating combat casualties and civilian trauma. Report of the Institute of Medicine. Washington: National Academy Press; 1999.

[40] Sun LL, Ruff P, Austin B, et al. Early up-regulation of intracellular adhesion molecule-1 and vascular cell adhesion molecule-1 expression in rats with hemorrhagic shock and resuscitation. Shock 1999;11:416–22.

[41] Alam HB, Sun L, Ruff P, et al. E- and P-selectin expression depends on the resuscitation fluid used in hemorrhaged rats. J Surg Res 2000;94:145–52.

[42] Chollet-Martin S, Jourdain B, Gilbert C, et al. Interactions between neutrophils and cytokines in blood and alveolar spaces during ARDS. Am J Respir Crit Care Med 1996;154: 594–601.

[43] Rhee P, Burris D, Kaufmann C, et al. Lactated Ringer's solution resuscitation causes neutrophil activation after hemorrhagic shock. J Trauma 1998;44:313–9.

[44] Alam HB, Stanton K, Koustova E, et al. Effect of different resuscitation strategies on neutrophil activation in a swine model of hemorrhagic shock. Resuscitation 2004;60:91–9.

[45] Rhee P, Wang D, Ruff P, et al. Human neutrophil activation and increased adhesion by various resuscitation fluids. Crit Care Med 2000;28:74–8.

[46] Junger WG, Hoyt DB, Davis RE, et al. Hypertonicity regulates the function of human neutrophils by modulating chemoattractant receptor signaling and activating mitogen-activated protein kinase p38. J Clin Invest 1998;101:2768–79.

[47] Stanton K, Koustova E, Alam H, et al. Effect of hypertonic saline dextran solution on human neutrophil activation. Shock 2001;5:79.

[48] Koustova E, Stanton K, Guschin V, et al. Effects of lactated Ringer's solutions on human leukocytes. J Trauma 2002;52:872–8.

[49] Gushchin V, Stegalkina S, Alam HB, et al. Cytokine expression profiling in human leukocytes after exposure to hypertonic and isotonic fluids. J Trauma 2002;52:867–71.

[50] Gushchin V, Alam HB, Rhee P, et al. cDNA profiling in leukocytes exposed to hypertonic resuscitation fluids. J Am Coll Surg 2003;197:426–32.

[51] Stanton K, Alam HB, Rhee P, et al. Human polymorphonuclear cell death after exposure to resuscitation fluids in vitro: apoptosis versus necrosis. J Trauma 2003;54:1065–74.

[52] Steller H. Mechanisms and genes of cellular suicide. Science 1995;267:1445–9.

[53] Burek MJ, Oppenheim RW. Programmed cell death in the developing nervous system. Brain Path 1996;6:427–46.

[54] Cohen JJ, Duke RC, Fadok VA, et al. Apoptosis and programmed cell death in immunity. Annu Rev Immunol 1992;10:267–93.

[55] Cohen JJ. Apoptosis: mechanisms of life and death in the immune system. J Allergy Clin Immunol 1999;103:548–54.

[56] Liaudet L, Soriano FG, Szabo E, et al. Protection against hemorrhagic shock in mice genetically deficient in poly(ADP-ribose) polymerase. Proc Natl Acad Sci U S A 2000;97: 10203–8.

[57] Eichhorst ST. Modulation of apoptosis as a target for liver disease. Expert Opin Ther Targets 2005;9:83–99.

[58] Deb S, Martin B, Sun L, et al. Resuscitation with lactated Ringer's solution in rats with hemorrhagic shock induces immediate apoptosis. J Trauma 1999;46:582–9.

[59] Deb S, Sun L, Martin B, et al. Lactated Ringer's and hetastarch but not plasma resuscitation after rat hemorrhagic shock is associated with immediate lung apoptosis by the upregulation of Bax protein. J Trauma 2000;49:47–55.

[60] Alam HB, Austin B, Koustova E, et al. Resuscitation induced pulmonary apoptosis and intracellular adhesion molecule-1 expression are attenuated by the use of ketone ringer's solution in rats. J Am Coll Surg 2001;193:255–63.

[61] Koustova E, Rhee P, Hancock T, et al. Ketone and pyruvate Ringer's solutions decrease pulmonary apoptosis in a rat model of severe hemorrhagic shock and resuscitation. Surgery 2003;134:267–74.

[62] Jaskille A, Koustova E, Rhee P, et al. Hepatic apoptosis following hemorrhagic shock in rats can be reduced through modifications of conventional Ringer's solutions. J Am Coll Surg 2006;202:25–35.

[63] Fink MP. Ethyl pyruvate: a novel treatment for sepsis and shock. Minerva Anesthesiol 2004;70:365–71.

[64] Shires GT, Browder LK, Steljes TPV, et al. The effect of shock resuscitation on apoptosis. Am J Surg 2005;189:85–91.

[65] Ayuste EC, Chen H, Koustova E, et al. Hepatic and pulmonary apoptosis following hemorrhagic shock in swine can be reduced through modifications of conventional Ringer's solutions. J Trauma 2006;60:52–63.

[66] Jaskille A, Alam HB, Rhee P, et al. D-Lactate increases pulmonary apoptosis by restricting phosphorylation of BAD and eNOS in a rat model of hemorrhagic shock. J Trauma 2004; 57(2):262–9.

[67] Lin T, Alam HB, Chen H, et al. Cardiac histones are substrates of histone deacetylase (HDAC) activity in hemorrhagic shock and resuscitation. Surgery 2006;139:365–76.

[68] Lin T, Koustova E, Chen H, et al. Energy substrate supplemented resuscitation affects monocarboxylate transporter levels and gliosis in rat model of hemorrhagic shock. J Trauma 2005;59:1191–202.

[69] Chen H, Inocencio R, Alam HB, et al. Differential expression of extracellular matrix remodeling genes in rat model of hemorrhagic shock and resuscitation. J Surg Res 2005; 123:235–44.

[70] Alam HB, Stegalkina S, Rhee P, et al. cDNA array analysis of gene expression following hemorrhagic shock and resuscitation in rats. Resuscitation 2002;54:195–206.

[71] Chen H, Alam HB, Querol RI, et al. Identification of expression patterns associated with hemorrhage and resuscitation: integrated approach to data analysis. J Trauma 2006;60: 701–23.

[72] Coimbra R, Porcides R, Loomis W, et al. HSPTX protects against hemorrhagic shock resuscitation-induced tissue injury: an attractive alternative to Ringer's lactate. J Trauma 2006;60:41–51.

[73] Macias CA, Kameneva MV, Tenhunen JJ, et al. Survival in a rat model of lethal hemorrhagic shock is prolonged following resuscitation with a small volume of a solution containing a drag-reducing polymer derived from aloe vera. Shock 2004;22:151–6.

[74] Van Way CW, Dhar A, Morrison D. Hemorrhagic shock: a new look at a new problem. Mo Med 2003;100:518–23.

[75] Szalay L, Shimizu T, Suzuki T, et al. Androstenediol administration after trauma-hemorrhage attenuates inflammatory response reduces organ damage and improves survival following sepsis. Am J Physiol Gastrointest Liver Physiol 2006;291(2):G260–6.

[76] Grunstein M. Histone acetylation in chromatin structure and transcription. Nature 1999; 389:349–52.

[77] Ruijteeer AJM. Histone deasetylases (HDACs): characterization of the classical HDAC family. Biochem J 2003;370:737–49.

[78] Marks PA, Miller T, Richon VM. Histone deasetylases. Curr Opin Pharmacol 2003;3: 344–51.

[79] Gonzales E, Chen H, Munuve R, et al. Valproic acid prevents hemorrhage-associated lethality and affects the acetylation pattern of cardiac histones. Shock 2006;25:395–401.

[80] Ahuja N, Ayuste E, Koustova E, et al. Acetylation of cardiac histones and expression of histone regulated genes can be modulated through fluid resuscitation in a swine model of hemorrhage. J Am Coll Surg 2005;201:S24.

[81] Velasco IT, Ponieri V, Rocha M, et al. Hyperosmotic NaCl and severe hemorrhagic shock. Am J Physiol 1980;239:H664.

[82] DeFelippe J Jr, Timoner IJ, Velasco IT, et al. Treatment of refractory hypovolemic shock by 7.5% sodium chloride injections. Lancet 1980;2:1002.

[83] Wade CE, Kramer GC, Grady JJ, et al. Efficacy of hypertonic 7.5% saline and 6% dextran-70 in treating trauma: a meta-analysis of controlled clinical studies. Surgery 1997;122: 609–16.

[84] Junger WG, Coimbra R, Liu FC, et al. Hypertonic saline resuscitation: a tool to modulate immune function in trauma patients? Shock 1997;8:235–41.

[85] Rotstein OD. Novel strategies for immunomodulation after trauma: revisiting hypertonic saline as a resuscitation strategy for hemorrhagic shock. J Trauma 2000;49:580–3.

[86] Bahrami S, Zimmermann K, Szelenyi Z, et al. Small volume fluid resuscitation with hypertonic saline prevents inflammation but not mortality in a rat model of hemorrhagic shock. Shock 2006;25:283–9.

[87] Pascual JL, Ferri LE, Seely AJ, et al. Hypertonic saline resuscitation of hemorrhagic shock diminishes neutrophil rolling and adherence to endothelium and reduces in vivo vascular leakage. Ann Surg 2002;236:634–42.

[88] Murao Y, Loomis W, Wolf P, et al. Effect of hypertonic saline on its potential to prevent lung tissue damage in a mouse model of hemorrhagic shock. Shock 2003;20:29–34.

[89] Murao Y, Hata M, Ohnishi K, et al. Hypertonic saline resuscitation reduces apoptosis and tissue damage of the small intestine in a mouse model of hemorrhagic shock. Shock 2003;20:23–8.

[90] Sheppard FR, Moore EE, McLaughlin N, et al. Clinically relevant osmolar stress inhibits priming-induced PMN NADPH oxidase subunit translocation. J Trauma 2005;58:752–7.

[91] Gonzales RJ, Moore EE, Ciesla DJ, et al. Hyperosmolarity abrogates neutrophil cutotoxity provoked by post-shock mesenteric lymph. Shock 2002;18:29–32.

[92] Staudenmayer KL, Maier RV, Jelacic S, et al. Hypertonic saline modulates innate immunity in a model of systemic inflammation. Shock 2005;23:459–63.

[93] Cuschieri J, Gourlay D, Garcia I, et al. Hypertonic preconditioning inhibits macrophage responsiveness to endotoxin. J Immunol 2002;168:1389–96.

[94] Resuscitation outcomes consortium. Available at: https://roc.uwctc.org/tiki/tiki-index. php. Accessed November 7, 2006.

[95] Uniformed Services University of the Health Sciences. Combat fluid resuscitation. Sponsored by US Office of Naval Research; US Army Medical Research and Material Command; Department of Surgery; Department of Military and Emergency Medicine. Bethesda, June 18–20, 2001.

[96] Defense and Civil Institute of Environmental Medicine. Fluid resuscitation in combat. Sponsored by Defense R & D Canada, Defense and Civil Institute of Environmental Medicine, Department of Surgery, University of Toronto, and the Office of Naval Research. Toronto, Ontario, October 25–26, 2001.

[97] Champion HR. Combat fluid resuscitation: introduction and overview of conferences. J Trauma 2003;54:7–12.

[98] Rhee P, Koustova E, Alam HB. Searching for the optimal resuscitation method: recommendations for the initial fluid resuscitation of combat casualties. J Trauma 2003;54:52–62.

[99] Gwande A. Casualties of war: military care for the wounded from Iraq and Afghanistan. N Engl J Med 2004;351:2471–5.

[100] Holcomb JB, Stansbury LG, Champion HR, et al. Understanding combat casualty statistics. J Trauma 2006;60:397–401.

[101] Hess JR, Holcomb JB, Hoyt DB. Damage control resuscitation: the need for specific blood products to treat the coagulopathy of trauma. Transfusion 2006;46:685–6.

[102] Martin M, Salim A, Murray J, et al. The decreasing incidence and mortality of acute respiratory distress syndrome after injury: a 5-year observational study. J Trauma 2005;59: 1107–13.

ELSEVIER
SAUNDERS

SURGICAL
CLINICS OF
NORTH AMERICA

Surg Clin N Am 87 (2007) 73–93

Damage Control in Trauma: Laparotomy Wound Management Acute to Chronic

Timothy C. Fabian, MD

Department of Surgery, University of Tennessee Health Science Center, 956 Court Avenue, Suite G228, Memphis, TN 38163, USA

Background

The concept of damage control laparotomy for seriously injured trauma patients was promulgated in 1983 [1]. At the Grady Memorial Hospital, Stone and colleagues documented improved outcomes in those patients who sustained intra-abdominal injury with associated blood loss by rapidly terminating the surgical procedure. They described managing life-threatening blood loss and vascular injury quickly followed by immediate closure of the abdomen without completing definitive management of bowel and other intra-abdominal injuries. Bowel ligation and packing were recommended with return to the operating room for definitive management of hollow viscus injuries after a patient's physiology had been corrected. Those clinical investigators recognized that hemorrhagic shock led to a progressive downward spiral that could be interrupted in some patients by stopping major bleeding and closing the abdomen to diminish the loss of body heat. This unremitting, cataclysmic event subsequently has been referred to as the "bloody vicious cycle" [2]. Moore and coworkers described this chain of events with major torso trauma leading to active hemorrhage progressing to metabolic acidosis, core hypothermia, and progressive coagulopathy (Fig. 1) [2].

Subsequent to this early description of rapid termination of laparotomy, Rotondo and coworkers coined the term, "damage control laparotomy" [3]. They reinforced the important concepts explored initially by Stone and demonstrated improved outcomes in the face of acidosis, hypothermia, and coagulopathy. As time has passed, all trauma centers have adopted these principles of management, and surgical techniques for acute and definitive management have been refined. Gauze packing of liver injuries and

E-mail address: tfabian@utmem.edu

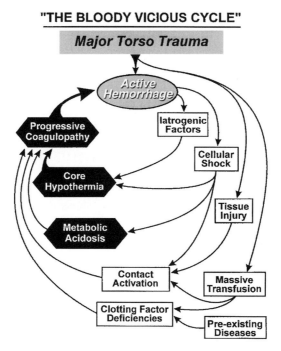

"THE BLOODY VICIOUS CYCLE"

Fig. 1. Pathogenesis of the "blood vicious cycle" after severe injury is multifactorial, but progressive core hypothermia and persistent metabolic acidosis are pivotal. (*From* Moore EE. Staged laparotomy for the hypothermia, acidosis, and coagulopathy syndrome. Am J Surg 1996;172:405; with permission. © Copyright 1996 Excerpta Medica, Inc.)

pelvic injuries has become standard procedure for managing blunt and penetrating injuries. Like so many areas in medicine and surgery, techniques that have been abandoned from the past are continuing to be rediscovered, refined, and reapplied as knowledge develops combined with advances in surgical management and critical care progress.

As damage control concepts disseminated, the important entity of abdominal compartment syndrome (ACS) was recognized as a major cause of morbidity and mortality in patients who are critically injured. As management techniques have evolved, the fundamental issues of wound management have been central to the advance of damage control laparotomy. The intent of this article is to define the scenarios and pathophysiology of ACS further, consider the varied methods of management of the open abdominal wound, and address issues surrounding definitive abdominal wall closure and current techniques for reconstruction.

Compartment syndromes

The majority of cases in which the abdomen is left open after trauma laparotomy are those associated with ACS. Compartment syndromes can develop in nearly every part of the body. These include increased intracranial pressure from closed head injury, renal failure from shock-associated acute tubular necrosis, the more commonly recognized compartment syndromes of the lower extremity, and the recently recognized entity of ACS. Compartment syndromes of the lower extremity usually are associated primarily with ischemia from arterial occlusion. These include acute popliteal artery thrombosis or embolus, iliac artery occlusion, and ileofemoral acute arterial injury with shock requiring proximal clamping for vascular control. Critical warm ischemia times are highly variable in these various clinical scenarios depending on extent of collateral blood flow and the metabolic demands of the compartmental tissues. Perhaps the most important variable that has an impact on the rapidity and severity of any compartment syndrome is that of associated hemorrhagic shock combined with vascular occlusion.

Etiologies of compartment syndome

Although the anatomy of compartment syndromes is highly variable, the pathophysiology remains similar. Fig. 2 outlines some of the basic processes involved with development of compartment syndrome. Although ischemia always is involved, soft tissue injury frequently is an accompanying insult. Ischemia and soft tissue injury lead to edema and increasing tissue pressures, which cause decreasing tissue perfusion that results gradually in critical capillary closing pressures. Further cellular ischemia with edema ensues until this continuing sequence ultimately leads to tissue death. Although compartment syndromes can occur anywhere in the body, they are most prone to develop in anatomic compartments with low compliance. Conversely, they are less likely to occur when there is room for expansion. Because of the current status of global cataclysm, extremity compartment syndrome, secondary to crushing injuries, is the most common worldwide. And, although

Compartment Syndrome

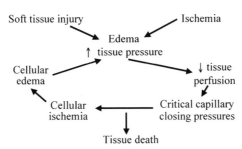

Fig. 2. The diagram illustrates the pathophysiologic processes involved with development and progression of compartment syndromes.

there is a wide variety of causes of compartment syndromes, including burn eschar, snakebites, iatrogenic sources (forearm intravenous infusion, pneumatic tourniquets, and Lloyd Davies positioning), for the purposes of this article, compartment syndromes caused by ischemia reperfusion (I/R) injury are discussed in detail.

Ischemia reperfusion injury

Endothelial damage incites the progressive cellular insult of I/R injury. In the tissue beds, the endothelial cells develop a proinflammatory phenotype and express cell surface adhesion molecules, which lead to neutrophil migration into the tissues producing cellular damage and swelling. Widened endothelial junctions simultaneously lead to increasing interstitial edema. This combination of interstitial edema and cellular swelling produces increased tissue pressures that ultimately end in a compartment syndrome. Reperfusion activates neutrophils and the production of free oxygen radicals, producing a simultaneous double-hit injury that causes damage and dysfunction of cellular membranes and further acceleration of intracellular and extracellular edema. The greatest damage occurs during this cascade of events after reperfusion. The end results of I/R are loss of membrane integrity with development of edema, leading to compromised blood flow and, ultimately, organ dysfunction and failure (Fig. 3). There have been many investigative avenues pursued to alleviate or prevent I/R injury. Although these endeavors have been successful in various animal models, there has been no significant advance relative to clinical applications.

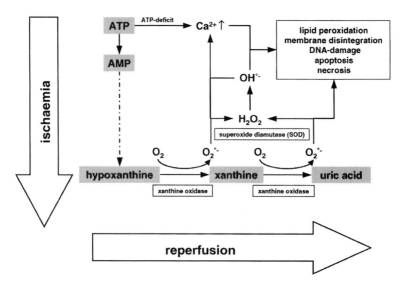

Fig. 3. Diagramatic illustration of I/R injury.

Abdominal compartment syndrome

The development of ACS can be looked on as the result of total body I/R injury. It generally begins as an insult resulting in either massive intracavitary or external hemorrhage. The hemorrhage component leads to hypoperfusion—the ischemic component of injury. In the face of prolonged shock acidosis, hypothermia and coagulopathy result. Splanchnic hypoperfusion with resultant gut mucosal acidosis, bowel edema, and hepatic ischemia follow. The gut edema is exacerbated markedly during the time of reperfusion associated with fluid resuscitation—events that visually are apparent in the operating room. The ischemia of muscle and gut leads to excessive systemic activation of the innate immune system, resulting in damage to essentially every organ, with the lung involved nearly uniformly by acute lung injury. As gut mucosal injury leads to bowel edema, there is a resultant increase in intra-abdominal hypertension, leading to the continued cycle of increasing ischemia, edema, and acidosis. The development of ACS is insidious and progressive. If not treated, ACS ends in the multiple organ dysfunction syndrome and, ultimately, death of the patient. The treatment of ACS is the same as treatment of most other compartment syndromes. The compartment must be decompressed.

Compartment syndromes result from intracompartmental hypertension. This hypertension produces dysfunction, which is inversely proportional to the compliance of the effected compartment. Compliance is represented by the formula, $C = \Delta V/\Delta P$ (C is compliance, Delta V is change in volume and Delta P is change in pressure).

Anatomic compartments with high compliance expand their volume (stretch) more readily with pressure increases than do low compliant systems. Fig. 4 illustrates this relationship conceptually. Increasing intracranial pressure from brain injury develops rapidly because of the inability to expand the cranium, whereas lower extremity compartments have a higher compliance because of limited capacity for fascial stretching to increase compartmental volume. In contrast, hypertension develops gradually in

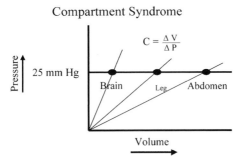

Fig. 4. The relationship of increasing volume and increasing pressure as they relate to compliance of three different body compartments.

the peritoneal cavity (abdominal compartment), as there is a greater cavitary volume compared with volume of contents. Although the figure is not meant to deal with exact relationships, it does call attention to the fact that the approximate pressure of 25 mm Hg is the critical compartment pressure for significant alterations in microvascular blood flow to the compartmental contents in essentially all parts of the body. At this pressure, therapies of either expansion of the compartment or reduction of volume (contents) have been used as the mainstay of therapy for many years. When compartment pressures in the lower extremity approach 25 mm Hg, fasciotomies are performed to expand the volume. For the brain, it is widely appreciated that at approximately a pressure of 25 mm Hg, significant alterations in flow occur, and, although diuresis has been a mainstay for many years in an attempt to decrease the intracranial swelling, frontal lobotomy also has been used to decrease the compartmental volume. In recent years, there has been a tendency toward craniectomy to increase the volume for expansion of the brain. This approach has developed simultaneously with concepts of decompressing the abdomen by leaving it open for the treatment of ACS.

Although urgent decompressive laparotomy has become the standard of care for treatment of ACS, understanding of these pathophysiologic processes has became appreciated more widely, and there has been a widespread movement toward a prophylactic approach to the management of ACS. Rather than closing the abdomen in the face of significant hemorrhage and abdominal injury, most trauma surgeons have begun leaving the abdomen open rather than risk further insult of intra-abdominal hypertension and ACS that often is lethal in this scenario.

The clinical picture of ACS is characterized by three physiologic perturbations: respiratory compromise, decreased splanchnic flow, and renal insufficiency. This pathophysiology has been delineated nicely in several laboratory experiments. In 1976, Richardson and Trinkle devised a series of experiments that were elegant in their simplicity [4]. They used an animal model of increased intra-abdominal pressure in which dogs had their peritoneal cavities insufflated with air in gradual increments. They noted that as the intra-abdominal pressure gradually went up as more air was instilled, the inspiratory pulmonary pressures rose in a gradual fashion until there was a marked increase when the intra-abdominal pressure approached 25 mm Hg. With the widespread application of laparoscopy for elective surgical procedures, 25 mm Hg is approximately the pressure at which cardiopulmonary compromise occurs. In addition, in this same model, there was a linear correlation of increasing vena caval and renal vein pressures with increased intra-abdominal pressure, and cardiac output had a linear decrease associated with increasing intra-abdominal pressures. A similar series of experiments was performed by Diebel and colleagues, in 1992 [5], in a swine model using instillation of lactated Ringer's solution to produce intra-abdominal hypertension. Systemic and splanchnic hemodynamics were investigated. It was noted that going from baseline up to 40 mm Hg in increments of 10 mm Hg that the mean arterial pressure did not change. This is similar to what is observed clinically in the scenario of ACS. Similarly, the pulmonary capillary wedge pressure did not change substantially. The cardiac output fell 30%, however, from 5.4 L per minute at baseline to 4.0 L per minute at 40 mm Hg. Also, the superior mesenteric artery flow dropped to 30% of baseline at 40 mm Hg, and, similar to the previous experiments, the drop occurred most abruptly when the intra-abdominal pressure was raised above 30 mm Hg. Using tonometry, the mucosal pH dropped from 7.21 at baseline to 6.98 at 40 mm Hg intra-abdominal pressure. These laboratory observations correlate well with what is seen in patients in operating rooms and ICUs who develop intra-abdominal hypertension and ACS.

Although ACS generally is believed to be associated with trauma, one of the first clinical descriptions of the syndrome clinically was made as a complication of ruptured abdominal aortic aneurysm repair [6]. That report documented the occurrence of ACS with ruptured aneurysms, and a subsequent report by Oelschlager and coworkers demonstrated that delaying primary closure of the abdomen resulted in improved survival [7]. Subsequently, Ivatury and colleagues documented significantly improved survival in a group of severely injured trauma patients who had mesh closure as a primary prophylactic measure versus a group of patients who had fascial closure [8]. The mortality in the prophylactic mesh group was 10.6% versus 36% in the group with the fascial closure ($P = .003$). That report and the clinical observations of surgeons in other trauma centers led to the current widespread practice of prevention of ACS by leaving the abdomen opened.

The early descriptions of ACS were from patients who had abdominal injury associated with major blood loss and shock. ACS, however, has been noted in patients who have no significant abdominal injury but require massive fluid resuscitation for extra-abdominal injuries. ACS has been seen in severe soft tissue and skeletal trauma and after burn resuscitation. Maxwell and colleagues reported seven patients who had ACS occurring after massive fluid resuscitation from extra-abdominal injuries and coined the term, "secondary ACS" [9]. It was found that emergent decompressive laparotomy significantly reduced peak inspiratory pressures, immediately yielded significant diuresis, and was associated with rapid improvements in base deficit. An important part of therapy is to administer sodium bicarbonate immediately before decompression in those patients who develop ACS. At my institution in Memphis, there were deaths associated with decompression, which was the result of a massive return of anaerobic by-products from the abdomen and lower extremities when the abdomen was opened. The patients who died became acutely hypotensive. Since institution of prophylactic sodium bicarbonate immediately before opening the abdomen, this adverse event has been avoided.

Open abdomen techniques

Although ACS has been reduced significantly since prophylactic open abdomen management has been adopted, a new set of problems has arisen, resulting in several controversial areas of management. Novel challenges, acute and chronic, have emerged. The acute problems involve managing the large open wounds and potential collateral damage, including the disastrous complication of intestinal fistulae. The chronic problem created by the successful avoidance of ACS is the challenge of definitive reconstruction of the large abdominal wall defects in those patients who recover from their acute traumatic insult. To address these difficult tasks, institutions have arrived at local approaches that are developed by trial and error techniques. Although art and science always are balanced in surgery, it seems that the approach to managing large abdominal wounds after these major traumatic events has developed with more art than science. In Memphis, this is an area where my colleagues and I certainly have learned a lot more from mistakes than from successes.

At my institution, a fairly standardized staged approach for managing the abdominal wound has been developed. The three stages are stage I—prosthetic insertion; stage —split-thickness skin grafting for a "planned ventral hernia"; and stage III—definitive reconstruction (Fig. 5). It seems that most trauma institutions have adopted similar strategies. In the remaining portion of this article, staged reconstruction methods are discussed, including alternatives to the various elements of each stage and analysis of complications associated with acute and definitive management plans.

The staged approach to the open abdomen was evaluated in 274 consecutive patients [10]. During the 8-year interval of this study, there were 2664 laparotomies performed for trauma. Thus, approximately 10% of all laparotomies were managed with open abdomen techniques because of the severity of abdominal injury, blood loss, and shock. All of these wounds

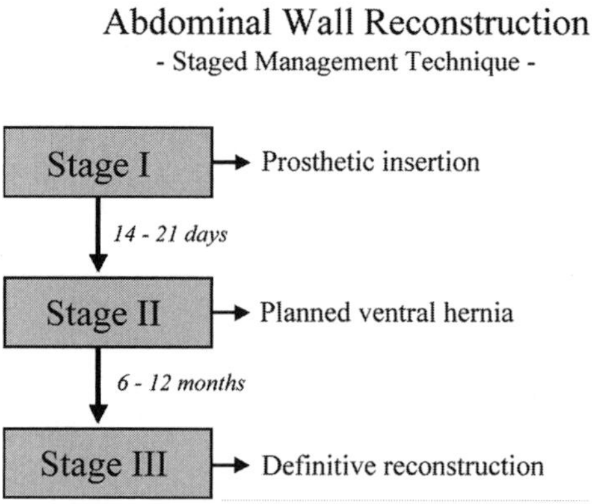

Abdominal Wall Reconstruction
- Staged Management Technique -

Fig. 5. This is an algorithm demonstrating the three-staged management of the open abdomen.

were incisions from xyphoid to pubic symphysis. Of the 274 open abdomen patients, there were 108 deaths (39%) within the first several days of injury resulting from complications associated with massive injury and shock.

Stage I

There are many methods described for acute management of the open abdominal defect. The technique of towel clip closure of the abdomen was used widely in the early days of damage control via rapid termination of laparotomy before definitive surgical procedures and to permit resuscitation of the clotting system, shock, and hypothermia in ICUs. Initially, surgeons used towel clipping of the fascia, whereas subsequently the technique was modified to clipping of the skin with multiple clips approximately 1 to 2 cm apart. The towel clip method was effective for rapid termination of surgery with tamponade maintained in the gauze-packed abdomen. Several patients developed ACS, however, regardless of whether or not the fascia or skin was clipped, because of the inability of the abdominal cavity to expand with increasing edema or blood and clot that developed. Thus, towel clip closure largely has been abandoned with the onset of the widespread practice of open abdominal wound management for damage control and prophylaxis against ACS.

Varying techniques have been promulgated for acute management of the open abdominal wound. Most surgeons have believed that it is important to place some type of prosthesis in the widely open abdomen to prevent evisceration and associated complications from bowels unprotected from gauze dressings. The Bogota bag was one of the early devices used and remains a practical tool. This approach is attributed to surgeons in Colombia who have had vast experience in the management of catastrophic penetrating abdominal wounds for many years. The technique uses sterile polyvinyl chloride solution bags that can be sewn to skin or fascia. Large genitourinary irrigation bags work well. X-ray cassette covers are used in a similar fashion and seem equally effective. Advantages of both are that they are widely available and inexpensive. Other materials used for acute management of the open wound include polypropylene mesh, polytetrafluoroethylene (PTFE) patches, the Wittmann Patch (Star Surgical), and absorbable meshes, including polyglycolic acid and polyglactin 910 meshes. Under ideal circumstances, omentum is inserted between the intestines and the prosthesis, but often the omentum either is inadequate or destroyed to such an extent that it is not available for coverage. I insertion of omentum in this space decreases the complication of intestinal fistula.

As part of the first stage of management, an attempt is made to pleat the prosthetic material gradually, as patients' hemodynamic status recovers to maintain midline tension to attain a potential secondary fascial closure. It has been my colleagues and my institutional policy to take patients back to the operating room within 24 to 48 hours of the initial operation for definitive repair of viscera and removal of packs. Polyglactin 910 woven mesh is inserted at that time, if it had not been placed at the primary operation. I find that attempts at pleating polyvinyl chloride have a tendency to tear the material, whereas the absorbable mesh maintains its integrity from pleating without having to replace the material at the fascia or skin edges where it has been attached. If the pleating process is begun but the patient deteriorates because of sepsis, with further swelling and abdominal distention, then occasionally the mesh is left in place, but additional mesh is sutured to expand the pleated area.

There is some disagreement as to whether or not prosthetic material should be sutured to the skin or to the fascia. The argument in favor of attaching it to the skin is that it reduces the incidence of fascial loss, which can be an important issue during definitive reconstruction. The argument for sewing it to the fascia is that there is a reduced tendency to lose abdominal domain by preventing the continuing retraction of the fascia. My general policy is to sew the prosthetic to the skin initially. If it becomes apparent that the abdomen is not be able to be closed, however, a fascial attachment is converted to, to minimize the loss of domain over the several months that pass before definitive reconstruction (Fig. 6). Using the staged approach with gradual pleating of the polyglycolic acid mesh has permitted 22% of 166 patients in my colleagues' and my experience to undergo a secondary fascial closure. Pleating also can be used with other materials that are used for acute abdominal wound management. The Wittmann Patch was designed specifically to allow gradual pleating in ICUs. The patch consists of two pieces of burr-type material that stick together like Velcro. A piece is sewn to each side of the abdomen, which allows for either expanding the abdominal cavity in the face of increasing intra-abdominal edema or for pleating to allow for gradual wound closure.

Polypropylene mesh was used extensively in the past but has fallen out of popularity because of the concern over development of enterocutaneous

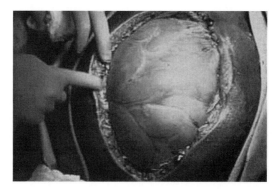

Fig. 6. The picture demonstrates placement of woven polyglactin 910 mesh for open abdomen management in stage 1.

fistulae. From a summary of 14 reports in the literature involving 128 patients, Jones and Jurkovich reported a 23% fistula rate [11]. These enterocutaneous, or perhaps more appropriately termed "enteroatmospheric" fistulas, are difficult to manage and associated with substantial morbidity and mortality. Although comparative data are not available on other materials, it is widely believed that the fistula rate is higher for polypropylene mesh than all the other techniques discussed.

An alternative technique to bridging a wound with prosthetic material is the use of the vacuum pack technique. This technique was described by Brock and coworkers in 1995 (Fig. 7) [12]. A plastic drape was inserted in the peritoneal cavity covering the viscera and on top of this was placed a surgical towel along with two sump drains covered with an adhesive-backed plastic drape attached to the skin. The sump drains are placed on continuous suction. This provided the theoretic advantages of evacuating the abdominal cavity of edema fluid, allowing for maintenance of tamponade to counteract bleeding and possible prevention of loss of domain. As opposed to my experience, in which 22% of abdomens could be closed progressively, Miller and colleagues reported being able to secondarily close approximately 80% of abdomens that were managed by a similar vacuum pack

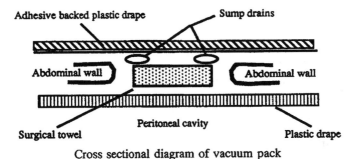

Cross sectional diagram of vacuum pack

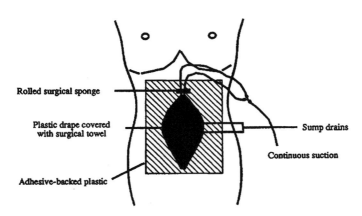

Fig. 7. Cross-section diagram of vacuum pack and completed vacuum pack.

technique [13]. It remains unclear, however, if the indications for managing patients who had the open abdomen are uniform among reported series. Institutions that are more liberal about leaving abdomens open after laparotomy for trauma likely have a much higher rate of closure than institutions that have less experience. Other factors could be reflected in referral patterns where institutions have a large number of patients who come at more prolonged intervals. Other patients may experience a greater level of shock after their injury and may have greater degrees of cellular insult prohibiting early closure resulting from prolonged time to resolution of the I/R injury. Regardless, it is important for investigators to report the total number of laparotomies in their series in addition to those managed by open abdomen so that a denominator is available to permit reasonable comparisons among institutional outcomes.

Since the early descriptions of the vacuum pack technique, commercially produced products have been developed for managing these open abdominal wounds (Kinetic Concepts, Inc.). There also is concern that the vacuum technique might promote dehiscence of intestinal suture lines in those patients who undergo intestinal repair or resection. To date, however, that complication has not been documented in the literature in association with this vacuum technique. Clinical trials would be valuable and are indicated in addressing these various techniques and products. Standard entry criteria and prospective stratification and evaluation would allow for addition of a little science to the art of open abdominal wound management.

Stage II—planned ventral hernia

When prosthetic material is inserted in stage I, patients either recover and mobilize fluids over the next several days, allowing for gradual closure of the abdomen, or develop varying degrees of multiple organ dysfunction or sepsis. In my experience, in the latter group, they rarely are able to get their fascia closed via progressive approximation. In that circumstance, the viscera granulate and adhere to the abdominal wall laterally and to the prosthesis. When absorbable mesh is used as the acute prosthetic material, granulation occurs through the mesh. Although conventional wisdom suggests that absorbable mesh would be absorbed completely and not have to be removed, that has not been my experience using the woven variety of polyglactin 910. Usually within 2 to 3 weeks, granulation occurs and a suppurative interface between mesh and viscera develops, which begins to separate the two. At this point of healthy granulation, the viscera are stuck laterally and patients are taken to an operating room. The mesh is removed easily because of the suppurative interface (Fig. 8). After removal of the mesh, a pulsatile pressure irrigation system is used to reduce colonization of the granulation tissue and a split-thickness skin graft is harvested and applied to "close" the abdominal wound.

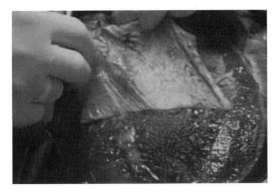

Fig. 8. The photograph demonstrates the removal of woven polyglactin 910 at stage 2 followed by placement of split-thickness skin graft for planned ventral hernia.

Intestinal fistulae

From my experience, excluding those cases of early mortality resulting from catastrophic injury, 14 fistulae developed in the 166 survivors for a fistula rate of 8.4% [10]. A root cause analysis of the fistulas was done. Ten were of small bowel origin, three were from the colon, and one was gastric. The timing of fistula development was one before insertion of the vicryl mesh resulting from suture line breakdown of a destructive small bowel injury, 10 after mesh insertion but before skin grafting, and the remaining three after split-thickness skin grafting. There were important findings that can be used to reduce fistula development in management of these large open wounds. It is important to get the skin graft on the open wound as soon as the prosthetic material is removed. When I evaluated the days of mesh insertion on patients who had and did not have fistula, those who did not have fistula had the mesh on for 18.1 days versus 26.5 for those who had fistula ($P < .04$); the longer the wound is left to granulate without coverage of the bowel, the more likely erosion of the bowel wall through the granulation tissue is to develop and instigate a fistula. One would not think that a skin graft necessarily would give much support to the wound and that this sort of coverage would not necessarily prevent a fistula. But, in my experience, it seems that skin grafting does stabilize the wound significantly. Besides bowel erosion from prolonged exposure of the uncovered, open granulating bed, I have had a few patients develop fistulae from coughing during suctioning or while on a ventilator. The presence of a skin graft seems to add a degree of integrity and reduces splitting of the bowel during sporadic increases in intraintestinal pressure. Closure of open granulating wounds also is important to decrease the proteinaceous losses through the wound and is similar to the benefit of early grafting of large surface burns. These prodigious open wounds act as major third-degree burns to the abdominal wall and produce a tremendous ongoing catabolic drain.

Regardless of how attentively the wound management care is provided, occasional fistulae develop. These can range from relatively minor irritants to life-threatening catastrophes. Sometimes, small fistulas develop on the lateral aspects of the wound. In that circumstance, wounds often granulate and contract over the top of these lateral fistulas with resolution of the fistula. Those small fistulas that do not close often can be handled as semiformal ostomies with bags placed over them until definitive reconstruction.

Those fistulas that occur away from the lateral wall in the midportion of the wound are problematic, however. For fistulae in the midst of the wound from distal small bowel, my colleagues' and my institutional approach is to constipate the patient (diphenoxylate/atropine) and to skin graft the entire wound around the fistula. Bed rotation and patient positioning are helpful adjuncts. After the graft adheres, the fistula is converted to a controlled ostomy. Although not always successful, this approach works better than might be anticipated. In contrast, midwound proximal, high-volume small bowel fistulas have significant morbidity and mortality and are the most challenging. My usual approach is to operate early to prevent the complications secondary to metabolic derangements and nutritional depletion. High-volume fistulas cannot be controlled as ostomies in these wounds. I prefer to operate within the first 7 to 10 days after they develop. Operation consists of incising the granulation tissue right at the osteum of the fistula with sharp and hemostat dissection. Generally, a relatively normal serosa is identified. Once the serosa is identified, the bowel loop is isolated gradually and resected back to nonindurated, nonedematous tissue. A primary anastomosis generally is performed. After anastomosis, an attempt is made to bury the anastomosis as deeply as possible in the abdomen beneath other bowel loops to minimize the likelihood of recurrent fistula. If recurrence develops, some fistulae may close if buried within loops of bowel, because the dehiscence is not exposed in the open wound. After resection, the large open wound is managed either with gauze abdominal dressings if the majority of the bowel is stuck, or if not, absorbable mesh once again is sewn to the skin edges laterally to maintain the viscera within the abdomen. Resection of these fistulas is an arduous task that takes many hours. It is my opinion, however, that patients do better with this early approach rather than waiting several weeks to months and having their nutritional status and overall recovery continue to erode while they are on total parenteral nutrition.

Stage III—definitive reconstruction of the abdominal wall

These giant abdominal wall defects can appear daunting (Fig. 9). An organized consistent approach, however, can provide excellent long-term outcomes. The appropriate timing for abdominal wall reconstruction is of paramount importance. If performed too early, dense adhesions make split-thickness skin graft removal difficult, often leading to multiple

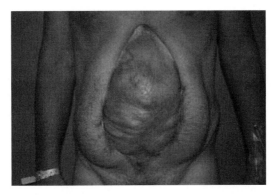

Fig. 9. Photograph of a patient 11 months after hospital discharge who is ready for abdominal wall reconstruction.

enterotomies or significant bowel deserosalization. When reconstruction is delayed for an excessive amount of time, the musculature of the abdominal wall tends to contract with a progressive loss of domain. In that circumstance, when autogenous tissue reconstruction is planned, mobilization of the components of the abdominal wall is difficult, leading to repairs under tension and an increased incidence of hernia formation over time.

Many techniques are advocated for repair of these defects. The most commonly applied approaches are with the use of prosthetic materials. Other options include the application of local myofascial advancement techniques, rotational muscle flaps, and, most recently, the use of biomaterials. There are advantages and disadvantages to each of these approaches. The most obvious advantages to the use of prosthetic materials, most commonly polypropylene mesh and PTFE, are their ready availability and the fairly simple techniques of implantation. Currently, long-term comparative outcomes are not available in this population of patients who have giant defects. The approach to repair with prosthetic materials is the same as for any ventral hernia. Mobilization of skin and subcutaneous fat is required beyond the myofascial edges bilaterally. Although there is a variety of suture methods available for attaching the prosthesis, it seems that the fascia underlay technique with attachment of the prosthetic with U-sutures placed 1 to 2 cm beyond the myofascial edge is associated with better long-term results, particularly regarding recurrent buttonhole-type hernias. The disadvantages to prosthetic materials are the risks of intestinal fistula, prosthetic infection, and recurrent hernias. Whatever material is used, it is advantageous to attempt to place an interface of omentum between the mesh and the underlying bowel. In these complex cases, however, that have had multiple abdominal injuries, the omentum generally is not of good quality or quantity. The use of PTFE, including the Dualmesh variety (W.L. Gore & Associates, Flagstaff, Arizona), is proposed to be associated with lower fistula rates. A major trade-off seems to be a higher incidence of seroma developing between the prosthesis and the large skin flaps that are required for these procedures. Overall, it is difficult to provide accurate data concerning morbidity and long-term outcomes with the various reconstructive techniques because of paucity of reported data.

Although construction of muscle flaps occasionally is reported in small series, there is no large experience with either free flaps or rotational flaps in the management of these abdominal wall defects. They have the advantage of being autogenous tissue. Disadvantages include the complexity of the techniques and complications associated with those cases in which the flap fails. Larger experiences hopefully will be reported in the near future.

The component separation technique was described by Ramirez and colleagues in 1990 [14]. A modification of that original description has become my preferred method of reconstruction in the majority of these cases. The original component separation technique was a description of local myocutaneous flap advancement after extensive relaxing incisions in the abdominal wall. This involved bilateral medial mobilization of the musculofascial units of the rectus abdominus muscles. It provides autologous continuity with dynamic support of the abdominal wall. The original technique provided for 3 to 5 cm of mobilization on each side. These large abdominal wall defects, however, usually cannot be repaired with this amount of mobilization. Therefore, prosthetic material generally is required to close the defect in a tension-free manner. After recognizing this drawback of limited mobilization, my colleagues and I added a modification of Ramirez's component separation technique [15].

Modified component separation

Fig. 10 demonstrates the application of this reconstructive approach. Although it seems complicated in the diagram, it actually is straightforward.

Step 1: Begin the operation by removing the split-thickness skin graft from the underlying abdominal viscera. As discussed previously, the timing for abdominal reconstruction is extremely important to ensure optimal results. My colleagues' and my plan for reconstruction when the intra-abdominal adhesion process has matured to the point of development of filmy adhesions between loops of bowel and skin graft. This can be ascertained simply by pinching the skin graft between the fingers, and, if the bowel falls away, the time for reconstruction is at hand. If the loops of bowel remain densely adhered to the underlying skin graft, reconstruction should be delayed. Experience suggests that most patients develop these flimsy adhesions in the 6- to 12-month interval after hospital discharge. Occasionally, patients resolve the dense inflammatory responses a little sooner and occasionally somewhat later, but the dense inflammatory process usually resolves at approximately 8 to 9 months. In an operating room, after wide preparation of the abdominal wall, the skin graft is grasped between the

Modified Components Separation

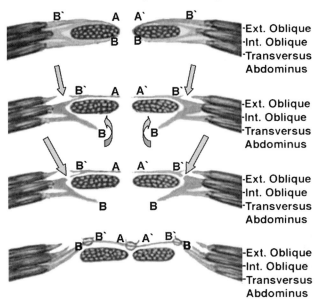

Fig. 10. Diagrammatic illustration of the modified components separation technique for reconstruction of abdominal wall defects.

fingers or with tissue forceps and sharply incised in an area that is obviously devoid of bowel. It is common for small areas of bowel to continue to have dense adhesions, so these areas are to be avoided when entering the abdomen. Once the incision is made, the flimsy adhesions are apparent and, with sharp and hemostat dissection, the skin graft is divided in its midportion from top to bottom. After this, adhesions of small bowel to the skin graft are mobilized bilaterally and dissection extends a few centimeters beyond the lateral edge of the rectus abdominus muscles bilaterally. Removal of the skin graft and satisfactory lyses of intra-abdominal adhesions generally take 45 to 60 minutes. The more dense adhesions generally are found at the medial myofascial edges bilaterally. Adhesions to the liver also generally are a little more dense then the flimsy adhesions to the loops of the bowel and caution must be exercised to avoid dissecting beneath Glisson's capsule and causing bothersome oozing of blood.

Step 2: After this mobilization, the full-thickness skin and subcutaneous fat are mobilized on each side of the wound to between the anterior and midaxillary lines, depending on the degree of abdominal wall contraction in order for lax skin closure.

Before completing description of the procedure, it is appropriate to review the anatomy of the rectus abdominus sheath. There are anterior and posterior rectus sheathes bilaterally. These are formed by the medial extensions of the fascia of the external oblique, internal oblique, and transversus abdominus muscles. The internal oblique aponeurosis splits just lateral to the rectus abdominus muscle and contributes to the anterior and posterior rectus sheaths. The external oblique fascial aponeurosis fuses with the anterior component of the internal oblique fascia, forming the anterior rectus sheath. In a similar fashion, the transverse abdominus aponeurosis and transversalis fascia fuse with the posterior element of the internal oblique aponeurosis just lateral to the lateral portion of the rectus abdominus, with this fusion producing the posterior rectus sheath. There is no posterior rectus sheath below the arcuate line. The following steps are for mobilization of the rectus abdominus myofascial flaps.

Step 3: The rectus abdominus muscle is grasped in the palm of the hand with the thumb on top and the fingers inside of the abdominal cavity. By rubbing the thumb and fingers back and forth, it is easy to identify the lateral border of the rectus abdominus muscle. The external oblique aponeurosis is divided approximately 1 cm lateral to the rectus abdominus muscle with use of hemostat to dissect the external oblique freely from the internal oblique component. The external oblique fascia then is divided superiorly and inferiorly, going over the lower costal region superiorly and down to the pubic symphysis inferiorly. In the diagram, that division is indicated by the line of incision at B′ bilaterally.

Step 4: After division of the external oblique aponeurosis, the posterior rectus fascia is separated from the rectus muscle with blunt dissection beginning at the superior aspect of the wound and continuing down below the arcuate line. In the diagram, this is indicated by the separation bilaterally at B, which indicates the medial extent of the posterior rectus fascia.

Step 5: The internal oblique component of the anterior rectus sheath is divided. This is done in a fashion similar to the division of the external oblique aponeurosis by initial sharp incision and then using hemostat dissection and cautery or knife to divide this fascia up over the lower rib cage superiorly. Inferiorly, it is imperative that the incision be stopped at the arcuate line. This can be seen from the peritoneal surface of the rectus sheath as a superiorly convex line approximately midway between umbilicus and pubic symphysis. This is the site of entry of the inferior epigastric artery into the rectus sheath and the site of spigelian hernia formation. If the internal oblique component of the anterior rectus sheath is divided below this point, a large hernia will develop, because there is no posterior fascia below the arcuate line. After these divisions of the internal and external oblique aponeuroses and mobilization of the posterior rectus sheath from the rectus muscles, mobile flaps of the rectus myofascial units have resulted bilaterally.

Step 6: The defect then is closed by suturing the medial components of the anterior rectus fascia (A to A′) (see Fig. 10), followed by closure of the medial aspect of the posterior rectus sheath to the lateral aspect of the anterior rectus sheath bilaterally (B to B′) (see Fig. 10). The suture technique used for closing these midline and lateral components of the abdominal wall is with three separate running #1 polypropylene sutures medially and bilaterally. Four flat closed suction drains then are inserted, two superiorly and two inferiorly bilaterally. The skin then is approximated in the midline to complete the procedure. (An audiovisual CD presentation of the modified components separation technique is available in the video collections of the American College of Surgeons [15a].)

This mobilization provides approximately 10 cm of medial advancement in the epigastrium, 20 cm in the midabdomen, and 8 cm in the lower abdomen. Generally, the most difficult mobilization of the myofascial units is in the superior aspect of the wound, which makes it important to carry the oblique incisions over the lower costal margin. Occasionally, a small piece of prosthetic material is required in this upper part of the incision to eliminate tension. Approximately 100 abdominal wall reconstructions have been performed at my institution using the modified component separation technique. The average follow-up of these patients is approximately 2.5 years. Long-term results have demonstrated recurrent hernias in 5% of these patients. The hernias usually are localized around one of the lateral suture lines. Results were analyzed for complications of recurrent herniation and the need for adjunctive mesh in the upper part of the wound versus timing of reconstruction. If reconstruction was performed less than 12 months after discharge, the complication rate was 7.6%, although of those who had reconstruction longer than a year after injury, complications occurred in 25% ($P = .10$). Adjunctive mesh was required in approximately 10% of my patients. The average time to reconstruction in those requiring adjunctive mesh was 20 months from the time of discharge. I believe that these are clinically relevant findings; they reinforce the concept that if reconstruction is undertaken much beyond the time of the development of loose intraabdominal adhesions that abdominal wall contraction progresses, resulting in loss of domain of the abdominal cavity; such loss leads to repairs under increased amounts of tension.

This experience with modified component separation technique remains the largest reported for management of large abdominal wall defects associated with damage control surgery. The complication rates have been low compared with experiences with repair of large ventral hernias in general. I have had no intestinal fistulas develop when using this approach. The hernia recurrence rate of 5% is low considering the size of these hernias. This technique remains my procedure of choice for definitive reconstruction in those patients who could not be closed during their initial hospitalization. In patients who require resection of significant amounts of rectus abdominus muscle resulting from necrosis associated with their original injury, however, the modified component separation technique is not possible. Patients usually should undergo abdominal wall reconstruction at less than 1 year to avoid the loss of domain that results in repairs under tension leading to higher recurrent hernia rates. In addition, the placement of permanent mesh is avoided with the attendant morbidities of foreign body infection and occasional production of intestinal fistula.

Biomaterials for abdominal wall reconstruction

Recently there have been reports of the use of human cadaveric acellular dermis for reconstruction (Alloderm, LifeCell Corporation Branchburg, NewJersey). Guy and colleagues report using this material acutely in a one-staged approach combined with local skin flaps advanced over the acellular dermis to avoid the need for extensive reconstruction [16]. Early results in that small series are promising. This material recently has been used in my institution in wounds that are not amenable to modified component separation reconstruction technique; the use of acellular dermis has provided good early results. Long-term follow-up, however, is required with larger numbers of patients to evaluate that approach adequately. It has been found that this material acts basically as a collagen matrix and allows for tissue ingrowth. In a few cases in which the material has been excised several months after implant, it appears histologically similar to the native tissue that it replaced.

Summary

Damage control surgery has become a fundamental component of operative trauma care. It undoubtedly has saved many lives that would have been lost in the not-too-distant past. In the development of these techniques, a great deal has been learned about intra-abdominal hypertension and ACS. Prophylactic application of open abdomen techniques evolved and led to avoidance of a great deal of the organ dysfunction associated with ACS. Additionally, in years past, many wounds were closed under considerable tension in the face of contamination that resulted in a high rate of necrotizing fasciitis, intestinal fistulization, and significant mortalities attributed to those dire complications. Surgeons now are learning a great deal about management of large open abdominal wounds. A wide variety of techniques has been adopted, but as time passes, there seems to be a general consensus developing regarding acute management of these wounds. Most institutions are adopting staged techniques of management similar to that described. It is recognized that getting the open wound closed as soon as possible leads to fewer complications, including lower fistula rates. The acute use of vacuum wound dressings is promising in that it may provide for early secondary closure of a significant portion these patients. Although we are continuing to learn about acute management, there has been less study focused on optimal definitive reconstructive techniques. The modified component separation technique has provided good results, with low recurrent hernia rates and long-term functional abdominal wall dynamics. Recently, the use of biomaterials for acute and chronic reconstruction shows promise in this area.

Further focus and study in all of these areas ultimately will lead to improved outcomes in this most seriously injured cohort of trauma patients.

References

[1] Stone HH, Strom PR, Mullins RJ. Management of the major coagulopathy with onset during laparotomy. Ann Surg 1983;197:532–5.
[2] Moore EE. Staged laparotomy for the hypothermia, acidosis, and coagulopathy syndrome. Am J Surg 1996;172:405.
[3] Rotondo MF, Schwab CW, McGonigal MD, et al. 'Damage control': an approach for improved survival in exsanguinating penetrating abdominal injury. J Trauma 1993;35:375–83.
[4] Richardson JD, Trinkle JK. Hemodynamic and respiratory alterations with increased intra-abdominal pressure. J Surg Res 1976;20:401–4.
[5] Diebel LN, Dulchavsky SA, Wilson RF. Effect of increased intra-abdominal pressure on mesenteric arterial and intestinal mucosal blood flow. J Trauma 1992;33:45–9.
[6] Fietsam R Jr, Villalba M, Glover JL, et al. Intra-abdominal compartment syndrome as a complication of ruptured abdominal aortic aneurysm repair. Am Surg 1989;55:396–402.
[7] Oelschlager BK, Boyle EM Jr, Johansen K, et al. Delayed abdominal closure in the management of ruptured abdominal aortic aneurysms. Am J Surg 1997;173:411–5.
[8] Ivatury RR, Porter JM, Simon RJ, et al. Intra-abdominal hypertension after life-threatening penetrating abdominal trauma: prophylaxis, incidence, and clinical relevance to gastric mucosal pH and abdominal compartment syndrome. J Trauma 1998;44:1016–23.
[9] Maxwell RA, Fabian TC, Croce MA, et al. Secondary abdominal compartment syndrome: an underappreciated manifestation of severe hemorrhagic shock. J Trauma 1999;47:995–9.
[10] Jernigan TW, Fabian TC, Croce MA, et al. Staged management of giant abdominal wall defects: acute and long-term results. Ann Surg 2003;238349–57.
[11] Jones JW, Jurkovich GJ. Polypropylene mesh closure of infected abdominal wounds. Am Surg 1989;55:73–6.
[12] Brock WB, Barker DE, Burns RP. Temporary closure of open abdominal wounds: the vacuum pack. Am Surg 1995;61:30–5.
[13] Miller PR, Meredith JW, Johnson JC, et al. Prospective evaluation of vacuum-assisted fascial closure after open abdomen: planned ventral hernia rate is substantially reduced. Ann Surg 204;239:608–16.
[14] Ramirez OM, Ruas E, Dellon AL. "Components separation" method for closure of abdominal-wall defects: an anatomic and clinical study. Plast Reconstr Surg 1990;86:519–26.
[15] Fabian TC, Croce MA, Pritchard FE, et al. Planned ventral hernia. Staged management for acute abdominal wall defects. Ann Surg 1994;219:643–53.
[15a] American College of Surgeons. Modified components separation technique. Available at: http://www.facs.org/education/videolibrary.html.
[16] Guy JS, Miller R, Morris JA Jr, et al. Early one-stage closure in patients with abdominal compartment sybndrome: fascial replacement with human acellular dermis and bipedicle flaps. Am Surg 2003;69:1025–9.

ELSEVIER
SAUNDERS

SURGICAL
CLINICS OF
NORTH AMERICA

Surg Clin N Am 87 (2007) 95–118

Thoracic Trauma:
When and How to Intervene

J. Wayne Meredith, MD*, J. Jason Hoth, MD

*Department of General Surgery, Wake Forest University School of Medicine,
Medical Center Boulevard, Winston-Salem, NC 27157, USA*

Trauma continues to be a significant source of patient morbidity and mortality, accounting for 140,000 deaths annually, and it is the leading cause of death in patients younger than 40 years of age [1]. Thoracic injuries are present after penetrating and blunt injury and are the primary or a contributing factor in up to 75% of all trauma-related deaths [2,3]. Most thoracic injuries can be managed with simple maneuvers such as tube thoracostomy [4]; however, 10% to 15% of patients who present with thoracic trauma require definitive operative repair [5].

The timing of intervention is oft debated but essentially takes place in one of three time periods mainly dictated by the patient's physiologic status upon arrival to the emergency room: immediate (emergency room thoracotomy), urgent (in the operating room, within 1–4 hours of arrival), and delayed (24 hours after admission) [6–8]. Once the need for intervention is apparent, the critical decision for an appropriate surgical approach is based on the location and nature of the injury. In this article, we review the common algorithm that applies to managing thoracic trauma patients. We discuss considerations and variables that enter into the decision-making process and describe various scenarios in which they are applicable.

Emergency department thoracotomy

Emergency department thoracotomy (EDT) is a drastic procedure with limited utility. Its primary use is in the management of patients in extremis after penetrating injury and, to a lesser extent, after blunt injury. The

---

* Corresponding author. Department of General Surgery, Wake Forest University School of Medicine, Medical Center Boulevard, Winston-Salem, NC 27157.

E-mail address: merediw@wfubmc.edu (J.W. Meredith).

therapeutic goals of EDT include control of hemorrhage, effective cardiac compression, cross-clamping the pulmonary hilum in the case of air embolism or massive bronchopleural fistula, relief of cardiac tamponade, and cross-clamping of the descending aorta for lower torso hemorrhage control [9]. Whenever possible, the patient should be stabilized and transported to the operating room where superior facilities are available for definitive care. The survival rate after EDT is approximately 7% [10,11,12].

When making a decision to perform an EDT, three factors must be taken into consideration: mechanism of injury, location of major injury, and signs of life. Better outcomes are seen when performed for penetrating (8%–10%) injuries rather than blunt injuries (approximately 1%), with greatest survival occurring when EDT is performed for stab wounds (18%–24%) rather than gunshot wounds (4%–5%) [12–16]. Likewise, patients with isolated penetrating chest injuries have the greatest chance of survival rather than patients with multi-cavity injuries [17,18]. The use of EDT in patients with isolated abdominal trauma or extremity trauma is controversial but has been demonstrated to be of some limited value [19,20]. Finally, the absence of signs of life (palpable pulse, pupillary or gag reflex, demonstrable blood pressure) must be considered. In general, patients most likely to respond favorably to EDT include victims of penetrating trauma with signs of life upon presentation to the emergency room or patients who lose signs of life within 10 minutes of arrival. Victims of blunt trauma with no signs of life upon arrival to the emergency room have poor survival rates, and EDT should not be performed in these patients. Current guidelines provided by the American College of Surgeons Advanced Trauma Life Support advocate the use of EDT in patients with penetrating chest trauma and cardiac electrical activity but not with pulseless blunt trauma or penetrating trauma without cardiac electrical activity [21]. It should be emphasized that EDT is a procedure for surgeons, and in the authors' experience there is no role for pericardiocentesis in these patients. Pericardiocentesis often is not effective in removing clotted blood from the pericardial space, it is not a risk-free procedure, it potentially delays the surgical procedure, and with the application of focused assessment with sonography for trauma (FAST) examination, the diagnostic use of this procedure is negligible.

Once the decision has been made to intervene, the standard incision is a left anterolateral thoracotomy that extends from the sternum below the nipple to the midaxillary line. After entering the pleural space, the hand is used to protect the lung, and scissors are used to open the intercostal space along the length of the incision. A chest retractor is then placed and opened. If required, additional exposure may be gained by using the scalpel to divide the costochondral junctions of the fifth, fourth, and third ribs, or alternatively, a Lebske knife or trauma shears may be used to divide the sternum transversely. After evacuating blood from the chest, attention is directed to the injury. If a great vessel is injured and bleeding, pressure is used to staunch hemorrhage. If air embolism is encountered, the pulmonary hilum is clamped or the affected lung may be twisted 180° and air in the aorta evacuated.

When hemopericardium is present, the pericardium may be divided longitudinally from the aortic root to the apex of the heart. At this point, care must be taken to identify and preserve the phrenic nerve. Once the hemopericardium is evacuated, the heart is delivered from the pericardial sac and digital pressure is applied to control hemorrhage. A temporary repair is performed using suture or staples. Alternatively, the hole may be "plugged" with a Foley catheter balloon held under tension [22]. After the cause of arrest has been addressed, a cross-clamp may be applied to the descending thoracic aorta after sweeping the lung anteromedially and exposing the posterior mediastinum. Momentarily arresting mechanical ventilation and nasogastric tube placement are helpful adjuncts to visualize and localize a flaccid descending aorta. The pleura along the posterior mediastinum is opened and the cross-clamp is applied. Intravascular volume is restored, and if the patient responds, he or she is transported to the operating room for definitive repair of injuries.

Urgent thoracotomy

For the purposes of this article, thoracotomy within the first few hours of injury is considered an urgent thoracotomy. Included in this category are compensated cardiac injuries, non-exsanguinating injuries to the great vessels of the aorta, tracheobronchial injuries, esophageal injuries, and, in some cases, traumatic rupture of the thoracic aorta. Indications for urgent thoracotomy include the presence of cardiac tamponade, high chest tube output, persistent air leak, and air embolism.

When deliberating whether a patient requires chest exploration based on chest tube output, the fundamental question is, "Will the bleeding stop?" If a hemothorax is suggested on physical examination or initial chest radiograph, a chest tube should be placed. The drainage of a massive amount of blood suggests the presence of major vascular injury that is unlikely to stop without surgical intervention. Many authors use 1500 mL of initial chest tube drainage as a trigger at which chest exploration becomes mandatory; however, we routinely use 1000 mL of chest tube drainage as an indication to consider chest exploration [23–25]. Ongoing bleeding after chest tube placement at a rate of 200 to 300 mL/h is also proposed to be an indication for chest exploration [6,24,25].

There are some caveats to these general guidelines. In some patients, however, this rule of thumb is not applicable. Some caveats to chest tube drainage as an indicator for chest exploration are (1) pulmonary parenchymal bleeding, (2) blunt chest trauma with delayed presentation, and (3) presence of a coagulopathy (medications in elderly patients or closed head injuries). In cases of pulmonary parenchymal bleeding, it is important to understand that the pulmonary circulation is a low pressure system, and complete expansion of the lung usually tamponades any parenchymal source of bleeding. Another scenario that is especially common in the setting of rural trauma is a patient presenting with blunt chest trauma in a delayed fashion. These patients may have a significant hemothorax that has accumulated in the time it has taken the patient to arrive in the emergency department. In these situations, evidence of ongoing bleeding rather than initial chest tube drainage may be a more reliable indication for chest exploration. This is in contradistinction to victims of penetrating trauma or blunt trauma occurring in close proximity to the trauma center. In these patients, 1000 to 1500 mL of chest tube drainage remains a reliable indicator for chest exploration. Another group of patients in whom caution should be exercised when considering thoracotomy are individuals with a coagulopathy and chest wall injury. Two common scenarios for this involve elderly patients on anticoagulant medications and coagulopathy in the presence of a closed head injury. In the authors' experience, operation in this setting is often not therapeutic and may add to the already present chest wall bleeding.

A second indicator for urgent chest exploration after injury is the presence of massive air leak defined as being present during all phases of respiration that is associated with an inability to fully expand the affected lung or impairing ventilation through the loss of effective tidal volume. These findings suggest major tracheobronchial injuries. The presence of cardiac tamponade, demonstrated using a combination of findings on physical examination (Beck's triad: muffled heart tones, distended neck veins, and hypotension) and, more recently, by the presence of a pericardial effusion on FAST examination, demands further evaluation with pericardial window or median sternotomy. Finally, air embolism, a rare entity associated with penetrating injury, occurs when a fistula develops between a bronchus and pulmonary vein; it requires urgent thoracotomy. Typically, the patient is stable until intubated and placed on positive pressure ventilation, when sudden cardiovascular collapse or the onset of lateralizing neurologic symptoms occurs [26]. To summarize, the major indicators for urgent thoracotomy include (1) chest tube output > 1000 mL (with noted exceptions as described above) (2) evidence of ongoing bleeding at a rate of 200 to 300 mL/h, (3) massive air leak, (4) cardiac tamponade, and (5) air embolism.

Given the indications for chest exploration, selecting the appropriate chest incision is critically important. What makes this decision difficult is that four different compartments must be considered: the right chest, left chest, mediastinum, and, in the case of concomitant abdominal injury, the peritoneal cavity. Several factors should be measured carefully before making a decision. Information regarding missile or injury trajectory, a thorough working knowledge of thoracic/mediastinal anatomy, and the exposures offered by each different incision are vital to choosing the appropriate incision. Surgical approaches for common traumatic injuries to thoracic viscera are summarized in Table 1. For example, a left parasternal

Table 1
Surgical approaches for traumatic injuries to thoracic viscera

Site	Sternotomy	Right thoracotomy	Left thoracotomy
Right atrium	+++	++	0
Right ventricle	+++	+	+
Left atrium	+++	+	+
Left ventricle	++	0	+++
SVC	+++	++	0
Azygos vein	++	+++	0
IVC	+++	++	0
Aortic root	+++	+	0
Aortic arch	+++	0	++
Right subclavian	++	++	0
Proximal right carotid	+++	+	0
Innominate	+++	++	0
Left subclavian	+	0	+++
Proximal left carotid	++	0	++
Descending aorta	0	+	+++
Main PA	+++	0	++
Right PA	++	+++	0
Left PA	++	0	+++
Right UL	++	+++	0
Right ML	++	+++	0
Right LL	+	+++	0
Left UL	+	0	+++
Left LL	0	0	+++
Right hilum	++	+++	0
Left hilum	++	0	+++
Pericardium	+++	++	++
Right IMA	++	+++	0
Left IMA	++	0	+++
Proximal esophagus	0	+++	0
Distal esophagus	0	++	+++
Proximal trachea	++	+	+
Carina	0	+++	+
Right main stem	0	+++	0
Left main stem	0	++	++
Right hemidiaphragm	+	+++	0
Left hemidiaphragm	+	0	+++
CPB	+++	++	++

Abbreviations: CPB, cardiopulmonary bypass; IMA, internal mammary artery; IVC, inferior vena cava; LL, lower lobe; ML, middle lobe; PA, pulmonary artery; SVC, superior vena cava; UL, upper lobe.

+++, preferred; ++, acceptable; +, with difficulty; 0, not accessible.

Data from Ritchie WP, Steele G, Dean RH, editors. General surgery. Philadelphia: JB Lippincott; 1995. p. 861.

gunshot wound may injure the anterior and posterior walls of the left ventricle. Of these two injuries, although the anterior injury is easily exposed and repaired through a median sternotomy or anterior thoracotomy, the posterior injury is more difficult to repair and is best approached with a left posterolateral thoracotomy.

Median sternotomy offers adequate exposure for most parasternal stab wounds because these injuries do not typically penetrate deeply and primarily involve the anterior mediastinum. Likewise, in the instance of right parasternal gunshot wound, a median sternotomy provides good exposure of structures that are likely to be injured, including the right atrium and ventricle, the superior vena cava, atrial appendage, right pulmonary artery, and lung. The incision for a sternotomy may be extended into the neck or supraclavicular fossa to enhance exposure of the great vessels (Fig. 1, see inset). Posterolateral thoracotomy provides superior exposure of the posterior

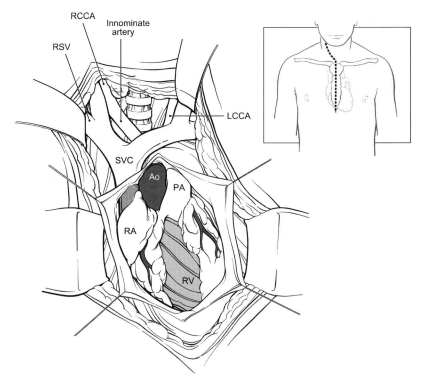

Fig. 1. Median sternotomy with optional extension. A median sternotomy provides excellent exposure for the right atrium and ventricle, the superior vena cava, atrial appendage, right pulmonary artery, and lung. If necessary, the incision may be extended into the neck or supraclavicular fossa (*inset*) to enhance exposure of the great vessels. Ao, aorta; LCCA, left common carotid artery; PA, pulmonary artery; RA, right atrium; RCCA, right common carotid artery; RSV, right subclavian vein; RV, right ventricle; SVC, superior vena cava.

heart and should be used in instances of left parasternal gunshot wound. For lateral wounds, depending on the side involved, a right or left posterolateral thoracotomy provides the best exposure because these injuries are more likely to be posterior. In cases of massive hemothorax, a posterolateral thoracotomy on the affected side offers excellent visualization of the great vessels, such as the subclavian artery or aorta. A left posterolateral thoracotomy (Fig. 2) is the incision of choice in instances of air embolism and massive air leak.

Right thoracotomy is an excellent approach for right lung, tracheal, and proximal left main stem bronchial injuries (a point that is often forgotten). Most esophageal injuries are best approached through a right thoracotomy, except in cases of distal esophageal injuries that are best accessed through the left chest. Right heart structures, such as the right atrium, right ventricle, atrial appendage, and left atrium, are also easily exposed with a right thoracotomy. Left thoracotomy provides adequate exposure of the left lung, left pulmonary hilum, aorta, proximal left subclavian artery, left heart chambers, distal esophagus, and distal left main stem bronchus. A "clam shell" incision, formed by extending a thoracotomy incision transversely across the sternum using the Lebske knife, a pair of trauma shears, or a saw,

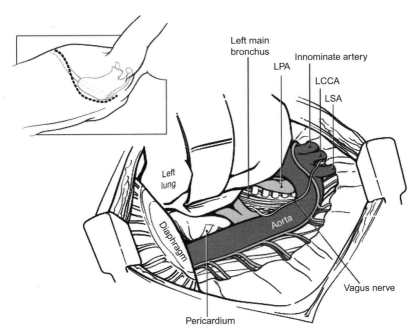

Fig. 2. Left posterolateral thoracotomy. A left posterolateral thoracotomy (*inset*) provides excellent exposure of the left pulmonary hilum, left lung, proximal left subclavian artery, descending aorta, distal esophagus, and left diaphragm. LCCA, left common carotid artery; LPA, left pulmonary artery; LSA, left subclavian artery.

provides excellent access but suboptimal exposure of every intrathoracic or mediastinal structure except the right ventricle and right atrium. When using this approach, the internal mammary arteries are divided and often do not bleed in the poorly perfused patient. Once blood pressure is restored, however, significant hemorrhage from these vessels may result. A more stable closure of the transverse sternotomy is achieved with sternal plates rather than wires.

Urgent exploratory thoracotomy

If the diagnosis is uncertain, then a posterior lateral thoracotomy along the fifth intercostal space on the injured side is the incision of choice. If time and circumstances permit, placement of a dual lumen endotracheal tube so that the lung may be collapsed is beneficial, but this is often not practical in a trauma setting. With a known diagnosis, the incision should be chosen to provide optimal exposure for the injury. Efforts to spare the latissimus dorsi, although commendable, rarely are practical in a trauma setting, although preservation of an intercostal flap is simple and advisable. The surgeon's thinking must remain flexible and insist on good exposure of the injury. Often an inexperienced surgeon attempts to repair an injury with less-than-optimal exposure. In most cases, after the immediately life-threatening issue has been addressed, even in a temporary fashion, the patient is better served by extending the initial incision or making a second incision so that definitive repair of the injury can be performed under optimal exposure. Finally, a damage control thoracotomy with packing of lung, bone, venous, or chest wall bleeding is a valid and commonly overlooked option.

The order of an exploratory thoracotomy should proceed in a logical and orderly fashion. If the diagnosis is uncertain, a posterolateral thoracotomy fashioned along the fifth intercostal space is the incision of choice. First, the thoracic cavity should be evacuated of clotted blood and then the lung packed out of the field, which may be facilitated by division of the inferior pulmonary ligament. Upon clearing the field, the mediastinum and pericardium should be evaluated carefully for bleeding. It is surprisingly difficult to detect the presence of blood in the pericardium by simple visual inspection. A small pericardiotomy that can be expanded as necessary is useful to exclude or confirm the presence of hemopericardium. Major vascular injuries require prompt proximal and distal control, which can be achieved effectively with hilar control in cases of pulmonary parenchymal bleeding. After hemorrhage is controlled, formal repair of injured vascular structures may proceed.

Cardiac injuries

Cardiac injuries may involve the myocardium, coronary arteries, valves, or septum or result in the late presentation of a ventricular aneurysm. Mortality rates range from 10% to 70%, reflecting various presentations and injury mechanisms [27–30]. Cardiac injuries usually cause either cardiac tamponade or hemorrhagic shock, depending on the nature of the pericardial injury and whether pericardial blood can escape into the pleural space [31]. Pericardial tamponade results from the accumulation of fluid within the pericardial space that compresses the heart and prevents cardiac filling. The sac-like pericardium has poor compliance, and as little as 50 mL of blood can effectively cause tamponade. Many patients with this condition die before arrival at the hospital. The presence of cardiac tamponade is usually made based on clinical findings of a distinctive dusky, plethoric facial complexion associated with distended neck veins, hypotension, and evidence of pericardial effusion on FAST examination [5]. It should be noted however, that the sensitivity of FAST in the detection of hemopericardium is markedly diminished in the presence of a massive hemothorax, in which blood may be escaping from the injured heart directly into the thoracic cavity, leaving only small amounts in the pericardium [32]. Muffled heart sounds are classically described with cardiac tamponade but are difficult to discern in the usually noisy emergency department. In patients who are in extremis, bilateral chest tubes should be placed, and if the patient's condition does not improve, immediate thoracotomy is warranted. In this situation, pericardiocentesis is ineffective in removing blood that is clotted in the pericardial space. Patients who are not in extremis should be taken to the operating room urgently for subxiphoid pericardial window or formal chest exploration, typically through a median sternotomy.

The incision for a subxiphoid pericardial window is made over the lower midsternum and upper abdomen, extending approximately 10 cm. The xiphoid process can be grasped with a clamp and either elevated out of the field, divided, or removed. A substernal plane is created using blunt dissection in the plane anterior to the peritoneum, detaching the muscle fibers between the diaphragm and the sternum. Once the pericardium is encountered and grasped with two Kocher clamps, a small incision is made between the clamps while lifting the pericardium so as to prevent injury to the underlying epicardium. An efflux of blood indicates cardiac injury and is an indication to proceed with definitive operation (most commonly through a sternotomy). When necessary, the pericardiotomy may be enlarged to relieve the tamponade. If no blood is encountered, then the incision should be enlarged sufficiently to visualize the epicardial surface of the heart and ensure that the pericardial sac truly has been entered. If negative, the incision may be closed with absorbable sutures [5].

Cardiac injuries that require immediate repair include wall defects, coronary artery injuries, and injuries to the great vessels. Injuries that can be repaired in a delayed fashion with the use of cardiopulmonary bypass include intracardiac lesions, such as septal defects, valve injuries, and ventricular aneurysms. If profound heart failure is present, however, cardiopulmonary bypass should be instituted and repair performed at the time of initial operation.

Atrial wounds are controlled by simple digital pressure or by exclusion with a curved vascular clamp and simple oversewing. Right or left ventricle free wall injuries that are remote from the coronary arteries are controlled with digital pressure. After hemostasis is restored, the injury is repaired using horizontal mattress polypropylene sutures (3.0 or 4.0) under the wound and reinforced with an epicardial running suture along the site of injury. Pledgeted sutures are an absolute requirement for repair of left ventricle wounds because they allow for compression and prevent the suture from tearing through the myocardium. Simple right ventricle wounds often may be closed without pledgets if the sutures are placed accurately. Injuries near the coronary arteries must be closed without encompassing the coronary artery. Horizontal mattress sutures are placed deep and lateral to the coronary artery across the injury and out the opposite side. This must be performed with awareness of the function of the myocardium distal to the repair and monitoring of the intraoperative electrocardiogram to prevent coronary artery occlusion and ischemia.

The possibility of coexistent intracardiac injury always must be considered by the surgeon [33–35]. Palpation of the pulmonary outflow tract or left ventricle for a thrill discloses the presence of a traumatic ventricular septal defect or aortic insufficiency, respectively. Digital palpation of the atrium or through atrial wounds should be used routinely to identify atrioventricular valvular insufficiency. Intraoperative transesophageal echocardiography is a useful adjunct and can facilitate diagnosis of intracardiac injuries. Postoperatively, chest auscultation should be used to exclude murmurs; if they are found, echocardiography is required.

Injuries to the great vessels

The great vessels of the aorta include the left subclavian, the left common carotid, and the innominate arteries. Great vessel injuries are rarely encountered after penetrating chest trauma, with a reported incidence of approximately 4% [36]. The principal reason for this low incidence is that victims typically exsanguinate into the chest or externally before arrival at the hospital; however, with improved prehospital care and decreased transit times, these injuries are increasingly encountered at trauma centers [28].

The detection of the presence of a great vessel injury can be overt or subtle in presentation, depending on multiple factors, including the mechanism and the vessel involved. The presence of a wound at the base of the neck or transmediastinal gunshot wound should alert the clinician to the possibility of great vessel injury. The patient may be pulseless or moribund at presentation, and diagnosis is confirmed at the time of EDT or urgent thoracotomy. In a stable patient or one who easily stabilizes with resuscitation, the diagnosis can be confirmed with angiography or CT angiography, if available [37]. Patients with proximal injuries may present with a massive hemothorax, pericardial tamponade or external bleeding. Pulse deficits in the affected vessel's distribution, brachial plexus injuries, stroke or coma, and the presence of a thrill or bruit in the base of the neck also support the diagnosis of a great vessel injury. Chest radiography may demonstrate the presence of an apical cap or widened mediastinum.

After a diagnosis has been made, the patient should be taken to the operating room for exploration. If possible, although frequently not feasible, the placement of a dual lumen endotracheal tube greatly facilitates exposure of the injuries. Many incisions have been described as providing adequate exposure for repair of great vessel injuries. For right subclavian injuries or right parasternal injuries, a median sternotomy with extension into the neck or a supraclavicular extension is recommended [38]. A median sternotomy provides excellent exposure of the ascending aorta and the proximal right subclavian, innominate, and common carotid arteries. A left thoracotomy provides optimal exposure of the descending aorta and adequate exposure of the proximal left subclavian and proximal left common carotid arteries. For distal control when dealing with left subclavian or left common carotid artery injuries, classically a supraclavicular or neck counter-incision is required. Alternatively, a mediansternotomy can be used to connect the incisions (trapdoor incision); however, this type of incision provides poor exposure and is associated with significant morbidity. It should be used only when necessary [39]. Comprehensive knowledge of chest and neck anatomy is required when exposing these vessels to prevent injury to the phrenic, vagus, and recurrent laryngeal nerves, which lie in close proximity to these vessels, and to protect the thoracic duct when approaching the left subclavian artery.

We would like to offer one recommendation regarding the approach used when a left infraclavicular stab wound with left subclavian artery injury is encountered. Anterior thoracotomy to expose the proximal subclavian artery for proximal control followed by a supraclavicular incision for distal control is the classical approach described for this type of injury. In the authors' experience, however, proximal control of the subclavian artery through this incision is difficult, and back bleeding from the vertebral and mammary arteries often can be profuse despite control of the proximal subclavian artery. We prefer preparing the entire chest, neck, and arm into the field followed by a posterolateral thoracotomy with the patient's arm extended and gaining exposure of the proximal subclavian artery. The subclavian artery may be followed distally from within the chest, exposing and controlling the vertebral and internal mammary arteries. After control is obtained, the arm may be dropped to the patient's side and a supraclavicular incision made to expose the distal subclavian artery. Repositioning of the operating room table after thoracotomy facilitates this approach.

Once proximal and distal control is obtained, many of these injuries lend themselves to lateral repair or end-to-end primary anastomosis. Interposition grafts composed of polytetrafluoroethylene or knitted Dacron are the conduits of choice. Caution must be exercised when subclavian arteries are repaired. In the authors' experience, these vessels are friable because of the lack of elastic fibers in the tunica media. End-to-end anastomosis is rarely possible because the anastomosis must be under no tension or the repair will fail. Interposition graft is desired when repairing these injuries. Associated venous injuries (superior vena cava, internal jugular, innominate) are common; if possible, they should be treated by lateral repair or patch venography. Internal jugular or innominate injuries can be ligated with little ill effect except in patients with closed head injury. Vena cava injuries can be shunted if repair is not feasible and ligated only as a measure of last resort.

Lung injuries

Lung injury that requires operative intervention is more common after penetrating rather than blunt injury [7,8]. Most cases of pneumothorax or hemothorax can be treated adequately with accurate chest tube placement and full re-expansion of the lung. It is estimated, however, that 20% to 40% of patients after penetrating injury and 15% to 20% of patients after blunt injury who require thoracotomy need some form of lung resection [7,40,41]. It must be noted that anatomic lung resection after blunt injury is distinctly uncommon but required in 0.5% of patients [7]. Trauma surgeons should remain familiar with the technique of anatomic lung resection, although most lung injuries that require thoracotomy can be dealt with successfully using lung-sparing techniques, such as nonanatomic stapled resections or tractotomies [42].

Operative indications for lung injury tend to fall into one of two categories: hemorrhage or persistent air leak impairing ventilation. The incision of choice for lung injury is a fifth intercostal space posterolateral thoracotomy on the involved side. The most common procedures performed are simple suture repair of superficial lung lacerations and wedge resection of the injured lung using a stapling device. In penetrating injuries, tractotomy is used as a definitive form of treatment for nonhilar injuries [43,44]. The principle of tractotomy is to open the tract of the bullet or knife wound (Fig. 3A) so that larger interior vessels may be identified and ligated individually. 3-0 polypropylene suture may be used to ligate the vessels individually or may be run along the length of the tractotomy (Fig. 3B). The practice of simply oversewing penetrating lung injuries should be discouraged. Oversewing entrance and exit sites may stop bleeding into the pleural cavity, but it does not stop intraparenchymal bleeding. Blood can be forced into the tracheobronchial tree and result in aspiration, pneumonia, acute respiratory distress syndrome, and further worsening of the functional lung injury. Simple maneuvers, such as tractotomy, wedge resection, and simple suturing, are more commonly performed after penetrating lung injury because more proximal lung injuries are often associated with concurrent fatal mediastinal injuries. Anatomic resections, such as lobectomy and

A   B

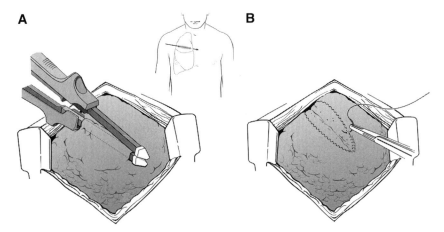

Fig. 3. Tractotomy for nonhilar injuries. (*A*) The principle of tractotomy is to open the tract of the bullet or knife wound (*inset*) so that larger interior vessels may be identified and ligated individually. (*B*) 3-0 polypropylene suture may be used to individually ligate the vessels or may be run along the length of the tractotomy. Oversewing penetrating lung injury is discouraged.

pneumonectomy, are more commonly performed if resection in needed after blunt injury. Blunt trauma often results in a more severe and diffuse lung injury that is typically more difficult to treat surgically and has worse outcomes when compared with penetrating trauma [39,45,46].

More extensive deep lobar and perihilar lung injuries frequently require anatomic lobectomy. Deep lobar injuries in patients with hemodynamic instability should be approached initially with tractotomy to expose the deep bleeding vessels. Simple oversewing may not suffice, in which case the edges of the tractotomy may be stapled or large, pledgeted mattress sutures may be used. If lung-sparing techniques fail or are not applicable, most of these patients require lobectomy.

Patients with perihilar injuries are typically in shock or have extensive parenchymal injury (as seen commonly after blunt injury). Hilar control should be the initial maneuver upon entering the chest if profuse lung bleeding is encountered. This procedure can involve placing a large clamp across the pulmonary hilum or dividing the pulmonary ligament to the level of the inferior pulmonary vein and twisting the mobilized lung. Occasionally, intrapericardial control of the pulmonary artery is required in cases of proximal injuries. If the artery and vein are injured, pneumonectomy is indicated. At this point, lung amputation can be performed using a stapler or, alternatively, the hilum may be oversewn. Animal models have demonstrated that each technique has similar bursting strength [47]. Traumatic pneumonectomy is associated with mortality rates of 50% to 100% and should be considered only if there is no alternative [41,48,49]. Sudden right heart failure contributes to the acute mortality after this procedure. If it occurs immediately, extracorporeal membrane oxygenation is an option, but it usually proves to be fatal. More insidious onsets that occur days after operation may be treated medically with oxygen and pulmonary vasodilators.

Tracheobronchial injuries

Injuries to the trachea or main stem bronchi are uncommon in patients who survive to reach the hospital and may occur after blunt trauma or, less commonly, after penetrating injury with an estimated incidence of 0.2% to 8% [50–53]. Blunt injuries typically occur as a result of a direct blow to the neck, shear forces on the trachea at its fixed points (ie, the cricoid and carina), or sudden increases in intratracheal pressure secondary to compression of the chest against a closed glottis. Gunshot wounds may occur at any point along the tracheobronchial tree; however, stab wounds almost exclusively involve the cervical trachea in patients who reach medical attention. Regardless of mechanism, most of these injuries occur within 2.5 cm of the carina, with main stem bronchial injuries present in 86%, distal bronchial injuries in 9.3%, and complex injuries in 8% [54]. Associated intrathoracic or mediastinal injuries are common [54].

Symptoms depend on the location of the injury and whether the injury communicates with the pleural cavity. Cervical injuries may present with stridor, hemoptysis, cervical subcutaneous emphysema, hoarseness, or respiratory distress secondary to an obstructed airway. Thoracic injuries with pleural communication present with pneumothorax that may or may not be under tension. A pneumothorax that persists after chest tube placement or has a continuous air leak indicates tracheobronchial damage. The "fallen lung sign" is a radiographic feature that is highly specific for tracheobronchial injury. On chest radiographs, the lung is falling away from rather than toward the hilum, as is the case with a simple pneumothorax [55]. In injuries with extrapleural communication, massive pneumomediastinum is typically encountered, occasionally without pneumothorax [55–57]. In this case, the diagnosis is more difficult to make on clinical grounds alone and often requires bronchoscopy. The injury may be initially missed and present later as tracheal or bronchial stenosis. Nonspecific symptoms of tracheobronchial injury can include subcutaneous emphysema and hemoptysis; however, most subcutaneous emphysema is a result of subpleural rupture of alveoli, not tracheobronchial injury, and hemoptysis is more often a result of aspiration of blood from facial and pharyngeal injuries. It has been reported that as many as two thirds of tracheobronchial injuries go unrecognized for more than 24 hours, and approximately 10% of patients may present weeks or months later, after stricture occurs [53,58,59]. The diagnosis of tracheobronchial injury is made based on clinical findings and radiographic findings (chest radiography and CT) and is confirmed with bronchoscopy [60,61]. Rigid or flexible bronchoscopy is essential to exclude reliably the diagnosis of tracheobronchial injury.

As with any trauma patient, the first priority is securing an adequate airway. Treatment of tracheobronchial injuries is directed at ensuring or establishing adequate ventilation. When safe, avoidance of positive pressure ventilation is recommended during the initial evaluation, but if necessary, bronchoscopic-guided intubation is suggested. Blind intubation in these patients is hazardous. In cases of small, well-contained tracheal injuries with minimal tissue loss, bronchoscopic guidance allows placement of the endotracheal tube safely past the injury with the cuff placed beyond the site of injury. Intubation past the site of injury alone for 48 to 72 hours occasionally may result in complete resolution of the injury in selected cases [54]. Nonoperative management is reserved only for highly selected patients who have lesions that involve less than one third of the bronchial wall with well-opposed edges and minimal tissue loss [61–64]. The lung must fully re-expand with chest tube placement, the air leak should stop soon after chest tube insertion, and positive pressure ventilation is not required [61]. These patients should be treated with prophylactic antibiotics, humidified air, frequent suctioning, and regular bronchoscopy and should be monitored for sepsis and airway obstruction.

Because most intrathoracic injuries occur within 2 cm of the carina, we recommend a right thoracotomy to approach virtually all of these injuries except in cases of distal left main stem bronchial injuries > 3 cm from the carina, where a left posterolateral thoracotomy is preferable. The incision should be placed over the fifth rib space, because we have found that resection of the fifth rib provides for optimal exposure and permits the intercostal muscle in this interspace to be saved for later use as a muscle flap to buttress the repair. Primary emphasis should be placed on maintaining an adequate airway, which may require advancing the endotracheal tube under direct vision beyond the level of injury or passing a sterile endotracheal tube through the operative field into one or both lungs. Tracheobronchial injuries should be repaired primarily using interrupted or running monofilament suture with the knots placed on the outside of the lumen to reduce granuloma or stricture formation. When limited tracheal resection is required, up to 2 cm of trachea can be excised easily and safely and primary repair performed. If needed, additional tracheal length may be gained by performing a pericardial release or by flexing the patient's neck intraoperatively and for a short period of time after operation, provided the cervical spine is without injury. Repairs should be buttressed with viable vascularized tissue, usually an intercostal muscle flap (as previously suggested), pericardium, omentum, or, rarely, rhomboid or latissimus muscle flaps.

Postoperatively, barring other contraindications, a thoracic epidural catheter should be placed to assist with pain control and ensure adequate pulmonary toilet. Patients on the ventilator should be extubated as soon as possible, ideally immediately after the operation is complete. If ongoing positive pressure ventilation is required, positioning of the endotracheal tube distal to the repair, jet ventilation, or, occasionally, extracorporeal membrane oxygenation may be necessary to allow the repair to heal. Routine postoperative use of proton pump inhibitors is recommended because acid and pepsin exposure promotes granuloma formation at the site of repair.

Esophageal injuries

Esophageal injuries are rare and primarily involve the cervical esophagus, typically as the result of gunshot wounds or iatrogenic trauma [65–68]. Intrathoracic esophageal injuries are present in approximately 1% of gunshot wounds to the chest [69]. Blunt esophageal injuries typically occur in the neck as a result of a direct blow or may occur in the chest just proximal to the esophagogastric junction. Blunt injuries are associated with increased intraluminal pressures against a closed glottis causing a bursting-type injury.

These wounds are usually diagnosed at the time of exploration for other injuries or on diagnostic studies that are obtained in stable patients because of the proximity of the wounding agent to the esophagus. Clinical manifestations may be present in 60% to 80% of patients depending on the location, size, amount of contamination, time to diagnosis, and presence of associated injuries [70]. Symptoms include odynophagia, dysphagia, and hematemesis. A small amount of mediastinal emphysema or small pleural effusion may be seen on chest radiograph. The presence of chest or back pain is also a clue to the presence of esophageal injuries [71,72]. Tracheal and vascular injuries are often found as associated injuries [73]. The diagnosis can be made definitively at the time of surgical exploration, on endoscopy, or with esophagoscopy. Our preference is to use CT to determine if the wound is in proximity to the esophagus followed by an esophagram. An esophagram with barium rather than water-soluble contrast is recommended for increased sensitivity, superior image quality, and decreased incidence of pneumonitis caused by aspiration [73,74]. Rapid diagnostic evaluation is desirable because the best surgical results are obtained when the duration of time between injury and repair is minimized [32,75].

Esophageal injuries should be treated early and aggressively. Cervical injuries should be approached through a neck incision along the anterior border of the left sternocleidomastoid muscle or with a collar incision. These injuries may be repaired primarily, whereas more complex wounds may require resection or combined tracheal repair. Upper and middle third thoracic injuries should be approached through a right posterolateral thoracotomy in the fourth or fifth interspace, depending on the level of the injury. Distal third esophageal injuries are best approached through left posterolateral thoracotomy through the sixth intercostal space. Once the wound is identified, the esophagus is mobilized sparingly but enough so that the injury can be defined completely. When diagnosed and operated on within 24 hours, most esophageal injuries lend themselves to primary repair with a single layer of absorbable monofilament suture [66,72,76].

Depending on the length of time before exploration, local inflammation, degree of contamination, and the severity of the injury, primary repair may not be feasible. Several techniques have been described in the literature, including esophageal diversion, esophageal exclusion, esophagectomy, and T tube drainage with later definitive repair. If the patient is in extremis, wide drainage with a chest tube and placement of a nasogastric tube above the injury is an option [77–79]. Regardless of the patient's condition, all esophageal repairs should be drained widely with a chest tube and buttressed with viable, vascularized tissue (intercostal muscle flap, pericardial fat pad, gastric wrap, or thickened pleura) [80,81].

Traumatic rupture of the thoracic aorta

Acute blunt rupture of the thoracic aorta is associated with a high death rate. Eighty percent to 90% of these patients die before reaching the hospital. Historically, of the individuals who reach the hospital, 50% die within the first 24 hours and 90% die within the first month if the injury is not repaired [82,83]. Acute rupture of the thoracic aorta may occur after any form of severe deceleration injury. A shearing effect is caused by different degrees of mobility of the aorta above and below the fixation point of the aortic isthmus by the ligamentum arteriosus and the intercostal vessels. Most ruptures occur at the aortic isthmus, distal to the origin of the left subclavian artery. Less commonly, the ascending aorta just above the aortic valve can be affected, but this occurrence is exceedingly rare. No signs or symptoms on physical examination are the rule. Chest radiography may provide the surgeon with several clues to the presence of this injury: a left apical cap, wide mediastinum, obscurity of the contour of the aortic knob and aortopulmonary window, depression of the left main stem bronchus, and deviation of the nasogastric tube to the right. Diagnosis is confirmed on chest CT angiography or, if it remains in doubt, by angiography. Once the diagnosis is made, a critical component of initial management is beta blockade, not just antihypertensive therapy. Beta blockade decreases the systolic ejection slope of the left ventricle, which decreases the tearing force on the aortic wall. Vasodilators given alone widen the pulse pressure by dropping the diastolic pressure and actually may increase the likelihood of rupture. In suitable candidates for immediate repair, the injury is best approached through a left posterolateral thoracotomy. Given the unpredictable nature of the aortic injury, which often requires complex repair and the lower reported rates of paraplegia, the use of cardiopulmonary bypass is highly recommended by the authors [84]. Most cases require an interposition graft, although 15% to 20% may be treated with primary anastomosis [84]. Alternatively, endovascular treatment of acute thoracic aortic rupture is gaining in popularity. Immediate outcome data in patients who undergo endovascular stent grafting seem at least as good as after conventional surgical repair [85]. Size mismatch and possible collapse of current large stent grafts when used in the young trauma population remain concerns. The long-term effectiveness of this management is still not known, but in the future, this technique may represent a viable alternative to surgery in patients with significant coexisting injuries that would preclude immediate repair.

Delayed thoracotomy

The indications for delayed thoracotomy (>24 hours) include missed tracheobronchial injuries, traumatic aortic rupture, intracardiac injuries, retained hemothorax, and posttraumatic empyema. Persistent air leak or tracheal/bronchial stenoses are typical manifestations of missed tracheobronchial injuries. The approach and principles of repair for these injuries are as previously described, although they are technically more demanding as a result of ensuing inflammation. The traditional management of acute traumatic rupture of the thoracic aorta endorses repair as quickly as possible. As we have gained a better understanding of the natural history of this injury and the role of pharmacologic treatment, however, the concept of delayed repair of this injury—often for hours or sometimes for days—has gained in popularity [54,86–88]. The principal use of delayed repair is to allow the more life-threatening injuries to be addressed initially and avoid systemic heparinization in the immediate posttraumatic setting [89]. In patients with major intra-abdominal or intracranial injuries or significant pulmonary contusions, adopting the practice of early beta blockade allows elective repair of their aorta anywhere from 2 to 29 months later [90]. Likewise, delayed repair of intracardiac injuries (atrioventricular valvular insufficiency, ventricular septal defects) is advocated by the authors, unless the patient develops severe congestive heart failure, in which case immediate repair is warranted [5].

Inadequately drained posttraumatic hemothorax and contamination of the pleural space are often the result of improper chest tube placement by a member of the trauma team with the least experience in sterile technique or proper placement. An incompletely drained hemothorax essentially has one of three possible outcomes: resolution, infection (posttraumatic empyema), or fibrothorax/entrapped lung [91]. Prophylactic antibiotic use does not reduce infectious morbidity [92]. Retained blood in the pleural space is a risk factor for the development of posttraumatic empyema. As a result, every effort should be made to place chest tubes correctly under sterile conditions and remove the tube as soon as possible after insertion. If chest tube drainage fails to evacuate a hemothorax, especially after penetrating trauma, video-assisted thoracoscopy or thoracotomy should be considered. Additional chest tube placement is often not effective in evacuating clotted blood from the pleural space [93–95]. Diagnosis of a retained hemothorax using plain chest radiography can be misleading, often underestimating the amount of fluid in the chest. Chest CT provides information about location and size of the hemothorax that can be used intraoperatively to make the appropriate incision [96]. Video-assisted thoracoscopy is minimally invasive, relatively easy to perform, and effective, especially when performed early after injury [97–99]. The best results are seen after penetrating injury [100]. Conversion to thoracotomy occurs in approximately 20% and is more common after blunt injury or when video-assisted thoracoscopy is performed later after injury [93–95]. A dual-lumen endotracheal tube and single lung ventilation are usually necessary. With the patient in decubitus position, typically two or three incisions approximately 2 cm in length are used as chest ports, and the clotted blood may be evacuated using suction catheters, ringed forceps, or a multitude of other instruments and techniques. The same ports then may be used for chest tube placement once the procedure is complete.

Thoracotomy is usually required in cases in which the hemothorax has been present for longer periods of time and dense adhesions have formed, which typically occurs after blunt trauma as continued oozing from rib fractures makes the timing of intervention in this group of patients more difficult to determine [100]. Often the hemothorax has become infected [91]. A posterolateral thoracotomy on the affected side through the fifth intercostal space typically provides adequate exposure. Often, the clotted hemothorax has a fibrous peel that necessitates decortication. Emphasis should be placed on completely removing the peel from the visceral surface of the pleural so that complete lung expansion may be obtained postoperatively. Ringed forceps or the scalpel may be required to remove the densely adherent peel from the lung, and moderate hemorrhage may be encountered during this part of procedure. Once decortication is complete and the retained hemothorax has been removed, wide drainage with chest tubes is required to prevent reaccumulation of blood and facilitate re-expansion of the involved lung. Postoperatively, a thoracic epidural greatly assists with pulmonary toilet. Chest tubes should be discontinued as soon as safely possible.

Summary

We have described the three windows of intervention in thoracic trauma dictated by the patient's physiologic status upon arrival to the emergency

Table 2
Thoracotomy in thoracic trauma

Thoracotomy	Immediate	Urgent	Delayed
Setting	Emergency room: upon arrival and assessment	Operating room: within 1–4 h	Operating room: >24 h
Injury	Patients in extremis after penetrating chest injury	Cardiac, lung esophagus, tracheobrochial, great vessel injuries, aortic rupture	Retained hemothorax, posttraumatic empyema, delayed tracheobronchial injuries, intracardiac injuries

room. As shown in Table 2, the time and setting of the thoracotomy primarily depend on the nature and site of the critical injuries. Many variables must be considered in this decision process, and each injury has unique issues to be addressed. We have characterized some of the most common injuries and scenarios that are likely to be encountered in thoracic trauma and report general methods for effective management. We also suggest and describe various surgical approaches that, in our collective experience, have proved useful for visualization, exposure, and repair of thoracic injuries. The thoracic trauma patient is at primary risk for trauma-related complications and, at worst, death. Thoughtful, effective, and timely surgical intervention is critical to favorable patient outcomes.

References

[1] Blansfield JS. The origins of casualty evacuation and echelons of care: lessons learned from the American Civil War. Int J Trauma Nurs 1999;5(1):5–9.
[2] Kemmerer WT, Eckert WG, Gathright JB, et al. Patterns of thoracic injuries in fatal traffic accidents. J Trauma 1961;1:595–9.
[3] Devitt JH, Pagliarello G, Simons J. The involvement of anesthetists in critical care medicine. Can J Anaesth 1990;37(4 Pt 2):S119.
[4] Cohn SM. Pulmonary contusion: review of the clinical entity. J Trauma 1997;42(5): 973–9.
[5] Hines MH, Meredith JW. Special problems of thoracic trauma. In: Ritchie WP, Steele G Jr, Dean RH, editors. General surgery. Philadelphia: JB Lippincott; 1995. p. 859–72.
[6] Karmy-Jones R, Jurkovich GJ, Nathens AB, et al. Timing of urgent thoracotomy for hemorrhage after trauma: a multicenter study. Arch Surg 2001;136(5):513–8.
[7] Karmy-Jones R, Jurkovich GJ, Shatz DV, et al. Management of traumatic lung injury: a Western Trauma Association Multicenter review. J Trauma 2001;51(6):1049–53.
[8] Karmy-Jones R, Jurkovich GJ. Blunt chest trauma. Curr Probl Surg 2004;41:211–380.
[9] Miglietta MA, Robb TV, Eachempati SR, et al. Current opinion regarding indications for emergency department thoracotomy. J Trauma 2001;51(4):670–6.
[10] Ivatury RR, Kazigo J, Rohman M, et al. Directed emergency room thoracotomy: a prognostic prerequisite for survival. J Trauma 1991;31(8):1076–81.
[11] Bleetman A, Kasem H, Crawford R. Review of emergency thoracotomy for chest injuries in patients attending a UK Accident and Emergency department. Injury 1996;27(2):129–32.
[12] Rhee PM, Acosta J, Bridgeman A, et al. Survival after emergency department thoracotomy: review of published data from the past 25 years. J Am Coll Surg 2000;190(3):288–98.
[13] Branney SW, Moore EE, Feldhaus KM, et al. Critical analysis of two decades of experience with postinjury emergency department thoracotomy in a regional trauma center. J Trauma 1998;45(1):87–94.
[14] Schwab CW, Adcock OT, Max MH. Emergency department thoracotomy (EDT): a 26-month experience using an "agonal" protocol. Am Surg 1986;52(1):20–9.
[15] Feliciano DV, Bitondo CG, Cruse PA, et al. Liberal use of emergency center thoracotomy. Am J Surg 1986;152(6):654–9.
[16] Velmahos GC, Degiannis E, Souter I, et al. Outcome of a strict policy on emergency department thoracotomies. Arch Surg 1995;130(7):774–7.
[17] Lewis G, Knottenbelt JD. Should emergency room thoracotomy be reserved for cases of cardiac tamponade? Injury 1991;22(1):5–6.
[18] Boyd M, Vanek VW, Bourguet CC. Emergency room resuscitative thoracotomy: when is it indicated? J Trauma 1992;33(5):714–21.

[19] Clevenger FW, Yarbrough DR, Reines HD. Resuscitative thoracotomy: the effect of field time on outcome. J Trauma 1988;28(4):441–5.
[20] Millham FH, Grindlinger GA. Survival determinants in patients undergoing emergency room thoracotomy for penetrating chest injury. J Trauma 1993;34(3):332–6.
[21] American College of Surgeons. Advanced trauma life support student manual. 6th edition. Chicago: American College of Surgeons; 1997.
[22] Rotondo MF, Bard MR. Damage control surgery for thoracic injuries. Injury 2004;35(7): 649–54.
[23] McNamara JJ, Messersmith JK, Dunn RA, et al. Thoracic injuries in combat casualties in Vietnam. Ann Thorac Surg 1970;10(5):389–401.
[24] Kish G, Kozloff L, Joseph WL, et al. Indications for early thoracotomy in the management of chest trauma. Ann Thorac Surg 1976;22(1):23–8.
[25] Mansour MA, Moore EE, Moore FA, et al. Exigent postinjury thoracotomy analysis of blunt versus penetrating trauma. Surg Gynecol Obstet 1992;175(2):97–101.
[26] Novitsky YW, Mostafa G, Sing RF, et al. Fatal cardiac air embolism. Injury 2006;37(1): 78–80.
[27] Demetriades D. Cardiac wounds: experience with 70 patients. Ann Surg 1986;203(3):315–7.
[28] Honigman B, Rohweder K, Moore EE, et al. Prehospital advanced trauma life support for penetrating cardiac wounds. Ann Emerg Med 1990;19(2):145–50.
[29] Demetriades D, Charalambides C, Sareli P, et al. Late sequelae of penetrating cardiac injuries. Br J Surg 1990;77(7):813–4.
[30] Henderson VJ, Smith RS, Fry WR, et al. Cardiac injuries: analysis of an unselected series of 251 cases. J Trauma 1994;36(3):341–8.
[31] Arreola-Risa C, Rhee P, Boyle EM, et al. Factors influencing outcome in stab wounds of the heart. Am J Surg 1995;169(5):553–6.
[32] Asensio JA, Chahwan S, Forno W, et al. Penetrating esophageal injuries: multicenter study of the American Association for the Surgery of Trauma. J Trauma 2001;50(2): 289–96.
[33] Asensio JA, Stewart BM, Murray J, et al. Penetrating cardiac injuries. Surg Clin North Am 1996;76(4):685–724.
[34] Simmers TA, Meijburg HW, de la Riviere AB. Traumatic papillary muscle rupture. Ann Thorac Surg 2001;72(1):257–9.
[35] Wall MJ Jr, Soltero ER. Trauma to cardiac valves. Curr Opin Cardiol 2002;17(2):188–92.
[36] Demetriades D. Penetrating injuries to the thoracic great vessels. J Card Surg 1997;12(2): 173–9.
[37] Wall MJ Jr, Hirshberg A, LeMaire SA, et al. Thoracic aortic and thoracic vascular injuries. Surg Clin North Am 2001;81(6):1375–93.
[38] Schaff HV, Brawley RK. Operative management of penetrating vascular injuries of the thoracic outlet. Surgery 1977;82(2):182–91.
[39] Stewart KC, Urschel JD, Nakai SS, et al. Pulmonary resection for lung trauma. Ann Thorac Surg 1997;63(6):1587–8.
[40] Borlase BC, Metcalf RK, Moore EE, et al. Penetrating wounds to the anterior chest: analysis of thoracotomy and laparotomy. Am J Surg 1986;152(6):649–53.
[41] Thompson DA, Rowlands BJ, Walker WE, et al. Urgent thoracotomy for pulmonary or tracheobronchial injury. J Trauma 1988;28(3):276–80.
[42] Demetriades D, Velmahos GC. Penetrating injuries of the chest: indications for operation. Scand J Surg 2002;91(1):41–5.
[43] Wall MJ Jr, Hirshberg A, Mattox KL. Pulmonary tractotomy with selective vascular ligation for penetrating injuries to the lung. Am J Surg 1994;168(6):665–9.
[44] Wall MJ Jr, Villavicencio RT, Miller CC III, et al. Pulmonary tractotomy as an abbreviated thoracotomy technique. J Trauma 1998;45(6):1015–23.
[45] Robison PD, Harman PK, Trinkle JK, et al. Management of penetrating lung injuries in civilian practice. J Thorac Cardiovasc Surg 1988;95(2):184–90.

[46] Carrillo EH, Block EF, Zeppa R, et al. Urgent lobectomy and pneumonectomy. Eur J Emerg Med 1994;1(3):126–30.

[47] Wagner JW, Obeid FN, Karmy-Jones RC, et al. Trauma pneumonectomy revisited: the role of simultaneously stapled pneumonectomy. J Trauma 1996;40(4):590–4.

[48] Jones WS, Mavroudis C, Richardson JD, et al. Management of tracheobronchial disruption resulting from blunt trauma. Surgery 1984;95(3):319–23.

[49] Bowling R, Mavroudis C, Richardson JD, et al. Emergency pneumonectomy for penetrating and blunt trauma. Am Surg 1985;51(3):136–9.

[50] Edwards WH Jr, Morris JA Jr, DeLozier JB III, et al. Airway injuries: the first priority in trauma. Am Surg 1987;53(4):192–7.

[51] Campbell DB. Trauma to the chest wall, lung, and major airways. Semin Thorac Cardiovasc Surg 1992;4(3):234–40.

[52] Grewal H, Rao PM, Mukerji S, et al. Management of penetrating laryngotracheal injuries. Head Neck 1995;17(6):494–502.

[53] Dowd NP, Clarkson K, Walsh MA, et al. Delayed bronchial stenosis after blunt chest trauma. Anesth Analg 1996;82(5):1078–81.

[54] Symbas PN, Justicz AG, Ricketts RR. Rupture of the airways from blunt trauma: treatment of complex injuries. Ann Thorac Surg 1992;54(1):177–83.

[55] Oh KS, Fleischner FG, Wyman SM. Characteristic pulmonary finding in traumatic complete transection of a main-stem bronchus. Radiology 1969;92(2):371–2.

[56] Hood RM, Sloan HE. Injuries of the trachea and major bronchi. J Thorac Cardiovasc Surg 1959;38:458–80.

[57] Spencer JA, Rogers CE, Westaby S. Clinico-radiological correlates in rupture of the major airways. Clin Radiol 1991;43(6):371–6.

[58] Barmada H, Gibbons JR. Tracheobronchial injury in blunt and penetrating chest trauma. Chest 1994;106(1):74–8.

[59] Stark P. Imaging of tracheobronchial injuries. J Thorac Imaging 1995;10(3):206–19.

[60] Baumgartner F, Sheppard B, de Virgilio C, et al. Tracheal and main bronchial disruptions after blunt chest trauma: presentation and management. Ann Thorac Surg 1990;50(4): 569–74.

[61] Hancock BJ, Wiseman NE. Tracheobronchial injuries in children. J Pediatr Surg 1991; 26(11):1316–9.

[62] Reece GP, Shatney CH. Blunt injuries of the cervical trachea: review of 51 patients. South Med J 1988;81(12):1542–8.

[63] Flynn AE, Thomas AN, Schecter WP. Acute tracheobronchial injury. J Trauma 1989; 29(10):1326–30.

[64] Hara KS, Prakash UB. Fiberoptic bronchoscopy in the evaluation of acute chest and upper airway trauma. Chest 1989;96(3):627–30.

[65] Sheely CH, Mattox KL, Beall AC Jr, et al. Penetrating wounds of the cervical esophagus. Am J Surg 1975;130(6):707–11.

[66] Attar S, Hankins JR, Suter CM, et al. Esophageal perforation: a therapeutic challenge. Ann Thorac Surg 1990;50(1):45–9.

[67] Armstrong WB, Detar TR, Stanley RB. Diagnosis and management of external penetrating cervical esophageal injuries. Ann Otol Rhinol Laryngol 1994;103(11):863–71.

[68] Demetriades D, Theodorou D, Cornwell E, et al. Transcervical gunshot injuries: mandatory operation is not necessary. J Trauma 1996;40(5):758–60.

[69] Cornwell EE III, Kennedy F, Ayad IA, et al. Transmediastinal gunshot wounds: a reconsideration of the role of aortography. Arch Surg 1996;131(9):949–52.

[70] Weigelt JA, Thal ER, Snyder WH III, et al. Diagnosis of penetrating cervical esophageal injuries. Am J Surg 1987;154(6):619–22.

[71] Nesbitt JC, Sawyers JL. Surgical management of esophageal perforation. Am Surg 1987; 53(4):183–91.

[72] White RK, Morris DM. Diagnosis and management of esophageal perforations. Am Surg 1992;58(2):112–9.

[73] Weiman DS, Walker WA, Brosnan KM, et al. Noniatrogenic esophageal trauma. Ann Thorac Surg 1995;59(4):845–9.

[74] James AE Jr, Montali RJ, Chaffee V, et al. Barium or gastrografin: which contrast media for diagnosis of esophageal tears? Gastroenterology 1975;68(5 Pt 1):1103–13.

[75] Glatterer MS Jr, Toon RS, Ellestad C, et al. Management of blunt and penetrating external esophageal trauma. J Trauma 1985;25(8):784–92.

[76] Ivatury RR, Rohman M, Simon RS. Esophageal injury. In: Maull KI, Wolfers HC, Rice C, et al, editors. Advances in trauma and critical care. St. Louis (MO): CV Mosby; 1994. p. 274.

[77] Abbott OA, Mansour KA, Logan WD Jr, et al. Atraumatic so-called "spontaneous" rupture of the esophagus: a review of 47 personal cases with comments on a new method of surgical therapy. J Thorac Cardiovasc Surg 1970;59(1):67–83.

[78] Urschel HC Jr, Razzuk MA, Wood RE, et al. Improved management of esophageal perforation: exclusion and diversion in continuity. Ann Surg 1974;179(5):587–91.

[79] Orringer MB, Stirling MC. Esophagectomy for esophageal disruption. Ann Thorac Surg 1990;49(1):35–42.

[80] Thal AO, Hatafuku T. Improved operation for esophageal rupture. JAMA 1964;188: 826–8.

[81] Grillo HC, Wilkins EW Jr. Esophageal repair following late diagnosis of intrathoracic perforation. Ann Thorac Surg 1975;20(4):387–99.

[82] Parmley LF, Mattingly TW, Manion WC, et al. Nonpenetrating traumatic injury of the aorta. Circulation 1958;17(6):1086–101.

[83] Gubler KD, Wisner DH, Blaisdell FW. Multiple vessel injury to branches of the aortic arch: case report. J Trauma 1991;31(11):1566–8.

[84] Miller PR, Kortesis BG, McLaughlin CA III, et al. Complex blunt aortic injury or repair: beneficial effects of cardiopulmonary bypass use. Ann Surg 2003;237(6):877–83.

[85] Amabile P, Collart F, Gariboldi V, et al. Surgical versus endovascular treatment of traumatic thoracic aortic rupture. J Vasc Surg 2004;40(5):873–9.

[86] Pate JW. Is traumatic rupture of the aorta misunderstood? Ann Thorac Surg 1994;57(3): 530–1.

[87] Pate JW, Fabian TC, Walker W. Traumatic rupture of the aortic isthmus: an emergency? World J Surg 1995;19(1):119–25.

[88] Zeiger MA, Clark DE, Morton JR. Reappraisal of surgical treatment of traumatic transection of the thoracic aorta. J Cardiovasc Surg (Torino) 1990;31(5):607–10.

[89] Karmy-Jones R, Carter YM, Nathens A, et al. Impact of presenting physiology and associated injuries on outcome following traumatic rupture of the thoracic aorta. Am Surg 2001;67(1):61–6.

[90] Symbas PN, Sherman AJ, Silver JM, et al. Traumatic rupture of the aorta: immediate or delayed repair? Ann Surg 2002;235(6):796–802.

[91] Hoth JJ, Burch PT, Bullock TK, et al. Pathogenesis of posttraumatic empyema: the impact of pneumonia on pleural space infections. Surg Infect (Larchmt) 2003;4(1):29–35.

[92] Maxwell RA, Campbell DJ, Fabian TC, et al. Use of presumptive antibiotics following tube thoracostomy for traumatic hemopneumothorax in the prevention of empyema and pneumonia: a multi-center trial. J Trauma 2004;57(4):742–8.

[93] Carrillo EH, Linker RW, Richardson JD. New technology in diagnosis and treatment of diseases of the pleural space. J Ky Med Assoc 1998;96(5):174–81.

[94] Carrillo EH, Schmacht DC, Gable DR, et al. Thoracoscopy in the management of posttraumatic persistent pneumothorax. J Am Coll Surg 1998;186(6):636–9.

[95] Carrillo EH, Richardson JD. Thoracoscopy in the management of hemothorax and retained blood after trauma. Curr Opin Pulm Med 1998;4(4):243–6.

[96] Hoth JJ, Burch PT, Richardson JD. Posttraumatic empyema. Eur J Trauma 2002;28: 323–32.

[97] Heniford BT, Carrillo EH, Spain DA, et al. The role of thoracoscopy in the management of retained thoracic collections after trauma. Ann Thorac Surg 1997;63(4):940–3.

[98] Sosa JL, Pombo H, Puente I, et al. Thoracoscopy in the evaluation and management of thoracic trauma. Int Surg 1998;83(3):187–9.

[99] Navsaria PH, Vogel RJ, Nicol AJ. Thoracoscopic evacuation of retained posttraumatic hemothorax. Ann Thorac Surg 2004;78(1):282–5.

[100] Richardson JD, Miller FB, Carrillo EH, et al. Complex thoracic injuries. Surg Clin North Am 1996;76(4):725–48.

SURGICAL
CLINICS OF
NORTH AMERICA

ELSEVIER
SAUNDERS

Surg Clin N Am 87 (2007) 119–156

Care of Central Nervous System Injuries

Randall M. Chesnut, MD

Department of Neurosurgery, University of Washington, Harborview Medical Center,
Box 359766, 325 Ninth Avenue, Seattle, WA 98104–2499, USA

In both adults and children, traumatic brain injury (TBI) is the single most important influence on outcome from trauma. It accounts for approximately half of on-site deaths. For patients who survive to hospital, TBI is directly or indirectly the major source of morbidity and mortality. In terms of outcome, TBI is generally the primary injury for patients discharged to long-term rehabilitation. As such, any improvement in the outcome from TBI has the potential profoundly to influence the effectiveness of trauma care in general.

In addition to having such a powerful influence on outcome from trauma, TBI management further integrates itself into overall trauma care because of its impact on critical care. Although the ability rapidly to perform neurosurgical procedures at any stage of TBI recovery (acute or subacute) is integral to proper care, most management of TBI is medical, not surgical. In many cases, including those with polytrauma, the intensive management of the injured brain is the primary director of critical care maneuvers for the term of the ICU stay, determining both therapeutic intensity and length of stay. In cases with multiple system dysfunction, modalities directed at optimizing cerebral perfusion or lower intracranial pressure (ICP) can collide with therapeutic goals focusing on problems with infection, ventilation, renal function, or even generalized perfusion. For this reason, integration of brain and systemic care is critical on all levels, from understanding the pathophysiologic principles to treatment through interdisciplinary communication.

Primary and secondary brain injury

Primary brain injury is the damage to the brain that occurs or is initiated at the time of trauma. Secondary brain injury covers those processes that

Dr. Chesnut is the recipient of an endowed professorship from the Integra Neuroscience Foundation and has received NIH, NCMRR, NINDS, and Fogarty Foundation support for national and international clinical outcome studies.

E-mail address: chesnutr@u.washington.edu

take place following the initial injury and either worsen that injury or negatively influence recovery. Although such a distinction is neither clean nor definitive, it is useful in directing TBI resuscitation and definitive treatment.

Primary brain injury

Primary brain injury may involve neurons, glia, and vascular tissue local to or remote from the site of injury. A blow to the head may produce one or a combination of forces that damage neural tissue. A skull fracture, particularly if displaced or comminuted, can produce or allow direct, focal damage to the brain underlying the lesion. Commonly, the brain is contused. This may be self-limiting or result in hematoma formation within the parenchyma or external to the brain (eg, subdural or epidural hemorrhage).

The brain reacts to an external force with different kinetics than the skull. As such, the initial blow occurs under the point of impact. Subsequently, as the brain decelerates against the contralateral skull, injury occurs to tissue on the opposite side. Such contrecoup injury is frequently worse than the coup injury underlying the impact.

Linear or rotational forces distributed throughout the brain can produce widespread primary injury (diffuse injury). In addition to injuring neural cells in the cortex or deep nuclei (eg, basal ganglia), axonal injury may occur, interrupting major conduction pathways. Such shear injury may produce immediate axonal disruption; alternatively, it may initiate a more protracted process wherein, over days to weeks, injured axons separate, retract, and form bulbous "retraction balls," the postmortem identification of which defines diffuse axonal injury. This formally pathologic term is frequently and somewhat incorrectly confused with diffuse injury, which simply describes widespread, immediate damage. The presence of small areas of high signal consistent with focal hemorrhage in white matter regions, such as the corpus callosum, centrum semiovale, and brainstem, is suggestive of widespread damage, indicates diffuse injury, and suggests diffuse axonal injury. Because the production of coma requires disruption of either the reticular activating system in the brainstem or diffuse damage to both hemispheres, diffuse injury frequently produces loss of consciousness of variable duration.

Rotational forces are common and extremely damaging, producing both diffuse injury and rupture of veins bridging from the brain to the venous sinuses producing subdural and subarachnoid hemorrhage. Rotational forces are the most likely forces to cause diffuse axonal injury, including damage to brainstem structures, such as the reticular activating system.

Penetrating injury damages tissue through direct interaction and more distally because of cavitation injury. Because the extent of cavitation injury can be extensive, it is generally responsible for most of the damage. Cavitation is related to the mass of the object in a linear fashion but to the velocity by a cubic function. It is not the size of a missile but its velocity that generally determines the extent of damage. Penetrating injury also causes vascular injury, including disruption or the formation of aneurysms or pseudoaneurysms.

Secondary brain injury

Primary brain injuries are presently not amenable to therapeutic intervention. As such, current care is directed at minimizing or preventing secondary injuries. Some of these are intrinsic consequences of the primary injuries. Others are caused by external factors occurring subsequent to the initial trauma.

Unfortunately, most of the intrinsic processes are also not treatable at present. Biochemical alterations include disruption of cellular homeostatic mechanisms, superoxide generation, excitotoxic consequences of glutamate and aspartate release, and energy failure. Abnormal genetic responses also play a role, including apoptotic cell death. Because these processes occur over time, they are exciting potential targets for therapy and generate most experimental agents. Unfortunately, no agents spawned from laboratory investigations have proved useful in the clinical arena.

Extrinsic secondary insults are more commonly treatable and often preventable. The primary secondary insult is hypotension. Hypotension has been operationally defined as a systolic blood pressure of <90 mm Hg. In the Traumatic Coma Data Bank, a single documented episode of hypotension occurring between injury and resuscitation occurred in one third of severe TBI victims and was independently associated with a doubling of mortality and a significant increase in morbidity [1]. Similar findings have been documented for the pediatric population [2]. Such hypotensive episodes are also surprisingly frequent and similarly injurious after admission, in the ICU setting [1,3]. The likelihood of intracranial hypertension is also markedly increased in patients who have suffered early hypotension. In consequence of these findings, the "old saw" of keeping TBI patients dry has been completely abandoned and replaced with evidence-based recommendations of full-volume resuscitation with isotonic solutions [4]. In select cases, pressors are also indicated as temporizing or supplemental agents, which are withdrawn as soon as the blood pressure can be maintained in their absence. At present, research continues to be needed to elaborate a physiologic definition of hypotension based on systolic and mean arterial parameters, optimal pressure values to target during treatment, and the proper agents to use.

Prehospital or in-hospital hypoxia (Pao_2 <60 mm Hg or apnea or cyanosis in the field) is also a strong predictor of poor outcome [1,3]. Advances in equipment and techniques since early reports seem to have decreased the frequency and magnitude of such episodes. Because the injury caused by hypoxia is presently unable to be reversed, prevention is the primary goal.

Pyrexia (core temperature ≥38.5°C) represents a third, primarily in-hospital secondary insult that is strongly correlated with worse outcome, both according to its duration and magnitude [3]. Although the precise mechanism has not been demonstrated, increased metabolism and recruitment of blood flow with resultant increases in ICP may play a role. Avoiding pyrexia is highly recommended but not to be confused with induced hypothermia.

The intermediary mechanisms through which secondary insults increase morbidity often involve two physiologic parameters central to TBI management: ICP and matching perfusion to demand. These are discussed in detail next.

Intracranial pressure and cerebral perfusion pressure

Understanding and treatment of ICP revolves around the Monro-Kellie doctrine [5,6]. This doctrine holds that, because the volume of the skull is fixed, the pressure is proportional to the volumes of the compartments within the skull. Under normal conditions, these compartments are brain; vascular (blood volume); and cerebrospinal fluid (CSF). Following trauma, there may also be mass lesions that need to be inserted into this equation. Brain volume can increase because of edema of any sort (eg, cytotoxic or vasogenic), both of which occur following trauma, although the cytotoxic form seems markedly to predominate. Vascular volume can increase if venous outflow is blocked or increased cerebral blood flow (CBF) is recruited for metabolic reasons (eg, seizures, pyrexia) or increases passively because of loss of autoregulation. CSF production is fixed so CSF volume increases generally occur because of blockage of outflow pathways or interference with reabsorption.

When the volume of one compartment changes slowly, compensatory decreases in the volume of other compartments may prevent a rise in ICP. When the volume change is rapid or the compensatory mechanisms are exhausted or dysfunctional, the ICP goes up.

Cerebral blood volume consists of arterial and venous side blood, the latter representing most cases. Drainage of venous blood from the brain into the cerebral sinuses and thence into the jugular system represents most of the vascular compliance mechanism. Compression of the veins bridging to the sinuses, thrombosis of the sinuses, or interference with jugular venous drainage (eg, by neck compression or increased intrathoracic pressure) interferes with venous compliance. Hyperventilation-induced vasoconstriction also lowers cerebral blood volume. Because hyperventilation works primarily on the delivery side, iatrogenic ischemia is a possible consequence.

Under normal conditions, CSF can be shunted into the lumbar subarachnoid space from the cerebral ventricular system. Interference with interventricular communication or compression in the posterior fossa interferes with CSF compliance. An external ventricular drain provides an artificial pathway for CSF compliance providing that there is CSF within the lateral ventricular system.

Although significant brain compliance can accommodate very large mass lesions if they grow sufficiently slowly (eg, frontal meningiomas), acute compliance of the brain is quite limited. At best, brain volume is fixed over the short term. Because of edema formation, brain volume generally increases following trauma, stressing the CSF and vascular compliance mechanisms. One can iatrogenically increase brain compliance by decreasing edema fluid by osmotic maneuvers. One can lower the brain volume by débriding contusions or by lobectomy (with the marginally acceptable consequence of removing normal brain). Surgical removal of mass lesions, such as subdural, epidural, or intracerebral hematoma, represents the most direct approach to improving intracranial compliance.

Finally, the Monro-Kellie relationship can be altered by changing the static and dynamic volume of the skull through decompressive craniectomy with expansion duraplasty. This can be done at the time of hematoma evacuation or later, as a direct approach to intracranial hypertension.

In aggregate, when intracranial compliance is good, small changes in compartmental volume result in little ICP elevation. When it is compromised, however, changes of even 1 mL of volume can result in elevations of ICP of 10 mm Hg or more. Optimizing compliance is an important adjunct to managing ICP. Unfortunately, quantitative measurement of intracranial compliance is presently primitive, although significant research is ongoing [7–9].

Intracranial hypertension can produce two deleterious consequences: herniation and ischemia. Herniation occurs when a pressure gradient across a fixed anatomic barrier causes shift of brain matter. Herniation can occur downward across the foramen magnum or laterally under the falx cerebri, but the most commonly involved barrier is the tentorial membrane separating the cerebral hemispheres from the posterior fossa. Downward tissue herniation exerts pressure on the brainstem and the third cranial nerve and tension on local vessels producing anisocoria, posturing, Duret's hemorrhage in the brainstem, autonomic disturbances, and death. Transtentorial herniation can occur at ICP values below 20 mm Hg, although this is uncommon [10]. The ICP at which a given patient herniates cannot presently be determined, so ICP thresholds of 20 to 25 mm Hg are used by convention.

The second mechanism through which intracranial hypertension can be deleterious is interference with perfusion by lowering the cerebral perfusion pressure (CPP). CPP is defined as the difference between the mean arterial pressure (MAP) and ICP (CPP = MAP − ICP). It represents the input pressure for and resistance to CBF.

Under normal circumstances, cerebral pressure autoregulation maintains CBF constant over a CPP range of approximately 50 to 150 mm Hg (Fig. 1). Following trauma, this relationship may be partially or totally disrupted [11]. Total disruption results in a pressure-passive system where CBF is directly proportional to CPP (straight dashed line in Fig. 1). Much more commonly, partial disruption alters autoregulatory behavior at the lower

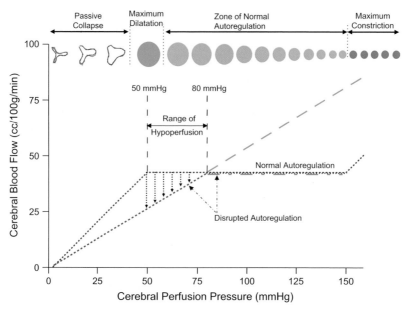

Fig. 1. Normal cerebral autoregulation is represented by the dark blue dotted line, with break-points at 50 and 150 mm Hg. Disrupted autoregulation is represented by the red dotted line and the green dot-dash line, depicting the resetting of the lower breakpoint with intact autoregulation above that value. The continuation of the red dotted line by the blue dashed line depicts complete loss of autoregulation. The circles at the top represent the cross-sectional diameter of the resistance vessels during normal autoregulation. The area of these circles depicts cerebral blood volume. Shifting the point of maximum dilation upward by 30 mm Hg represents disrupted autoregulation. Complete loss produces progressive dilation in parallel with increasing CPP. (Courtesy of Randall M. Chesnut, MD, Seattle, WA)

breakpoint but overall autoregulation remains (sigmoid dashed line in Fig. 1). The direct advantage of being within the zone of active pressure autoregulation is that the brain can weather limited changes in CPP without notable alterations of CBF. Because pressure autoregulation does not function when local ischemia exists, its presence argues against widespread hypoperfusion.

Autoregulation works by reactive changes in cerebral vascular resistance, which normally becomes active above 50 mm Hg. Increased cerebral vascular resistance is accomplished by vasoconstriction, with the consequence that a higher cerebral vascular resistance is accompanied by a lower cerebral blood volume, producing a lower ICP. When autoregulation is lost, cerebral blood volume (and ICP) is directly proportional to CPP. As such, multimodality monitoring must be used to balance delivery against metabolism while controlling ICP when a pressure-passive condition exists.

Approximately two decades ago, the relationship between CPP and ICP as a result of pressure autoregulation led to the concept of CPP therapy [12]. This promoted maintaining the CPP above 70 mm Hg, often significantly higher. Unfortunately, a growing body of evidence now suggests that such practice does not improve outcome [13–16] and may produce significant systemic complications [17,18]. Although the initial version of the Guidelines for the Management of Severe Traumatic Brain Injury reported evidentiary support for maintaining CPP >70 mm Hg [4], a subsequent revision lowered the recommended threshold to 60 mm Hg [19] and an as yet unpublished evidence-based update written by the author will further amend that to a range of 50 to 60 mm Hg.

The primary issue is that attention to CPP management probably works by avoiding ischemia and that there is no clear clinical benefit to further elevation [9,13,20]. As such, monitoring for ischemia should be considered to direct CPP elevation above 50 to 60 mm Hg when such is considered in an individual patient.

Much of the confusion has probably resulted from confounding of low CBF with ischemia in the literature. The flaw lies in the assumption of static and normal metabolic demands. In reality, cerebral metabolism is generally lower than normal following trauma in patients with all levels of recovery [21], normalizing only over time. How this relates to cellular responses to trauma versus induced sedation and analgesia is unclear but, in either case, the relationship between CBF and ischemia is clouded by such changes [22]. As illustrated in Fig. 2, where ischemia is defined by an elevation in the arteriovenous difference in oxygen measured in the jugular bulb, a given CBF may represent ischemia, coupled delivery, or hyperemia depending on metabolic demands [22]. As such, in cases where ischemia is suspected, multimodality monitoring is necessary to guide therapy. This becomes critical when ICP or CPP management is difficult or when systemic concerns interfere with TBI treatment.

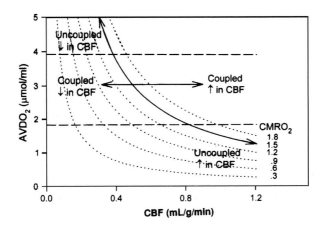

Fig. 2. The relationship between CBF, arteriovenous difference in oxygen (AVDO$_2$), and metabolism. Changes in CBF may produce AVDO$_2$ evidence of ischemia, coupling, or hyperemia, depending on the cerebral metabolic rate. (*Adapted from* Robertson CS, Cormio M. Cerebral metabolic management. New Horizons 1995;3:410–22.)

Monitoring for ischemia requires measuring both CBF and cerebral metabolism or the balance between the two. CBF can be measured (with varying degrees of accuracy) locally by laser Doppler flowmetry, near infrared spectroscopy, or thermal diffusion, or regionally by CT perfusion, cold or radiolabeled xenon studies, or single-photon emission CT. Unfortunately, direct cerebral metabolism measurement is not realistically available in the clinical setting. As such, one is left with monitoring the interaction between delivery and demand.

The relative balance between substrate delivery and demand can be estimated by evaluating cerebral oxygen extraction or lactate production, tissue oxygen tension, or the metabolic byproducts of oxidative glucose metabolism. Placing a sampling catheter into the jugular bulb allows intermittent or continuous sampling of venous blood exiting the brain before contamination with extracranial blood. Jugular venous desaturation ($J_V$so$_2$ < 50%) implies cerebral ischemia and has been associated with poor outcome [23]. Management based on optimizing the $J_V$so$_2$ may be associated with improved outcome in patients with diffusely swollen brains [14]. Unfortunately, this monitoring technique can be limited by technical issues regarding accuracy. In addition, it samples and averages a large but incomplete volume of the brain, which can mask focal areas of abnormality. In some instances, monitoring the brain for production of lactate (arteriovenous lactate difference) can be of value in detecting occult ischemia [24].

More recently, an implantable tissue oxygen tension electrode has allowed monitoring of focal oxygenation ($P_{Br}O_2$). As a direct, sensitive index of the balance between oxygenation and delivery, maintaining $P_{Br}O_2$ above 20 to 25 seems favorably to influence outcome [25,26]. This system takes up to an hour to stabilize following insertion and is very focal in its measurement.

Cerebral microdialysis is also evolving from a research tool into a clinical monitor, allowing intermittent assessment of markers of ischemia and cellular injury, such as the lactate/pyruvate ratio, glycerol, and glucose [27]. The ability favorably to influence outcome by treating based on microdialysis values remains to be adequately studied. Similar to $P_{Br}O_2$ monitoring, microdialysis is very focal and the results seem to reflect the location of the catheter with respect to areas of pathology as shown on imaging studies [28].

Targeted therapy

To date, the approach to the management of intracranial hypertension has been to escalate therapeutic interventions based on their efficacy in lowering ICP and their risk:benefit ratios. This has led to treatment algorithms that are either linear or "staircase," wherein the same approach is taken to all patients. This linear-approach philosophy dominates the literature such that treatment guidelines based on evidence-based medicine necessarily promote such algorithms.

Fortunately, this is changing as the understanding of the pathophysiology of TBI improves and monitoring systems become clinically available to allow the investigation of specific physiologic abnormalities. Targeted therapy is replacing linear algorithms. Targeted therapy supports a physiology-based, parallel processing approach. Instead of simply targeting the ICP level, one now should concentrate on such issues as blood flow, oxygen delivery, metabolism, compliance, and so forth as underlying processes that may need concomitant manipulation. Such an approach should facilitate effective treatment while avoiding overtreatment and unnecessary procedures. Under such a system, such values as ICP and CPP will most likely evolve into treatment variables rather than "magic numbers."

Clinical care

Patient assessment

The primary neurologic goal of assessment is not to miss a brain injury. Patients admitted with a Glasgow Coma Scale (GCS) score ≤8 generally are triaged as severe brain injuries and activate a full evaluation-resuscitation approach. It is important to remember that patients with unknown scores or with a GCS score >8 can also harbor a potentially devastating brain injury. It is this group that is most likely to include patients who "talk and die." As such, it is important to remember that intoxication can occur in parallel with brain injury and that it is hazardous to attribute a patient's global mental status changes to alcohol or drugs without imaging. Focal deficits should never be attributed to intoxication.

The goals of assessment include neurologic examination and imaging. Initially, it is critical to assess level of consciousness, pupillary response, and motor function. A more complete neurologic examination can then be performed as part of the tertiary survey.

Level of consciousness, Glasgow Coma Scale

The GCS is the most universal consciousness scale (Table 1). It is simple, it can be easily and rapidly obtained and repeated, it is widely understood, and it forms the basis of many trauma triage protocols. It has been widely criticized as frequently being incomplete or absent in prehospital records; being inconsistent with the use of sedation, neuromuscular blockade, and endotracheal intubation; and needing to be correctly performed [29]. All of these criticisms are relevant but addressable and there are no sufficiently accurate and sensitive scales available to justify replacing the GCS. Its use is recommended in the Guidelines for the Prehospital Management of Severe Brain Injury [30]. Special training has been developed by the Brain Trauma Foundation to optimize its accuracy (http://www.braintrauma.org/). Notably, the GCS is not a neurologic examination (eg, the motor score only reflects the best limb) and must not be substituted for such.

Table 1
Influence on outcome of secondary brain insults occurring during the interval from initial injury through resuscitation (n = 717)

Secondary insults	Number of patients	Number of patients	Outcome (%)		
			Good or moderate	Severe or vegetative	Dead
Neither	308	43	53.9	19.2	26.9
Hypoxia	161	22.4	50.3	21.7	28
Hypotension	82	11.4	32.9	17.1	50
Both	16	23.2	20.5	22.3	57.2

The GCS is useful for quantifying level of consciousness to drive resuscitation protocols and for serial assessment for deterioration. By convention, severe TBI has been defined as a GCS ≤8. Such patients require endotracheal intubation, mechanical ventilation, and full Advanced Trauma Life Support resuscitation. Moderate brain injury is defined as GCS 9 to 12 and mild TBI as GCS 13 to 15. Life-threatening intracranial injuries may exist in patients with higher GCS scores. A potentially confusing group is patients with initial GCS scores of 13 or 14 who, although classified as mild, may harbor intracranial lesions and deteriorate without imaging and close observation [31].

Pupils

Pupillary asymmetry, loss of light reaction, or unilateral or bilateral dilation should establish a working diagnosis of herniation until definitely proved otherwise. Although traumatic optic neuropathy can produce a unilaterally dilated, nonreactive pupil, the presence of local orbital trauma must not lead to missing intracranial mass lesions. With pupillary signs of herniation, immediate efforts should be initiated toward lowering ICP pending diagnostic studies.

Motor system

Although the GCS only indexes the response of the best limb, it is necessary to assess all four. Hemiparesis, monoparesis, quadraparesis, or paraparesis all may reflect intracranial or spinal cord injury and these are not mutually exclusive. In the patient not responsive to verbal cues, a noxious stimulus should be applied to a distal region of both arms and legs. If withdrawal is observed, the response to a central noxious stimulus should be checked to differentiate withdrawal from localization. Localization (GCS motor score of 5) reflects crossing the midline to a contralateral stimulus or when the arm raises above the jaw to a stimulus, such as supraorbital pressure. Hemiparesis caused by an intracranial mass lesion may be ipsilateral or contralateral in nearly equal proportions.

Imaging studies

The most important tool in neurotrauma is the CT scan. When expeditiously performed, it has eliminated the use of skull films, directed definitive operative management, provided hard data on which to base triage and resuscitation decisions, and allowed avoidance of much overtreatment and undertreatment. CT imaging should be considered whenever there is a possibility of TBI, with the urgency based on estimating the likelihood and risk of intracranial pathology and the relative resuscitation priorities for an individual patient. A list of indications is contained in Table 2. For the purposes of resource use and economics, arguments and algorithms have appeared trying to define groups with mild head injury who can be observed without imaging. Most neurosurgeons, however, argue for liberal use of CT scanning even in these patients to expedite diagnosis and treatment, stressing its sensitivity, the downside of missing intracranial pathology, and the ability safely and economically to discharge or downgrade patients based on the information produced [32]. Although clearly useful in predicting the presence of a surgical intracranial mass lesion [33], skull films are now essentially obsolete in the era of readily available CT imaging.

Follow-up surveillance CT scans at 4 to 6 hours following trauma are commonly recommended. Although they do not generally produce significant changes in management (one argument against them), they do influence management in terms of degree and duration of ICU observation and the implantation of ICP monitors in patients with marginal initial indications for monitoring. Particularly in cases that arrive at hospital shortly following trauma, follow-up CT imaging may show new lesions and frequently reveals evolution of contusions in older patients. Optimally, return to the radiology suite for follow-up CT is coordinated with obtaining other necessary extracranial imaging studies.

Because of the strong association between TBI and cervical spine trauma and the elimination of patient subjective data when their consciousness level is abnormal, early CT imaging of the cervical spine is recommended. Although the cervical spine can be reliably radiographically cleared with a complete set of plain films of good quality, it is difficult to obtain such in the comatose trauma patient and early CT imaging adds much efficiency to this process. It must be remembered, however, that the clinical examination is critical to clearing the spine at any level. Even in the comatose patient with normal films, there should be no evidence on examination of a movement deficit not clearly related to cerebral injury.

Table 2
Age-related values for hypotension (5th percentile of blood pressure for age) an normotension (50th percentile)

Age (y)	Systolic blood pressure (mm Hg)	
	Hypotension	Normotension
0–1	70	90
2–5	75	100
6–12	80	110
13–16	90	120

The level of cervical spine injury in children shifts toward the craniocervical segments. Given the desire to limit radiation exposure in children, it is reasonable for an early CT of the head to continue down to C3. Combined with a plain lateral image of the cervical spine, this should allow radiographically clearing the spine in children without undue radiation.

CT findings in trauma

Mass lesions

Hematoma in the brain generally shows up as high-attenuation collections on acute CT imaging. Blood that is not clotted, such as associated with chronic (several weeks) subdural collections or active bleeding, is lower in attenuation. An acute subdural or epidural collection comprised of mixed-density signal caused by ongoing bleeding is termed "hyperacute" (Fig. 3). Such collections, often occurring in patients with altered coagulation factors, tend to expand rapidly and require emergent surgical management.

An epidural hematoma is a blood collection between the dura mater and the skull (see Fig. 3). It may originate from an arterial source (most commonly the middle meningeal artery); venous bleeding (most commonly at the temporal tip or along one of the cerebral sinuses); or fracture bleeding. Arterial bleeding is frequently life threatening because of the pressure involved. Venous bleeding may also expand but does so less reliably. Epidural hematoma involving the temporal or lateral frontoparietal region should be considered arterial because fractures there often arise from the middle

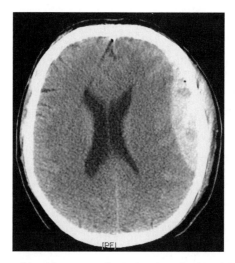

Fig. 3. CT image of an epidural hematoma, lenticular shaped, with minimal mass effect on the midline. The presence of high signal and lower signal areas within the clot suggest ongoing bleeding (hyperacute clot).

meningeal artery. CT appearance is a high-attenuation lesion with a smooth, lenticular shape. Epidural hematoma may cross the midline. Although classically associated with a lucid interval, this actually occurs in less than 50% of cases.

A subdural hematoma lies below the dura mater. Because they are distributed over the cortex, they appear as a high- or mixed-density signal with an irregular medial border (Fig. 4). They can arise from parenchymal bleeding from a contusion wherein they may be either arterial or venous, or from rupture of bridging veins. No matter what the source, they are very frequently associated with underlying parenchymal injuries, which strongly influence long-term outcome. The midline shift associated with a subdural hematoma may be larger than the thickness of the clot, signifying underlying brain swelling and predicting a worse prognosis [34].

Acute intracerebral contusions and hematoma appear as focal areas of high attenuation because of clotted blood, often interspersed with low-attenuation regions of injured tissue (Fig. 5). The most common locations for contusions are the temporal lobes and the base of the frontal lobes because of contact with the adjacent bony surfaces. They may increase in size over time early after trauma. Edema tends to develop around them over the first week or so, particularly in young patients, and contributes to their mass effect. Such evolution can result in delayed deterioration and death, particularly with deep frontal or temporal lesions. Patients with such injuries and evidence of edema progression must be observed very closely and imaged until their lesion progression and condition have stabilized because they may experience trouble as far out as 10 to 14 days. ICP monitoring should be considered when such progression is noted. Lesions of the temporal lobes

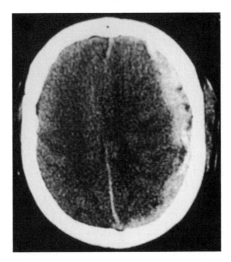

Fig. 4. CT image of a subdural hematoma. The medial border is concave and conforms to the surface of the underlying brain. There is significant mass effect on the falx cerebri.

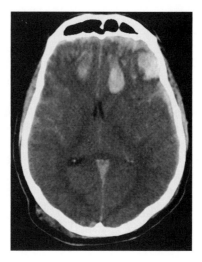

Fig. 5. CT image of intracerebral contusions and hematoma (with accompanying subdural collections) in both frontal regions.

are constrained by the bone of the middle cranial fossa, focusing most of any expansion toward the brainstem, increasing the risk of rapid herniation (Fig. 6). As such, the threshold for surgical management of temporal injuries, particularly those of the nondominant hemisphere, tends to be lower than for similar lesions in other areas.

Blood can also accumulate in the ventricular system and the subarachnoid space. In the ventricles, it is generally seen as a "hematocrit" level,

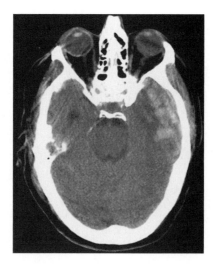

Fig. 6. CT image of a left temporal contusion, demonstrating its constraint by surrounding bone and proximity to the brainstem.

layering posteriorly in the lateral horns. Unless copious enough to interfere with the CSF circulation, intraventricular hemorrhage is usually an incidental finding.

Subarachnoid hemorrhage commonly appears over the convexities, within the sylvian fissure, or in the basal cisterns (Fig. 7). The presence of subarachnoid blood is of prognostic significance, although it is unclear if this role is caused by the blood itself or as a marker for significant parenchymal injury [4,35]. There is evidence that treating patients with posttraumatic subarachnoid hemorrhage with nimodipine may improve outcome [36]. It has also been suggested that posttraumatic subarachnoid hemorrhage–related vasospasm may induce late ischemia in some patients, allowing the use of monitoring them with transcranial Doppler [37]. Finally, in some cases (eg, single vehicle road accidents or falls) the subarachnoid hemorrhage may have been of aneurismal origin and precipitated the trauma. When such is suspected, CT angiography or a formal dye study may be indicated.

Cerebral edema appears as local or global loss of gray-white definition. It may be local (eg, surrounding contusions over time) or global. Vasogenic edema appears over days, whereas cytotoxic edema can occur rapidly and may account for much of the mass effect involved in acute brain swelling. Two of the most predictive CT findings are those of mass effect, with compressed or absent basal cisterns (Fig. 8), or midline shift of > 5 mm indicating severe swelling and being independently predictive of outcome [38]. These two findings mandate ICP monitoring. Shear injury may appear as widely distributed white matter and deep nuclear punctate areas of high attenuation (Fig. 9).

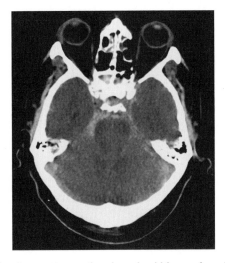

Fig. 7. CT image showing posttraumatic subarachnoid hemorrhage in the basal cisterns.

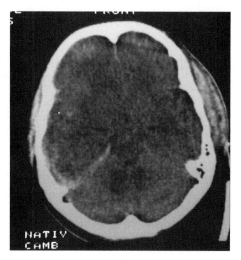

Fig. 8. CT image showing compression of the basilar cisterns caused by brain swelling.

Treatment of patients with traumatic brain injury

Evidence-based management

In 1996, the author published the first evidence report on TBI management, the Guidelines for the Management of Severe Traumatic Brain Injury [4]. These followed an explicit and rigorous evidence-based medicine approach to assessing the literature, classifying it into three levels of rigor, and producing Standards, Guidelines, and Options for treatment based

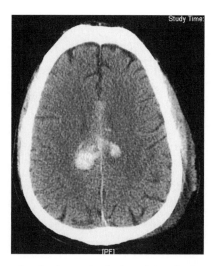

Fig. 9. CT image showing hemorrhagic shear injury in the corpus callosum.

exclusively on those levels. These guidelines were approved by the American Association of Neurological Surgeons and the Congress of Neurological Surgeons, endorsed by the World Health Organization, and recognized by numerous associations within disciplines related to trauma, critical care, and emergency medicine. Subsequently, these have been revised [19] and are currently in a concerted phase of revision and expansion. Additional guidelines have now been published in the area of prehospital care [30], pediatric TBI [39], penetrating TBI [40], and surgical management of TBI [41]. All of these are now linked to a regular revision pathway, coordinated by the Brain Trauma Foundation (www.braintrauma.org).

Consistent with the variable quality of the underlying literature, most recommendations in these guidelines remain limited to treatment options. Nevertheless, wherever possible, the following treatment recommendations directly reflect these guidelines.

Resuscitation

It is a truism that there is no brain recovery if a patient dies. The principles of trauma resuscitation remain entirely applicable to the patient with TBI. The ABCs are paramount, modified slightly to optimize comanagement of any intracranial pathology. To these have been added a "D," standing for disability and representing the importance of CNS injury.

Airway and breathing. Patients with GCS ≤8 require airway control, adequate oxygenation, and controlled or assisted ventilation (Fig. 10). Because of decreased level of consciousness and the likelihood of aspiration, airway control is critical. In adults, endotracheal intubation is the preferred method [30]. In children, the advantages of endotracheal intubation seem balanced by the difficulties inherent in intubating this population and the difficulty in staying in practice, and there is no clear advantage to any individual method until conditions are optimal (eg, arrival at an equipped hospital) [39]. Because coma does not represent a lack of physiologic response to noxious stimulation and such response can precipitate intracranial hypertension and herniation, adequate analgesia and sedation are necessary during airway manipulation whenever possible. Endotracheal intubation should be confirmed by demonstration of CO_2 return.

Initially, 100% oxygen should be delivered and ventilation should be directed at the lower end of eucapnia (eg, $Paco_2$ of approximately 35–38 mm Hg). Hyperventilation lowers ICP through hypocapneic vasoconstriction, which also lowers CBF. Prophylactic hyperventilation has been associated with diminished recovery [42]. As such, hyperventilation before implantation of an ICP monitor should be limited to a $Paco_2$ range of 30 to 35 mm Hg and only used when there are clinical signs of intracranial hypertension, such as pupillary changes, motor posturing, or neurologic deterioration not attributable to other causes (Fig. 11) [30]. Quantitative capnography is recommended in the absence of blood gas values.

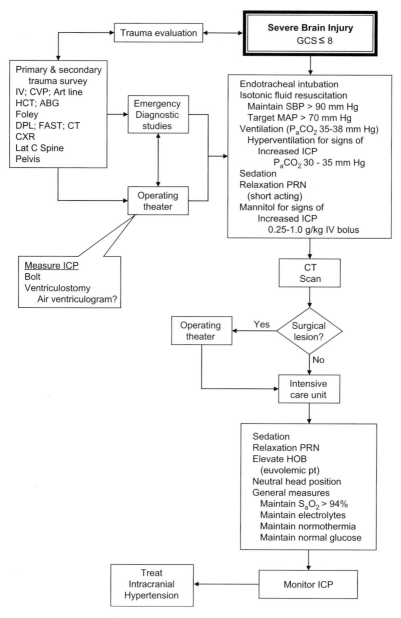

Fig. 10. An algorithm for evaluation and treatment of the severe TBI patient on arrival at the trauma center, based on the Guidelines for the Management of Severe Traumatic Brain Injury. The order of steps is determined by the risk:benefit ratio for individual treatment maneuvers. This algorithm should be viewed as expert opinion and used as a framework that may be useful in guiding an approach to initial hospital management of such patients before ICP monitoring. ABG, arterial blood gases; CVP, central venous pressure; CXR, chest radiograph; DPL, diagnostic peritoneal lavage; FAST, Focused assessment with sonography for trauma; GCS, Glasgow Coma Score; HCT, hematocrit; HOB, head of bed; ICP, intracranial pressure; IV, intravenous; MAP, mean arterial pressure; PRN, according to circumstances; SBP, systolic blood pressure. (Courtesy of Randall M. Chesnut, MD, Seattle, WA.)

Circulation. Hypotension is an independent predictor of morbidity and mortality in TBI and occurs in approximately one third of TBI patients [1,2]. A single measurement of a systolic blood pressure between injury and the end of resuscitation is associated with a doubling of the mortality rate (see Table 2) [1]. The recognition of the frequency and impact of hypotension has prompted completely discarding the old tenet of "keeping the patient dry" in TBI. Volume resuscitation should be directed toward normal perfusion and volume status. The tonicity of the solution seems to remain important. Free water may exacerbate cerebral edema. Isotonic solutions should be used whenever possible, making 0.9% normal saline somewhat preferable to Ringers lactate. The prehospital administration of hypertonic saline has been supported by the demonstration of improved resuscitation and short-term outcome in the TBI subgroup of three randomized controlled trials of prehospital hypertonic saline administration [43–45] and a meta-analysis of hypertonic saline use in TBI suggested an improvement in the odds ratio for survival to discharge of 2.12 [46]. Unfortunately, the only randomized controlled trials specific for hypertonic resuscitation of TBI patients did not show a positive effect [47], significantly dampening enthusiasm for this approach.

Although hypotension clearly needs to be avoided, optimal systemic pressures remain undetermined. To maintain a CPP of 50 mm Hg at the upper end of normal ICP requires a mean arterial pressure of 70 mm Hg. The likelihood of blood pressure fluctuations during the early posttraumatic period and the possibility of intracranial hypertension have prompted supporting targeting mean arterial pressure values of 80 to 90 mm Hg [19]. For children, age-related values should be used to define hypotension (fifth percentile of blood pressure for age – approximately 70 + 2[age]) and normotension (50th percentile – approximately 90 + 2[age]) (see Table 2) [48].

As with all trauma patients, volume is the primary method of resuscitation. Because of the exquisite sensitivity of the injured brain to even transient episodes of hypotension, however, the possible use of pressors as temporizing or supplemental agents has been supported. In general, alpha agonists are preferred and concomitant close monitoring of arterial and central venous pressure is suggested. Pressors should be discontinued as soon as possible consistent with adequate maintenance of perfusion with less toxic means.

Disability. Baseline neurologic status should be established early and frequently checked. Evidence of deterioration should prompt further investigation and immediate treatment (see Fig. 11). Hyperventilation should be initiated when signs of intracranial hypertension are noted. Such findings should also prompt osmotherapy. When the choice of osmotic agents is limited to mannitol, it should only be administered when the patient is euvolemic because mannitol-related hypotension has been implicated in poor recovery [49].

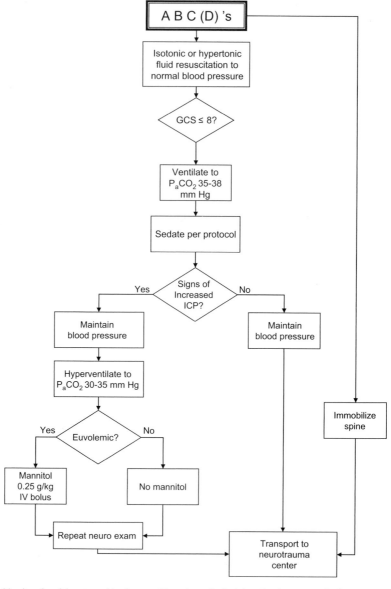

Fig. 11. An algorithm to guide the consideration of administering hyperventilation or mannitol during the initial management of the TBI patient before or on arrival at the trauma center, based on the Guidelines for the Prehospital Management of Severe Traumatic Brain Injury and the Guidelines for the Management of Severe Traumatic Brain Injury. The order of steps is determined by the risk:benefit ratio for individual treatment maneuvers. This algorithm should be viewed as expert opinion and used as a framework that may be useful in guiding an approach to prehospital or initial in-hospital management. GCS, Glasgow Coma Score; ICP, intracranial pressure; IV, intravenous. (Courtesy of Randall M. Chesnut, MD, Seattle, WA.)

General measures before intracranial pressure monitoring

Monitoring of ICP is indicated in all patients with severe TBI and any patient with moderate TBI thought to be at risk of intracranial hypertension (eg, cisternal compression on CT, midline shift, multiple contusions) or who are unavailable for serial examination because of anesthesia, neuromuscular blockade, or deep sedation. When indicated, an ICP monitor should be inserted as soon as possible. The following describes management during the pre-ICP interval.

Pre-ICU care

Consistent with Figs. 10 and 11, resuscitation should be rapid and vigorous in all TBI patients. In the absence of signs of intracranial hypertension, the $Paco_2$ should be maintained at the lower end of eucapnia. Hyperventilation should be avoided and no mannitol given. When clinical signs of intracranial hypertension are obtained (or the initial CT scan reveals cisternal compression, midline shift, or effacement of the sulci), the $Paco_2$ should be lowered to 30 to 35 mm Hg and mannitol given if the patient is euvolemic.

CT imaging of the brain should be accomplished as soon as possible. The hazards of transport are well known, so monitoring should be arranged before transport and maintained during scanning. Persons capable of continuing resuscitation and recognizing and responding to deterioration should attend the patient in the radiology suite with the requisite equipment and medications. In addition, someone capable of definitively reading the CT should be immediately available.

Patients with moderate or severe TBI should be scanned as soon as possible, consistent with resuscitation. In instances where resuscitation priorities preclude CT imaging of the brain (eg, the need for immediate, life-saving maneuvers, such as laparotomy or embolization), other means of assessment should be entertained. These include plain skull films; insertion of an intraparenchymal ICP monitor; insertion of a ventriculostomy (with air ventriculography, if desired); transcranial Doppler examination; or exploratory burr holes. In particular, insertion of an intraparenchymal ICP monitor should be considered to assist in temporizing or guiding further maneuvers when the brain CT is delayed. Findings suggestive of intracranial hypertension may alter anesthetic management and assist the trauma surgeon in setting damage control priorities. In some cases, burr hole exploration may lead to the diagnosis of surgical intracranial mass lesions, which can be immediately evacuated [50]. As such, the inability to obtain an admission CT in a patient suspected to have a brain injury should prompt immediate neurosurgical consultation for consideration of performing such alternative maneuvers during the other procedure. The existence of such alternatives to CT imaging render meaningless algorithms for guessing which trauma patients requiring immediate surgery have low likelihood of intracranial mass lesions [50,51]. At the least, ICP monitoring should never be delayed by extracranial surgery.

Unless surgery is necessary, the patient should be transported to the ICU as soon as possible for the initiation of definitive care and placement of an ICP monitor (unless such can be placed in the emergency department). When immediate craniotomy is indicated, the trauma surgeon should amend the systemic work-up accordingly so the unnecessary delay does not attend in the CT suite. When immediate craniotomy and extracranial surgery are simultaneously necessary, the two services should work in parallel, with two scrub teams.

Surgical management of intracranial pathology is rarely definitive and almost universally requires meticulous ICU care to optimize outcome. As such, it should be rare that surgery for non–life-threatening injuries follows craniotomy. When delay in transport to ICU is necessary, ICP monitoring should be initiated immediately on closure of the scalp.

Initial ICU care

Fig. 10 represents an algorithm for management before ICP monitoring, which has been developed based on the previously mentioned evidence reports [4,19,30,39]. An ICP monitor should be inserted as soon as possible so that this algorithm can be expanded to definitive TBI care.

The initial goals for resuscitation should be continued in the ICU. Euvolemia and normotension should be maintained with isotonic fluids. Central venous and arterial pressures should be continuously monitored. Ventilation should target a $Paco_2$ of 35 to 38 mm Hg in the absence of clinical or CT evidence of intracranial hypertension. End tidal CO_2 monitoring is useful for following ventilation trends. The initial blood pressure goals should continue to be the absolute avoidance of hypotension and the maintenance of age-adjusted normotension.

Head-of-bed elevation to 30 degrees is recommended to lower ICP by facilitating venous drainage of the brain. Reverse Trendelenburg position should be used until the thoracolumbar spine is cleared. Raising the head-of-bed higher than 30 degrees may exacerbate intracranial hypertension if it increases intra-abdominal pressure so should not be performed until an ICP monitor is placed. Raising the head-of-bed in underresuscitated patients may lower the CPP by dropping the systemic pressure so patients should be euvolemic before head-of-bed elevation.

Venous drainage can also be facilitated by avoiding jugular venous compression (eg, by cervical orthoses or tracheostomy ties) and by minimizing intrathoracic or intra-abdominal pressures. When positive end-expiratory pressure is necessary, its effect on ICP is difficult to predict.

Pain and agitation raise ICP, making both analgesia and sedation necessary. Short-acting agents are preferred because they facilitate monitoring of the neurologic examination. To avoid peaks and troughs using short-acting agents, administration by continuous intravenous infusion is preferred.

Agents, such as propofol (in adults), that decrease cerebral metabolism generally should be favored, particularly during the early postinjury period.

Neuromuscular blockade for the purposes of treating ICP should only be initiated for documented intracranial hypertension. When necessary, short-acting agents are preferred.

Fever seems to be an independent predictor of poor outcome from TBI [3]. Systemic temperatures of greater than 38.5°C should be rapidly lowered. The use of lower temperature treatment thresholds is recommended in patients with intracranial hypertension; indications for their use in the general TBI population are unclear.

Transfusion after trauma has repeatedly been shown to increase the risk of acute respiratory distress syndrome and multisystem organ failure [52–54]. The exquisite sensitivity of the injured brain to hypoperfusion, however, is well recognized [1,2,55,56]. There is presently no evidence that the transfusion threshold of a hematocrit of 30 commonly recommended in neurosurgical circles improves outcome from TBI. In patients with unstable blood pressures or CPP issues, higher hematocrit values may be considered or the need for transfusion may be guided by the use of intraparenchymal oxygen tension or jugular venous oxygen monitoring.

Hypertonic saline infusion is frequent used as prophylaxis for intracranial hypertension, albeit without significant research support. Maintaining serum sodium at the upper border of normal or slightly above normal with a continuous infusion of 3% NaCl at 0.5 to 1 mL/kg/h is of little risk and may decrease the likelihood of cerebral edema and intracranial hypertension. Hyperchloremic acidosis should be avoided.

Neither the Guidelines for the Management of Severe Traumatic Brain Injury nor the Guidelines for the Management of Penetrating Brain Injury recommend the administration of anticonvulsants for the prophylaxis of late epilepsy [4,40]. There is evidence that early treatment prevents seizures during the period of drug administration, although without an effect on outcome, so prophylactic treatment is left to the discretion of the physician. A reasonable approach is to limit such treatment to situations where a seizure might compromise tenuous ICP control or when neuromuscular blockade prevents clinical diagnosis of early epilepsy. Patients with penetrating brain injury should receive prophylaxis during the first week because of the high incidence of seizures [40].

Treatment of intracranial hypertension

Figs. 12–14 represent algorithms for managing intracranial hyperventilation in adults and children, respectively. They are based on the adult Guidelines for the Management of Severe Traumatic Brain Injury [4,41] and the Guidelines for the Acute Medical Management of Severe Traumatic Brain Injury in Infants, Children, and Adolescents [39]. Individual treatments are based on the relative risk:benefit ratios as perceived by the authors of these guidelines. Note, too, that these algorithms represent linear treatment,

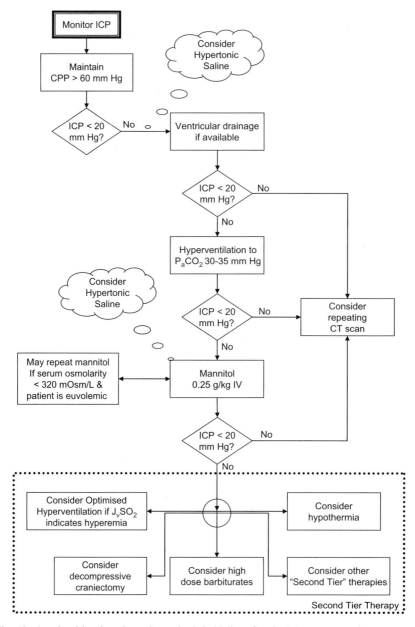

Fig. 12. An algorithm based on the revised Guidelines for the Management of Severe Trau-matic Brain Injury to guide management of intracranial hypertension in adults. The order of steps is determined by the risk:benefit ratio for individual treatment maneuvers. This algorithm should be viewed as expert opinion and used as a framework that may be useful in guiding an approach to ICP management in adults. CPP, cerebral perfusion pressure; ICP, intracranial pressure. (Courtesy of Randall M. Chesnut, MD, Seattle, WA.)

as opposed to the growing role for targeted therapy, which is organized in parallel fashion.

Fever is an independent predictor of decreased recovery from TBI [3]. In addition, metabolism-related recruitment of CBF raises ICP. Temperature control should be a primary mechanism for ICP control. Lowering the treatment threshold for fever to 37.5° or 38°C decreases ICP. When simple measures, such as acetaminophen, cooling blankets, and a fan, are not effective, such agents as indomethacin (50 mg every 6 hours) or intravenous cooling catheters may be considered.

For established intracranial hypertension, a continuous infusion of 3% NaCl should be considered, starting at 0.5 to 1 mL/kg/h. Serum sodium values of 150 mEq/L or greater and serum osmolarities of 320 to 340 mOsm/L may be targeted. Serum sodium and osmolarity limits should be 160 mEq/L and 360 mOsm/L, respectively. Rarely, rebound intracranial hypertension may occur on withdrawal of hypertonic osmotherapy, so it is wise to taper the 3% infusion off and normalize the serum sodium before removing the ICP monitor.

When a ventricular drain is available or can be inserted, CSF drainage is a relatively safe and easy method of lowering ICP [57]. The major risks are hemorrhage and infection, which can be minimized by careful insertional and management technique and serial monitoring for colonization [41]. Because ICP monitoring is inaccurate when the drain is open, CSF drainage for ICP control should be accomplished by intermittent drainage to a slightly positive gradient.

Neuromuscular blockade may lower ICP. It prevents neurologic examination and has treatment and systemic complications that should limit its use to established intracranial hypertension not amenable to less hazardous treatments [31]. If not readily effective, it should be discontinued. A reasonable target is blockade to one to two out of four twitches on a train-of-four monitor.

Hyperventilation is an excellent method of acutely lowering ICP. Because of the risk of inducing ischemia, its use should be limited [42,58]. Its position in the algorithms in Figs. 12 and 13 is based on such a risk:benefit ratio [4]. Initial hyperventilation should target a $Paco_2$ of 30 to 35 mm Hg. Levels lower than that are more hazardous, warrant increased monitoring for ischemia, and are considered second-tier therapy. Because the body compensates for the alkalosis produced by hypocapnia, the duration of effect of hyperventilation is unclear but is certainly limited.

Hyperosmolar therapy at this level may consist of higher dose continuous infusion of hypertonic saline solutions or the rapid intravenous administration of mannitol or sodium chloride solutions ranging from 3% to 23.4% [59–63]. Hypertonic saline infusion has been best studied in children and, as such, is recommended for consideration in parallel to mannitol in the Guidelines for the Acute Medical Management of Severe Traumatic Brain Injury in Infants, Children, and Adolescents [39]. Bolus dosing of

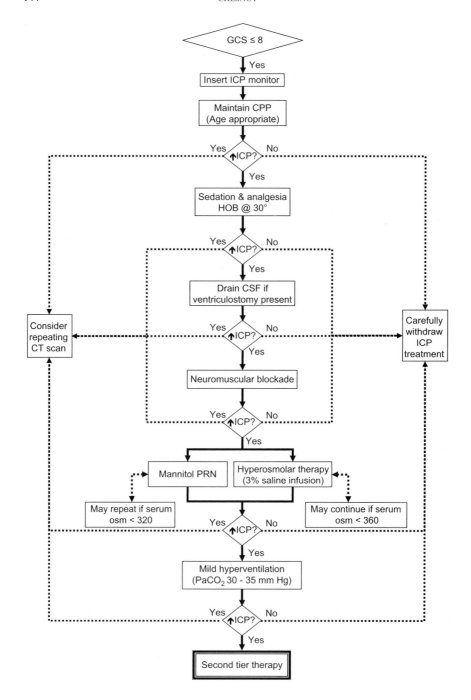

hypertonic saline is less well studied in either population and rigorous outcome studies are lacking. Two randomized controlled trials using ICP control as the dependant variable have suggested that bolus doses of 7.5% saline is more effective than equimolar mannitol [61,62]. Nevertheless, mannitol is readily available, has a long clinical history, and is effective in ICP control. Mannitol may be administered in doses ranging from 0.25 to 1 g/kg. A recent Cochrane review found evidence that higher doses may be more effective [64]. Dosing should be limited to serum osmolarity ≤ 320 mOsm/L. Because mannitol may be sequestered in areas of disrupted blood-brain barrier and thereby increase edema, other agents should be considered when repeated doses are frequently necessary. Hypertonic saline should be limited to serum sodium levels of 160 mEq/L and osmolarity of 360 mOsm/L. The risk of rebound intracranial hypertension suggests not removing the ICP monitor and avoiding major nonemergent surgical cases until the serum sodium has returned to within normal limits. When mannitol is used, intravascular volume must be maintained against its diuretic effect. Dehydration does not play a role in therapeutic osmotherapy.

Second tier therapy

When ICP control proves refractory to the treatments listed previously, second tier therapies may be considered (see Figs. 12 and 14). These are treatments that may have higher risks, be more invasive, or be less well established, but which have some support for salvage. They have not been tested against each other, so choice of second tier treatments is generally based on the perceived pathophysiology of the lesion or applicability of the treatment in each individual case. At the point of entering the second tier of treatment, it is reasonable to ask whether the refractory nature of the intracranial hypertension represents an ongoing secondary injury to a potentially salvageable brain or is a proxy for an extremely severe injury with minimal hope of recovery even with ICP control. If the latter case is highly suspected, a decision to not proceed to the second tier might be considered.

Pentobarbital coma is the most established second tier therapy. It has randomized controlled trials data supporting its efficacy in the setting of refractory intracranial hypertension [65]. Unfortunately, it is quite toxic, with a high incidence of hypotension and cardiac suppression and serious infection often attends the general 5- to 7-day course. The dosing goal of treatment is

Fig. 13. An algorithm based on the Guidelines for the Acute Medical Management of Severe Traumatic Brain Injury in Infants, Children, and Adolescents to guide management of intracranial hypertension. Second tier therapies are represented in Fig. 14. The order of steps is determined by the risk:benefit ratio for individual treatment maneuvers. This algorithm should be viewed as expert opinion and used as a framework that may be useful in guiding an approach to ICP management in pediatric patients. CPP, cerebral perfusion pressure; CSF, cerebral spinal fluid; GCS, Glasgow Coma Score; HOB, head of bed; ICP, intracranial pressure; PRN, according to circumstances. (Courtesy of Randall M. Chesnut, MD, Seattle, WA.)

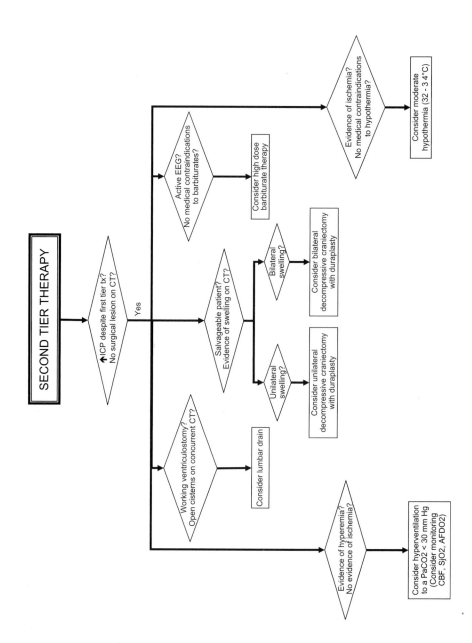

SECOND TIER THERAPY

↑ICP despite first tier tx?
No surgical lesion on CT?

Yes

Active EEG?
No medical contraindications
to barbiturates?

Consider high dose
barbiturate therapy

Evidence of ischemia?
No medical contraindications
to hypothermia?

Consider moderate
hypothermia (32 - 3 4°C)

Salvageable patient?
Evidence of swelling on CT?

Bilateral
swelling?

Consider bilateral
decompressive craniectomy
with duraplasty

Unilateral
swelling?

Consider unilateral
decompressive craniectomy
with duraplasty

Working ventriculostomy?
Open cisterns on concurrent CT?

Consider lumbar drain

Evidence of hyperemia?
No evidence of ischemia?

Consider hyperventilation
to a PaCO2 < 30 mm Hg
(Consider monitoring
CBF, SjO2, AFDO2)

burst suppression on continuous EEG. Barbiturate withdrawal is initiated after 24 hours of ICP control, at 50% per day. Because of the high complication rate, this therapy is not indicated in patients with cardiovascular risks; ongoing infections, such as pneumonia or sepsis; or unstable blood pressure.

Optimized hyperventilation involves adjusting the level of hypocapnia to achieve a jugular venous saturation at the lower margin of normal (approximately 60%). It is only applicable in patients with a degree of hyperemia where the decrease in CBF is tolerated. As such, it requires close monitoring. When carefully applied to the proper patient group (eg, hyperemic patients with diffuse swelling of the brain without evidence of widespread contusion or primary parenchymal injury), it is associated with significant benefit [14]. The major concern is inducing ischemia in areas not well represented by the monitored jugular saturation in patients with heterogeneous CBF.

Although randomized controlled trial evidence has demonstrated no beneficial effect of hypothermia on severe TBI in general [66], mild (34°C) hypothermia (but not moderate hypothermia [31°C]) can be effective in lowering ICP refractory to first tier therapy with beneficial outcome [67,68]. Such treatment is attended by hypothermia-induced anergy, electrolyte disturbances, and coagulation abnormalities. It is potentially particularly useful for patients with intracranial hypertension plus marginal perfusion, where lowering the metabolic rate improves the perfusion:demand balance.

Decompressive craniectomy has recently become very popular as second tier therapy in large part because of its rapidly definitive effect on ICP. Properly performed, intracranial hypertension should no longer be an issue. This means a very wide bony decompression accompanied by a generous expansion duraplasty. Because decompressive craniectomy interferes with autoregulation, CPP should not be pushed after surgery. Because decompression should be effective regardless of the underlying cause of intracranial hypertension (other than swelling from unsalvageable cellular damage), it has become a treatment of choice.

Reports on outcome following decompressive craniectomy have been variable. Historically, initial enthusiasm [69] was tempered by reports of increased vegetative survival by the same group [70]. Subsequent reports have suggested favorable outcomes in patients with more diffuse injury who have not suffered many secondary insults before surgery [71–73]. This supports avoiding decompression in patients with significant hypoxic or hypotensive-ischemic insults and performing the decompression before the refractory intracranial hypertension has caused much further damage.

Fig. 14. An algorithm based on the Guidelines for the Acute Medical Management of Severe Traumatic Brain Injury in Infants, Children, and Adolescents to guide second tier management of intracranial hypertension. This algorithm should be viewed as expert opinion and used as a framework that may be useful in guiding an approach to ICP management in pediatric patients. $AFDO_2$, arteriovenous difference in oxygen; CBF, cerebral blood flow; EEG, electroencephalogram. (Courtesy of Randall M. Chesnut, MD, Seattle, WA.)

Special considerations

Early decompressive craniectomy

Although initially regarded as a second tier approach to refractory intra-cranial hypertension, early decompressive craniectomy seems to have a grow-ing role in TBI management. The goal of such surgery is to treat the intracranial hypertension definitively, thereby eliminating the need for further ICP treatment. This procedure is of relatively low risk. As such, it is useful in two situations: when ICP is becoming increasingly difficult to control (eg, an-ticipation of subsequent refractory intracranial hypertension); and when ICP management collides with the treatment of extracranial abnormalities.

Pre-emptive decompression should be considered in patients with diffuse unilateral or bilateral swelling where ICP control is initially difficult, requir-ing rapid escalation of therapy. Because many such patients go on to a re-fractory state, suffering pressure- and perfusion-related secondary insults on the way, early decompression should be considered.

An example of the second indication is the patient with chest trauma or the respiratory distress syndrome where ventilatory problems obtain and mean intrathoracic pressures are often high. Because attempting to balance often conflicting treatments may limit the ability to manage both issues, de-compressive craniectomy may be performed simply to eliminate the need for ICP treatment and facilitate unrestricted management of the extracranial disease. Given that most treatment modalities for intracranial hypertension have some degree of systemic toxicity, decompressive craniectomy may not only shorten ICU stay but also decrease iatrogenic complications.

Burr holes

Burr holes have two roles in the neurosurgical treatment of TBI: explo-ration and temporizing. Exploration involves placing burr holes in patients with evidence of mass effect who have not been imaged for whatever reason. It is relatively sensitive for extra-axial hematoma if six holes (bilateral tem-poral, frontal, and parietal) are drilled before declaring the exploration neg-ative [50]. They are not sensitive to mass effect from intraparenchymal lesions. Given the modern ready availability and rapidity of helical CT scan-ners, however, burr hole exploration is presently rarely indicated.

Burr hole drainage may be life saving in patients herniating from an epi-dural hematoma. It is much less effective in lowering ICP in subdural hema-toma because they are generally lower pressure and clotted, requiring exposure and evacuation for decompression. In epidural hematoma, where there is often a component of active bleeding producing liquid clot, the ICP can be decreased by performing a temporal burr hole and allowing egress of the blood. This is, of course, most effective if it immediately leads to evac-uation by craniotomy and direct management of the bleeding source.

Much interest in burr hole drainage is expressed by emergency depart-ment physicians and general and trauma surgeons who may occasionally encounter a herniating patient with an epidural hematoma in the absence of immediate neurosurgical consultation. The mechanics of such a procedure are simple enough that, in general, the most limiting factor is the willingness of the practitioner to perform a rarely done procedure outside of their specific expertise under difficult circumstances. As such, before operating, the willing physician should directly contact a neurosurgeon for support in the choice to proceed and for back-up, both for possible complications and for definitive management of the clot.

To perform a simple trephination, the scalp is opened in a linear fashion, from just above the zygoma to the mid-lateral skull. The incision is extended down through the temporalis muscle. The temporal artery lies between the scalp and the fascia of this muscle and bleeds vigorously if transected. Optimally, it can be identified and tied off or cauterized with bipolar electrocautery before being cut. If it is simply divided, the bleeding can be stopped by clamping both ends and tying it off later. Opening the skull is best performed with a cutting burr under irrigation. Because the epidural hematoma separates the dura from the skull, burring the bone is relatively protected. Once the intracranial cavity is entered, the hole can be expanded with the burr or rongeurs. If definitive craniotomy is not to follow directly, the hole should be made large enough to support continued egress of blood, the wound gently packed with loose gauze, and the patient transferred immediately for ultimate management.

Intracranial pressure monitoring

The management of severe TBI mandates ICP monitoring and there are frequent indications for monitor insertion in moderate TBI patients. Optimally, every TBI patient should be directly attended by a neurosurgeon that is available to place ICP monitors rapidly whenever they are indicated. In some instance, unfortunately, this may not be possible. In circumstances where such a situation may not infrequently arise, it is likely in the patient's interest to have a trauma surgeon or intensivist available and trained in the insertion of an ICP monitor with the blessing of the neurosurgical consultant. The ease of insertion and very low complication rate of intraparenchymal ICP monitors makes them a good choice for placement by nonneurosurgeons.

In the interest of accuracy, intraparenchymal and intraventricular monitoring devices are preferable to subdural, subarachnoid, or epidural monitors [39,41]. The benefits of simple, rapid insertion and very low clinical complication rate associated with intraparenchymal monitors should be balanced against the inability to drain CSF with such systems.

Cerebral spinal fluid rhinorrhea and otorrhea

Over 85% of CSF leaks following TBI close spontaneously within 7 to 10 days with head-of-bed elevation and avoidance of sneezing, coughing, and the Valsalva maneuver [74]. The incidence of infection seems to increase markedly when leaks persist beyond this interval, suggesting that lumbar CSF drainage should be considered if leaks persist beyond the first several days following fracture. Surgical closure should be considered for persistent otorrhea or rhinorrhea. A recent Cochran review reported no efficacy for prophylactic antibiotics in patients with basilar skull fractures with or without CSF leaks with respect to preventing meningitis [75].

Observation of traumatic brain injury patients

TBI patients admitted for observation because of concerns for neurologic worsening should generally not be admitted to a general floor bed. Modern floor staffing ratios rarely permit hourly neurologic examination. If the risk of deterioration is believed to warrant admission for monitoring, the proper setting is an ICU, high dependency unit, or an observation unit.

Patients with lesions in the temporal lobe or deep frontal lobe are at risk of late deterioration because of the development of edema. Such patients may seem awake and alert, although they generally complain of headache, and do not seem to need ICU care soon after admission. ICP monitoring may not reveal intracranial hypertension. If edema seems to be progressing on serial CT imaging or there is CT evidence of mass effect (cisternal compression or midline shift), these patients warrant close observation for up to 10 to 14 days or until resolution of symptoms and imaging abnormalities is clearly evident. Rebound from osmotherapy can be particularly hazardous in this group.

Surgical issues

Epidural hematoma

Aggressive management has reduced the overall mortality of epidural hematoma to less than 10% [41,76]. Outcome varies significantly with level of consciousness at the time of surgery, mandating haste in surgical management. Epidural hematoma of >30 mL volume, clot thickness >15 mm, or midline shift >5 mm should be emergently surgically evacuated regardless of the patient's GCS score. Hematoma not meeting these criteria should also be considered for evacuation in patients with a GCS ≤8. Such lesions in patients with higher GCS scores may be considered for nonoperative management under close observation.

Subdural hematoma

Mortality from subdural hematoma [41] continues to run at up to 50%. A significant percentage of this mortality and morbidity is caused by associated parenchymal injuries.

An acute subdural hematoma with a thickness >10 mm or midline shift >5 mm should be surgically evacuated, regardless of the patient's GCS score. Evacuation should be emergent if the GCS score is less than eight and as soon as reasonably possible in the rest. Hematoma not meeting these criteria should also be considered for evacuation in patients with a GCS ≤8 if their GCS score deteriorates ≥2 points, they have pupillary abnormalities, or the ICP is >20 mm Hg.

The limited available evidence regarding timing of surgery and outcome suggests that emergent evacuation should be within 4 hours of trauma [77]. The option of leaving the bone out and performing an expansion duraplasty is left to the surgeon.

Intraparenchymal lesions

The surgical management of intraparenchymal lesions [41] is very controversial. In general, surgery should be considered for mass lesions >50 mL in volume and for mass lesions of lesser size that are associated with

- Signs of progressive neurologic deterioration referable to the lesion
- Refractory intracranial hypertension
- CT evidence of mass effect
- Midline shift >5 mm
- Cisternal compression

Patients with small intraparenchymal lesions and depressed levels of consciousness should be considered for ICP monitoring. Progressive edema development may increase the mass effect of parenchymal lesions over time, particularly in younger patients.

Posterior fossa lesions

Lesions of the posterior fossa [41] do not reliably produce classic signs of progressive mass effect. Instead, patients with such lesions may simply rapidly deteriorate into coma and die, even under observation. In addition, there is presently no method for measuring posterior fossa pressures. Signs of mass effect include obscuration of the fourth ventricle and basal cisterns and the development of obstructive hydrocephalus. Urgent surgery should be considered when significant mass effect is seen on CT or when the patient shows any signs of deterioration. Lesions of >3 cm diameter are also candidates for evacuation. Obstructive hydrocephalus not responsive to surgery should be treated with a ventricular drain with careful attention to the drainage gradient to prevent upward herniation.

Depressed skull fractures

Indications for the surgical management of closed skull fractures [41] are generally the management of underlying intracranial injury or cosmesis. The general rule is to elevate fractures that are displaced beyond the inner table of the skull, although there is little basis for such an arbitrary threshold. Fractures that cross large venous sinuses and are not associated with hemorrhage are often best left alone unless elevation is necessary to restore sinus patency.

Open fractures are generally managed for the purpose of avoiding infection. Fractures driven below the inner table of the skull are considered potentially surgical. Other indications include

- Gross wound contamination
- Significant intracranial hematoma
- Dural penetration
- Depression >1 cm
- Gross cosmetic deformity
- Frontal sinus involvement
- Wound infection

Surgery should consist of elevation and debridement, exenteration and isolation of air sinus involvement, and absolute avoidance of external CSF leakage. Replacement of fracture fragments in noninfected wounds is at the surgeon's discretion. Open fractures should be treated with broad-spectrum antibiotics regardless of the nature of management. In the absence of hard evidence, the general duration is 1 to 2 weeks.

Penetrating brain injury

Management of penetrating injuries involves treatment of intracranial hypertension, avoidance of infection, addressing the risk of vascular injuries, and the prophylaxis of seizures [40]. Mass lesions should be evacuated for indications similar to those in closed injuries: management of intracranial hypertension, mass effect, and patient deterioration. As such, ICP monitoring is useful in patients with depressed levels of consciousness.

There is a growing body of evidence that débriding bone or missile fragments does not improve outcome. Debridement of the missile tract is only performed when surgery is indicated for other reasons and is limited to removal of debris easily at hand. There is no evidence that removal of such foreign bodies alters the incidence of infection.

Outside of removal of significant mass lesions, the primary goal of surgery is wound management so that there is no CSF leak. Small wounds without much tissue loss may be managed by irrigation and closure. More extensive disruption of skin, skull, dura, or brain requires surgical management followed by meticulous wound closure or grafting to achieve a watertight closure.

Ninety percent of infections occur within 6 weeks. The major risk factors for meningitis or abscess are wound dehiscence, CSF leaks, or air sinus involvement. Antibiotic prophylaxis seems to lower the infection rate but there is little systematic information as to drug type or duration of treatment. At present, broad-spectrum aerobic and anaerobic coverage is recommended for 7 to 14 days.

Conventional or CT angiography should be performed for most penetrating injuries, particularly when the wound's trajectory passes through or near the sylvian fissure, supraclinoid carotid, cavernous sinus, or a major venous sinus, because of the increased risk of traumatic aneurysm or arteriovenous malformation. Large hematoma or the delayed appearance of subarachnoid blood suggests vascular injury. The time course of development of such lesions is unclear so that repeating the study in a delayed fashion should be entertained in suspicious injuries.

Thirty percent to 50% of patients with penetrating brain injury develop seizures, approximately 10% within the first week and 80% within the first 2 years. At 15 years, approximately half of the patients stop having seizures. Because of these high incidence values, the Guidelines for the Management of Penetrating Brain Injury recommended prophylaxis (eg, phenytoin, carbamazepine, valproate, or phenobarbital) for the first postinjury week. Thereafter, the long-term incidence is not influenced by prophylaxis and the recommendation is to stop medication, restarting it only for proved seizure activity.

References

[1] Chesnut RM, Marshall LF, Klauber MR, et al. The role of secondary brain injury in determining outcome from severe head injury. J Trauma 1993;34:216–22.
[2] Pigula FA, Wald SL, Shackford SR, et al. The effect of hypotension and hypoxia on children with severe head injuries. J Pediatr Surg 1993;28:310–4 [discussion: 315–6].
[3] Jones PA, Andrews PJ, Midgley S, et al. Measuring the burden of secondary insults in head-injured patients during intensive care. J Neurosurg Anesthesiol 1994;6:4–14.
[4] Bullock R, Chesnut R, Clifton G, et al. Guidelines for the management of severe head injury. J Neurotrauma 1996;13:639–734.
[5] Kellie G. An account of the appearances observed in the dissection of two of the three individuals presumed to have perished in the storm of the 3rd, and whose bodies were discovered in the vicinity of Leith on the morning of the 4th November 1821 with some reflections on the pathology of the brain. Trans Med Chir Sci Edinburgh 1824;1:84–169.
[6] Monro A. Observations on the structure and function of the nervous system. Edinburgh: Creech and Johnson; 1783.
[7] Howells T, Elf K, Jones PA, et al. Pressure reactivity as a guide in the treatment of cerebral perfusion pressure in patients with brain trauma. J Neurosurg 2005;102:311–7.
[8] Maset AL, Marmarou A, Ward JD, et al. Pressure-volume index in head injury. J Neurosurg 1987;67:832–40.
[9] Steiner LA, Czosnyka M, Piechnik SK, et al. Continuous monitoring of cerebrovascular pressure reactivity allows determination of optimal cerebral perfusion pressure in patients with traumatic brain injury. Crit Care Med 2002;30:733–8.
[10] Marshall LF, Barba D, Toole BM, et al. The oval pupil: clinical significance and relationship to intracranial hypertension. J Neurosurg 1983;58:566–8.
[11] Lang EW, Chesnut RM. A bedside method for investigating the integrity and critical thresholds of. Br J Neurosurg 2000;14:117–26.
[12] Rosner MJ, Rosner SD, Johnson AH. Cerebral perfusion pressure: management protocol and clinical results. J Neurosurg 1995;83:949–62.
[13] Chesnut RM. Avoidance of hypotension: condition sine qua non of successful severe head-injury management. J Trauma 1997;42(5 Suppl):S4–9.
[14] Cruz J. The first decade of continuous monitoring of jugular bulb oxyhemoglobinsaturation: management strategies and clinical outcome. Crit Care Med 1998;26:344–51.
[15] Juul N, Morris GF, Marshall SB, et al. Intracranial hypertension and cerebral perfusion pressure: influence on neurological deterioration and outcome in severe head injury. The Executive Committee of the International Selfotel Trial. J Neurosurg 2000;92:1–6.

[16] Robertson CS, Valadka AB, Hannay HJ, et al. Prevention of secondary ischemic insults after severe head injury. Crit Care Med 1999;27:2086–95.

[17] Clifton GL, Miller ER, Choi SC, et al. Fluid thresholds and outcome from severe brain injury. Crit Care Med 2002;30:739–45.

[18] Contant CF, Valadka AB, Gopinath SP, et al. Adult respiratory distress syndrome: a complication of induced hypertension after severe head injury. J Neurosurg 2001;95:560–8.

[19] Bullock R, Chesnut RM, Clifton G, et al. Guidelines for the management of severe head injury: revision. J Neurotrauma 2000;17:451–553.

[20] Downard C, Hulka F, Mullins RJ, et al. Relationship of cerebral perfusion pressure and survival in pediatric brain-injured patients. Journal of Trauma-Injury Infection and Critical Care 2000;49:654–8 [discussion: 658–9].

[21] Obrist W, Gennaralli T, Segawa H, et al. Relationship of cerebral blood flow to neurologic status and outcome in head injured patients. J Neurosurg 1979;51:292–300.

[22] Robertson CS, Cormio M. Cerebral metabolic management. New Horizons 1995;3:410–22.

[23] Robertson CS, Contant CF, Gokaslan ZL, et al. Cerebral blood flow, arteriovenous oxygen difference, and outcome in head injured patients. J Neurol Neurosurg Psychiatry 1992;55:594–603.

[24] Robertson CS, Narayan RK, Gokaslan ZL, et al. Cerebral arteriovenous oxygen difference as an estimate of cerebral blood flow in comatose patients [see comments]. J Neurosurg 1989;70:222–30.

[25] Stiefel MF, Spiotta A, Gracias VH, et al. Reduced mortality rate in patients with severe traumatic brain injury treated with brain tissue oxygen monitoring. J Neurosurg 2005;103:805–11.

[26] van den Brink WA, van Santbrink H, Steyerberg EW, et al. Brain oxygen tension in severe head injury. Neurosurgery 2000;46:868–76 [discussion: 876].

[27] Bellander BM, Cantais E, Enblad P, et al. Consensus meeting on microdialysis in neurointensive care. Intensive Care Med 2004;30:2166–9.

[28] Engstrom M, Polito A, Reinstrup P, et al. Intracerebral microdialysis in severe brain trauma: the importance of catheter location. J Neurosurg 2005;102:460–9.

[29] Marion DW, Carlier PM. Problems with initial Glasgow Coma Scale assessment caused by prehospital treatment of patients with head injuries: results of a national survey. J Trauma 1994;36:89–95.

[30] Gabriel EJ, Ghajar J, Jagoda A, et al. Guidelines for prehospital management of traumatic brain injury. J Neurotrauma 2002;19:111–74.

[31] Hsiang JN, Yeung T, Yu AL, et al. High-risk mild head injury. J Neurosurg 1997;87:234–8.

[32] Stein SC, Ross SE. Mild head injury: a plea for routine early CT scanning. J Trauma 1992;33:11–3.

[33] Mendelow AD, Teasdale G, Jennett B, et al. Risks of intracranial haematoma in head injured adults. BMJ 1983;287:1173–6.

[34] Zumkeller M, Behrmann R, Heissler HE, et al. Computed tomographic criteria and survival rate for patients with acute subdural hematoma. Neurosurgery 1996;39:708–12 [discussion: 712].

[35] Servadei F, Murray GD, Teasdale GM, et al. Traumatic subarachnoid hemorrhage: demographic and clinical study of 750 patients from the European brain injury consortium survey of head injuries. Neurosurgery 2002;50:261–7 [discussion: 267].

[36] Harders A, Kakarieka A, Braakman R. Traumatic subarachnoid hemorrhage and its treatment with nimodipine. German tSAH Study Group [see comments]. J Neurosurg 1996;85:82–9.

[37] Martin NA, Doberstein C, Zane C, et al. Posttraumatic cerebral arterial spasm: transcranial Doppler ultrasound, cerebral blood flow, and angiographic findings. J Neurosurg 1992;77:575–83.

[38] Marshall LF, Bowers-Marshall S, Klauber MR, et al. A new classification of head injury based on computerized tomography. J Neurosurg 1991;75:S14–20.

[39] Adelson PD, Bratton SL, Carney NA, et al. Guidelines for the acute medical management of severe traumatic brain injury in infants, children, and adolescents. Pediatr Crit Care Med 2003;4(3 Suppl):S1–71.

[40] Aarabi B, Alden TD, Chesnut RMD, et al. Guidelines for the management of penetrating brain injury. J Trauma 2001;51(2 Suppl):S1–86.

[41] Bullock MR, Chesnut R, Ghajar J, et al. Guidelines for the surgical management of traumatic brain injury. Neurosurgery 2006;58(3 Suppl):S1–60.

[42] Muizelaar JP, Marmarou A, Ward JD, et al. Adverse effects of prolonged hyperventilation in patients with severe head injury: a randomized clinical trial. J Neurosurg 1991;75:731–9.

[43] Vassar MJ, Fischer RP, O'Brien PE, et al. A multicenter trial for resuscitation of injured patients with 7.5% sodium chloride: the effect of added dextran 70. The Multicenter Group for the Study of Hypertonic Saline in Trauma Patients. Arch Surg 1993;128:1003–11 [discussion: 1011].

[44] Vassar MJ, Perry CA, Gannaway WL, et al. 7.5% sodium chloride/dextran for resuscitation of trauma patients undergoing helicopter transport. Arch Surg 1991;126:1065–72.

[45] Vassar MJ, Perry CA, Holcroft JW. Prehospital resuscitation of hypotensive trauma patients with 7.5% NaCl versus 7.5% NaCl with added dextran: a controlled trial. J Trauma 1993;34: 622–32 [discussion: 632].

[46] Wade CE, Grady JJ, Kramer GC, et al. Individual patient cohort analysis of the efficacy of hypertonic saline/dextran in patients with traumatic brain injury and hypotension. J Trauma 1997;42(5 Suppl):S61–5.

[47] Cooper DJ, Myles PS, McDermott FT, et al. Prehospital hypertonic saline resuscitation of patients with hypotension and severe traumatic brain injury: a randomized controlled trial. JAMA 2004;291:1350–7.

[48] Horan MJ, Sinaiko AR. Synopsis of the Report of the Second Task Force on Blood Pressure Control in Children. Hypertension 1987;10:115–21.

[49] Chesnut RM, Gautille T, Blunt BA, et al. Neurogenic hypotension in patients with severe head injuries. J Trauma 1998;44:958–63 [discussion: 963].

[50] Andrews BT, Pitts LH, Lovely MP, et al. Is computed tomographic scanning necessary in patients with tentorial herniation? Results of immediate surgical exploration without computed tomography in 100 patients. Neurosurgery 1986;19:408–14.

[51] Fulton RL, Everman D, Mancino M, et al. Ritual head computed tomography may unnecessarily delay lifesaving trauma care. Surg Gynecol Obstet 1993;176:327–32.

[52] Dutton RP, Lefering R, Lynn M. Database predictors of transfusion and mortality. J Trauma 2006;60(6 Suppl):S70–7.

[53] Hebert PC, Wells G, Blajchman MA, et al. A multicenter, randomized, controlled clinical trial of transfusion requirements in critical care. Transfusion Requirements in Critical Care Investigators, Canadian Critical Care Trials Group. N Engl J Med 1999;340:409–17.

[54] Napolitano L. Cumulative risks of early red blood cell transfusion. J Trauma 2006;60(6 Suppl):S26–34.

[55] Fearnside MR, Cook RJ, McDougall P, et al. The Westmead Head Injury Project. Physical and social outcomes following severe head injury. Br J Neurosurg 1993;7:643–50.

[56] Pietropaoli JA, Rogers FB, Shackford SR, et al. The deleterious effects of intraoperative hypotension on outcome in patients with severe head injuries. J Trauma 1992;33:403–7.

[57] Ghajar J. Intracranial pressure monitoring techniques. New Horizons 1995;3:395–9.

[58] Bouma GJ, Muizelaar JP, Bandoh K, et al. Blood pressure and intracranial pressure-volume dynamics in severe head injury: relationship with cerebral blood flow. J Neurosurg 1992;77: 15–9.

[59] Khanna S, Davis D, Peterson B, et al. Use of hypertonic saline in the treatment of severe refractory posttraumatic intracranial hypertension in pediatric traumatic brain injury [comment]. Crit Care Med 2000;28:1144–51.

[60] Peterson B, Khanna S, Fisher B, et al. Prolonged hypernatremia controls elevated intracranial pressure in head-injured pediatric patients [comment]. Crit Care Med 2000;28:1136–43.

[61] Battison C, Andrews PJ, Graham C, et al. Randomized, controlled trial on the effect of a 20% mannitol solution and a 7.5% saline/6% dextran solution on increased intracranial pressure after brain injury. Crit Care Med 2005;33:196–202 [discussion: 257].

[62] Vialet R, Albanese J, Thomachot L, et al. Isovolume hypertonic solutes (sodium chloride or mannitol) in the treatment of refractory posttraumatic intracranial hypertension: 2 mL/kg 7.5% saline is more effective than 2 mL/kg 20% mannitol. Crit Care Med 2003;31:1683–7.

[63] Ware ML, Nemani VM, Meeker M, et al. Effects of 23.4% sodium chloride solution in reducing intracranial pressure in patients with traumatic brain injury: a preliminary study. Neurosurgery 2005;57:727–36 [discussion: 736].

[64] Wakai A, Roberts I, Schierhout G. Mannitol for acute traumatic brain injury. Cochrane Database Syst Rev 2005;4:CD001049.

[65] Eisenberg H, Frankowski R, Contant C, et al. The Comprehensive Central Nervous System Trauma Centers: high-dose barbiturate control of elevated intracranial pressure in patients with severe head injury. J Neurosurg 1988;69:15–23.

[66] Clifton GL, Miller ER, Choi SC, et al. Lack of effect of induction of hypothermia after acute brain injury. N Engl J Med 2001;344:556–63.

[67] Shiozaki T, Nakajima Y, Taneda M, et al. Efficacy of moderate hypothermia in patients with severe head injury and intracranial hypertension refractory to mild hypothermia. J Neurosurg 2003;99:47–51.

[68] Shiozaki T, Sugimoto H, Taneda M, et al. Effect of mild hypothermia on uncontrollable intracranial hypertension after severe head injury. J Neurosurg 1993;79:363–8.

[69] Ransohoff J, Benjamin MV, Gage ELJ, et al. Hemicraniectomy in the management of acute subdural hematoma. J Neurosurg 1971;34:70–6.

[70] Cooper PR, Rovit RL, Ransohoff J. Hemicraniectomy in the treatment of acute subdural hematoma: a re-appraisal. Surg Neurol 1976;5:25–8.

[71] Gaab MR, Rittierodt M, Lorenz M, et al. Traumatic brain swelling and operative decompression: a prospective investigation. Acta Neurochir Suppl 1990;51:326–8.

[72] Piek J. Decompressive surgery in the treatment of traumatic brain injury. Curr Opin Crit Care 2002;8:134–8.

[73] Schneider GH, Bardt T, Lanksch WR, et al. Decompressive craniectomy following traumatic brain injury: ICP, CPP and neurological outcome. Acta Neurochir Suppl 2002;81: 77–9.

[74] Brodie HA. Prophylactic antibiotics for posttraumatic cerebrospinal fluid fistulae: a meta-analysis. Arch Otolaryngol Head Neck Surg 1997;123:749–52.

[75] Ratilal B, Costa J, Sampaio C. Antibiotic prophylaxis for preventing meningitis in patients with basilar skull fractures. Cochrane Database Syst Rev 2006;1:CD004884.

[76] Fearnside MR, Cook RJ, McDougall P, et al. The Westmead Head Injury Project outcome in severe head injury. A comparative analysis of pre-hospital, clinical and CT variables. Br J Neurosurg 1993;7:267–79.

[77] Seelig JM, Becker DP, Miller JD, et al. Traumatic acute subdural hematoma: major mortality reduction in comatose patients treated within four hours. N Engl J Med 1981;304:1511–8.

ELSEVIER
SAUNDERS

SURGICAL
CLINICS OF
NORTH AMERICA

Surg Clin N Am 87 (2007) 157–184

Lessons Learned from Modern Military Surgery

Alec C. Beekley, MD*, Benjamin W. Starnes, MD,
James A. Sebesta, MD

*US Army Medical Corps, Madigan Army Medical Center, 9040 Fitzsimmons Avenue,
Fort Lewis, WA 98431, USA*

The terrorist attacks of September 11, 2001 on the United States marked the beginning of the "Global War on Terror." The United States military responded with the first massive deployment of troops from all branches of service since the Persian Gulf War of 1991. Unlike that conflict, in which prewar casualty estimates far exceeded the actual number of casualties sustained, Operations Iraqi and Enduring Freedom have generated casualties in the largest numbers the United States military has sustained since the Vietnam War. As of June 23, 2006, a total of 18,572 United States military personnel have been wounded in Operation Iraqi Freedom, and another 773 have been wounded in Operation Enduring Freedom. Of these 19,345 casualties, 8975 of them have been wounded seriously enough to warrant evacuation out of the theaters of operations. In addition, 2511 soldiers or Department of Defense civilians have been killed in Operation Iraqi Freedom; 528 of these deaths were from non-hostile causes. An additional 302 personnel have been killed in and around Afghanistan [1].

The collection of combat casualty data from these operations has resulted in the largest combat trauma database in existence, dubbed the Joint Theater Trauma Registry (JTTR). Data from deployed medical and surgical units are pooled in a central databank at the United States Army Institute of Surgical Research at Brooke Army Medical Center in San Antonio. These data are currently being linked across three continents so that casualty data from point of injury to ultimate outcome in stateside military

---

The views expressed in this paper are those of the authors and do not reflect the official policy or position of the Department of the Army, the Department of Defense, or the United States Government.

* Corresponding author.
E-mail address: alec.beekley@amedd.army.mil (A.C. Beekley).

medical facilities can be tracked. The logistic, administrative, and technical hurdles involved in this undertaking are obviously enormous, and the process and ease by which individual casualties or groups can be tracked is still somewhat cumbersome. Nevertheless, data analysis and actionable research findings continue to be generated from this extraordinary set of trauma data.

The evolution of a streamlined trauma system in the theaters of operations [2], the introduction of an in-theater institution review board process, and dedicated personnel to collect combat casualty data have resulted in improved data capture and real-time, on-the-scene research (personal communication, John B. Holcomb, MD COL, US Army Medical Corps, 2006). The result has been the generation of a tremendous body of research on multiple facets of combat casualty care; only a handful of topics are touched on in the current article.

This article first identifies how new or improved devices, dressing, or drugs have impacted prehospital care of casualties, and how prehospital triage guidelines and resuscitation strategies have been changed. The second section focuses on lessons learned at the level of surgical care of combat casualties, and how these concepts are crossing back into civilian practice and training initiatives. The authors conclude with a brief look at the future of combat casualty and, by extension, civilian trauma patient care.

Prehospital devices, dressings, and drugs

Improved helmets and body armor

There is overwhelming evidence that most survivable war injuries since the beginning of recorded time have been predominantly extremity injuries. This observation remains true of the current conflict [3]. Truncal injuries in prior conflicts carried an initial high mortality rate and many casualties did not survive to receive surgical treatment. Lethality of truncal injuries and effectiveness of modern body armor predict that a thorough understanding of the management of extremity injury to include complex vascular repair is paramount for successful outcome in most cases. The Israeli Trauma Group evaluated 669 recent terror-related firearm injuries and found that not only did body armor have a protective effect against high-velocity gunshot wounds but it also reduced the actual severity of injuries sustained to the chest and abdomen [4]. Current operational security restrictions prohibit detailed discussion of modern United States military body armor and resultant changes in wound patterns. Nevertheless, already published data suggest that because of the effectiveness of body armor, distinct new patterns of combat injuries are being encountered [5–7].

The combat casualty often presents to a treatment area with full body armor and armed with weapons or other ordnance, which may have been carried by the soldier or may be embedded in tissue (Figs. 1 and 2). Knowledge

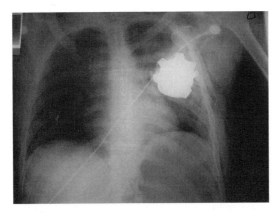

Fig. 1. Portable AP chest radiograph of patient who was hit during a firefight. The radiograph generated initial concern regarding the possibility that the patient had unexploded ordnance in his chest.

in the safe removal of this body armor and safe disarmament and storage of weapons and ordnance remains of paramount importance in protecting the casualty and the health care provider from grave injury. All United States military body armor has favorable photon attenuation characteristics. When medically advantageous, patients wearing standard military body armor can be examined radiographically with standard plain films or computed tomography [8].

Tourniquets

Prehospital tourniquet use, at times a matter of debate in trauma circles [9,10], plays a central role in hemorrhage control on the modern battlefield. Data from Bellamy's [11] landmark paper on causes of death on the modern

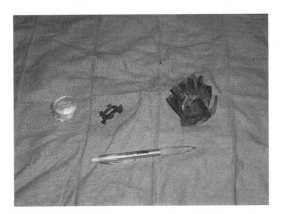

Fig. 2. Operation revealed tail-piece fragments from an explosive munition.

battlefield demonstrated that 9% of soldiers killed in action during the Vietnam War died of extremity hemorrhage. Initial evaluation of those killed in action in Iraq demonstrates a similar rate of soldiers dying from compressible extremity hemorrhage [12].

Analysis of casualties who arrived at a single combat support hospital (CSH) in Iraq with major vascular injuries or traumatic amputations treated with prehospital tourniquets demonstrated significantly improved hemorrhage control over those casualties who did not have prehospital tourniquets applied for the same injuries [13]. Although no survival benefit of tourniquets was identified in this data set (the data are notably biased to those casualties who survived to reach the CSH), analysis of the seven soldiers who did die of their wounds in this data set found that four of the deaths potentially could have been prevented if properly applied tourniquets had been used. Anecdotal reports of soldiers dying from hemorrhage from isolated extremity wounds potentially amenable to tourniquets have been published in national media outlets [14]. Finally, average prehospital tourniquet time was only 70 minutes, and no complications directly related to tourniquet use (secondary amputation, peripheral nerve injury) were identified in this group of patients.

The results of the cause of death analyses from the Vietnam War and Operation Iraqi Freedom, combined with the early experience described above, have resulted in fielding of individual tourniquets to each soldier. As of August 2005, more than 275,000 tourniquets had been deployed overseas to combat theaters (personal communication, John B. Holcomb, MD, COL, US Army Medical Corps, 2005) Current military doctrine mandates use of a tourniquet as a first-line treatment for casualties who have extremity hemorrhage when care is administered under hostile fire. Once the casualties are removed from hostile fire, the need for the tourniquet may be reassessed to determine if a lesser form of hemorrhage control (eg, a pressure dressing) would be sufficient [15]. In practice, this doctrine has resulted in many casualties arriving to a level of surgical care with tourniquets in place for extremity injuries, even when subsequent evaluation revealed that the tourniquets were not necessary (personal communication, Matthew J. Martin, MD, LTC, US Army Medical Corps, 2006). This current doctrine and the resulting liberal practical application are similar to those described by Lakstein and colleagues [16] in the Israeli Defense Forces study on prehospital tourniquet use. In the Israeli experience, 47% of tourniquets applied subsequently were deemed non-indicated.

The substantial number of casualties arriving to hospitals with prehospital tourniquets has provided lessons for surgeons treating these casualties. First, casualties who sustained traumatic amputations, mangled extremities, or major vascular injuries may have had substantial hemorrhage before first responder treatment and tourniquet application. Bleeding may have slowed or stopped spontaneously because of hypotension combined with vessel spasm and retraction. The cues the medic looks for to know if a tourniquet has been tightened enough (cessation of bright red bleeding) may not be present, or the pressure required to stop arterial bleeding may not be very high. The tourniquets thus may not be tight enough to control hemorrhage once resuscitation begins and higher blood pressures are restored. An only venous tourniquet can lead to more rapid exsanguination, which may not be noted immediately by providers if the patient is covered by blankets, warming devices, or surgical drapes. To prevent this rebleeding phenomenon, our practice is to bring pneumatic tourniquets from the OR to the ER and immediately replace a patient's field tourniquets with pneumatic tourniquets. We also recommended that surgical units' emergency bays stock pneumatic tourniquets so they are available immediately if needed.

Second, current military prehospital doctrine and training now emphasize that casualties who have hemorrhage control, normal mentation, and stable vital signs (even mild hypotension, or systolic blood pressure at 90), should have intravenous access established in the field but fluid administration withheld or minimized [17]. Casualties who have abnormal mental status, signs of intracranial injury, or profound hypotension are administered fluids, although in certain instances (eg, mass casualty situations) these casualties may be triaged into an expectant category. The practice of permissive hypotension is designed to decrease the incidence of rebleeding from quiescent or partially controlled hemorrhage sites. Receiving physicians must be aware that casualties may have received little or no resuscitation. Our strategy in patients who have proximal or multiple tourniquets, who present with hypotension, is to initiate a massive transfusion protocol emphasizing hemostatic products and early use of fresh whole blood. This strategy is discussed in greater detail later in this article.

Finally, the liberalized use of tourniquets must be studied to ensure that tourniquet-related ischemic or neurologic injuries are not occurring at unacceptably high rates, particularly in those patients on whom tourniquet use was retrospectively identified as unnecessary. Our series demonstrated no ischemic or peripheral neurologic injuries that could be related clearly to tourniquet use. The assessment of the causative factors for ischemia and peripheral neurologic deficits can be difficult in these patients because frequently adjacent nerves along with major vascular structures are injured by the wounding agent.

Hemostatic dressings

Hemostatic dressings are designed to treat battlefield injuries to proximal vascular structures not amenable to tourniquet control but nevertheless compressible with manual pressure. This type of proximal vascular injury was graphically illustrated in the film *Black Hawk Down*, in a scene with medics attempting to control bleeding from a soldier's transected external iliac/common femoral artery in a dark field environment. The scene demonstrated the success of direct manual pressure and the difficulty of attempting to place surgical clamps on the bleeding vessel without appropriate lighting, anesthesia, and retraction. This event and others like it have guided research toward advanced dressings that could be applied to such a wound in a similar fashion to standard dressings but would have hemostatic products incorporated in the dressing to enhance or augment the body's own clotting mechanisms.

Although multiple products are available on the market, two products have been deployed by the United States military in large numbers into battlefield settings. These two products are zeolite (QuikClot, Z-Medica Corporation) and chitosan (HemCon, HemCon Hemorrhage Control Technologies, Inc.). The choice to deploy these products was based on their relative ease in application, portability, durability, and demonstrated success in controlling hemorrhage in animal models.

Zeolite, a granular mineral-based product, causes an exothermic reaction when exposed to water or blood, thereby concentrating blood-clotting factors and accelerating hemostasis [18,19]. Compared with standard gauze dressings, zeolite has been demonstrated to provide superior hemostasis, decreased blood loss, and decreased resuscitation requirements in several animal injury models, including a grade V liver injury [20] and a lethal groin injury model in swine [21]. Currently, only anecdotal reports regarding its use in humans exist [22], although a clinical series of casualties who had zeolite used on their wounds on modern battlefields has been collected and is being prepared for publication (personal communication, Matthew J. Martin, MD, LTC, US Army Medical Corps, 2006). Several concerns have been raised regarding the amount of heat generated by the dressing [22] and its stability during movement and transport of casualties. As a result, the company that produces QuikClot has recently marketed a product that contains the zeolite granules inside a gauze sack that is applied to the wound rather than pouring the free zeolite granules themselves into the wound [23,24]. As this product evolves it will require continued evaluation in carefully controlled animal studies and review of clinical uses in prehospital and hospital settings.

Another hemostatic product currently deployed in battlefield settings is the chitosan-based hemostatic dressing, HemCon. Chitosan is a nontoxic, biodegradable, complex carbohydrate derivative of chitin, a naturally occurring substance. In its acid salt form, chitosan has mucoadhesive properties that augment hemostasis [25]. The current deployed dressing product is lightweight and flexible and has no special storage requirements. It comes in a package similar to other standard dressings and can be opened rapidly and applied to a wound. It has a nonadhesive surface on the inactive side of the dressing to avoid sticking to the care provider's gloves, hands, or other standard gauze dressings and dislodging. Both the liquid forms of chitosan and the dressing that has been deployed in battlefield settings have demonstrated superiority in hemorrhage control over standard dressings in multiple animal models [26–28]. In addition, Wedmore and colleagues [29] recently reported on the use of chitosan-based hemostatic dressings (Hem-Con) in 64 patients in a combat casualty setting. In 66% of these uses, chitosan dressings were used after standard gauze had failed and the chitosan dressings were successful 100% of the time. In 62 cases (97%), use of the chitosan dressing resulted in cessation of bleeding or improved hemostasis. The two failures of the chitosan dressings occurred in patients who had large cavitational wounds in which the bleeding sites were multiple or in which the chitosan was placed blindly into the cavity [29]. Anecdotal reports from medics and observations during live tissue training revealed similar pitfalls in the use of HemCon dressing. Like QuikClot, these limitations include rebleeding with resuscitation or dislodging of the dressing during transport of the casualty.

Overall, the animal injury models and early clinical experience demonstrate a clear superiority of these dressings over standard gauze dressings in providing hemorrhage control, particularly in injuries not amenable to tourniquet use. Further study and refinement of these dressings is necessary and ongoing.

Needle thoracostomy

In a review of the Vietnam Wound Data and Munitions Effectiveness Team study, tension pneumothorax was found to be the cause of death in 3% to 4% of fatal combat wounds [30]. In this review, 15 of the 26 casualties who had tension pneumothorax survived long enough to receive first aid from a medic or other medical personnel. These data confirm the need for proper training of medics and other care providers in early echelons of care to prevent these deaths. The use of needle thoracostomy in urban trauma systems has come under fire recently by some who believe that it is overused and ineffective [31–34]. This belief should not be applied to combat situations in which the most common mechanism of trauma is penetrating injuries. In addition, tactical situations and other factors may delay transportation of these patients to treatment facilities capable of diagnosing and definitively treating the tension pneumothorax.

Medics throughout the army are trained to identify and treat a tension pneumothorax. In the combat environment, however, the identification of a tension pneumothorax in the field may be nearly impossible. Most of the casualties have body armor that covers the entire chest and neck and surrounding noise prevents any possibility of auscultation of breath sounds. Medics are instructed to treat any patient who is hypotensive and has chest injury with needle thoracostomy. In addition to the standard placement of a needle in the second or third intercostal space, midclavicular line, medics are also taught to place a needle one hand's width below the axilla in the midaxillary line. This position allows placement without having to remove the soldier's body armor. This is also the thinnest area of the chest, which may prevent improper placement because of inadequate catheter length.

To date, there are no published combat outcomes related to the use of needle thoracostomy or complications recorded.

Intraosseous access

Acute hemorrhage is the leading cause of battlefield deaths in modern warfare, accounting for more than 50% of fatalities [11]. Standard resuscitation of casualties involves the variable administration of fluids or blood products to sustain blood pressure and perfusion of vital organs until hemorrhage can be arrested. More often than not, casualties presenting in overt shock have difficult intravenous access and a more technically demanding surgical venous cut-down is required. Some data suggest that the placement of an intravenous line in a trauma patient in a moving ambulance takes 10 to 12 minutes and has a 10% to 40% failure rate [35]. Translation of these ideal circumstances into a combat situation adds the complexity of a tactically hostile environment often in the dark of night with the need for extreme light discipline. Standard intravenous access often can seem nearly impossible under these circumstances.

Drinker and colleagues [36] introduced the concept of intraosseous infusion in 1922 as a result of a study of circulation of the sternum. Intraosseous vascular access devices are reemerging as an important field treatment option in a military setting [37–39]. Commonplace in the management of civilian pediatric trauma, the advantages of intraosseous infusion over conventional means of vascular access are ease and rapidity of insertion (114 seconds or less in one study [39]) and ability to infuse large amounts of either saline or colloid until better vascular access can be obtained. The adult sternum has distinct advantages as an intraosseous infusion site. The sternum is usually easy to expose in trauma patients and the cortical bone and marrow space are uniform, resisting collapse of the vascular space in the face of shock [38]. Johnson and coworkers [38] recently evaluated the First Access for Shock and Trauma system (Pyng Medical Corp., Vancouver, Canada) in 106 cadavers and found infusion rates of greater than 100 mL/min for either saline or colloid solutions. Rates of up to 250 mL/min could be delivered with single syringe infusion. In this study, a liter of fluid could be infused in less than 10 minutes and insertion force was similar to that of other devices at a mean of 8.5 kg. This system relied on the authors' finding that the thickest part of the manubrium was routinely in the midline of the sternum 15 mm below the sternal notch and this became the preferred insertion site [38].

Other infusion sites are possible and include the adult tibia, femur, iliac crest, humerus, radius, and clavicle [38]. These sites in adults have a large portion of the less vascular yellow marrow, which is inferior to the sternum regarding infusion rates. The entire concept of intraosseous infusion is extremely attractive in a combat setting given the potential number of casualties and long evacuation times, allowing for a stretching of the envelope of resuscitation when minutes are a matter of life and death because of exsan-guinating hemorrhage.

Pain medications and antibiotics by medics

Effective analgesia is an essential part of casualty management. Fewer options exist for relief of pain in a combat situation than in routine civilian medical care. Before the current conflict in Iraq, several Special Operations physicians instituted a protocol of providing each soldier with a wound pack of oral medications containing acetaminophen, rofecoxib, and a fluoroqui-nolone. Soldiers were instructed to take these medications if wounded to decrease the level of pain and potentially reduce the potential for wound in-fections in a battlefield environment [40]. Historically, morphine has been administered on the battlefield by way of auto-injectors (10–20 mg intra-muscularly) to relieve severe pain [41]. Limitations of intramuscular mor-phine administration revolve around uncertain rates of absorption. Intravenous morphine provides for rapid pain relief but requires the inser-tion of a simple intravenous catheter, which often may be delayed by tactical requirements. With newer availability of oral transmucosal fentanyl citrate or "fentanyl lollipops," up to 1600 μg of fentanyl may be self-administered by a casualty and provide rapid analgesia. Only 25% of the drug is absorbed by the oral mucosa and the remainder is absorbed through the gastrointes-tinal tract [42]. Kotwal and colleagues [42] described the use of fentanyl lol-lipops on 22 casualties from Operation Iraqi Freedom. Side effects were few but did include nausea and vomiting, suggesting that an antiemetic may be of benefit for simultaneous administration. Advantages of this analgesic technique include the ability of the casualty to titrate to effect. When ade-quate pain relief is assumed, the soldier can remove the lollipop from his mouth.

Other evolving techniques of battlefield analgesia involve the concept of continuous peripheral nerve block (CPNB). This technique was successfully used by Buckenmaier and coworkers [43] to treat a severely injured soldier's extremity in the current conflict. The technique involves simultaneous con-tinuous lumbar plexus block and sciatic nerve block. Standard epidural catheters are inserted in juxtaposition to the relevant neural plexus after first localizing the nerve with 0.5 mA or less of current transmitted through a pe-ripheral nerve stimulator. The lumbar plexus and sciatic catheters are then infused first with 1% lidocaine as a test dose followed by infusion of 0.2% ropivacaine at 6 mL/hr and 10 mL/hr, respectively [43]. The catheters placed in Iraq were maintained for 16 days without signs or symptoms of infection. Unfortunately, the soldier eventually required below-knee amputation be-cause of ischemic compromise from his war wound. The authors recom-mend exercising caution with the use of CPNB for potentially ischemic extremities as it may cloud examination findings consistent with an advanc-ing compartment syndrome.

Antibiotics have advanced the successful management of war wounds. Since 1943, when systemic penicillin was introduced onto the battlefield, the risk for wound myonecrosis and gas gangrene has decreased dramatically [44]. Although a useful adjunct, antibiotic treatment cannot replace adequate debridement of devitalized and dead tissue from a war wound. Timing of antibiotic therapy is critical. In an extensive review of the value of antibiotics on the battlefield, Konrad Hell stated in 1991 [45]:

> For prophylaxis for wound sepsis, a single injection of a long-acting, broad-spectrum antibiotic should be given as soon as possible after injury. It should remain at sufficiently high levels in tissues for 24 hours, or over the whole period of risk of infection from the moment of injury until surgical debridement is completed.

Hell suggested that this antibiotic be ceftriaxone; however, today armed forces carry an oral fluoroquinolone for self-administration.

Complications from antibiotic therapy for war wounds also are well described. Current casualty statistics reveal an increased incidence of war wound infection and osteomyelitis, especially caused by multi-drug–resistant *Acinetobacter* species [46]. In fact, many military treatment facilities have reported dramatic increases in the rate of multi-drug–resistant *Acinetobacter* infections. Treatment aimed at these infections poses considerable challenges and at many military treatment facilities involves dual therapy with Imipenem (500 mg every 6 hr) in combination with high-dose Amikacin (15–20 mg/kg daily) [46]. Recent investigation by the military medical community suggests that these are nosocomial infections; however, their exact source remains unclear (Fig. 3).

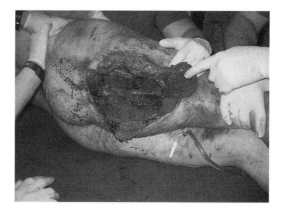

Fig. 3. Casualty who had severe contamination with mud and dirt from fragment wounds. Patients such as this are at high risk for infection even with aggressive surgical debridement and broad-spectrum antibiotic use. (Courtesy of Lowell W. Chambers, MD, Westerville, Ohio.)

Hextend

Hextend (BioTime, Inc) has replaced lactated Ringer as the fluid carried by medics in the field. It is storable at room temperature and has no recommended refrigeration requirements. Hextend is a hydroxyethyl starch in a solution of electrolytes, physiologic levels of glucose, and a lactate buffer. It is believed to provide a more favorable acid–base balance compared with other colloids. It has been shown to reduce resuscitative fluid requirements [47]. Hextend is effective in hypotensive resuscitations and potentially has a benefit as the sole resuscitation fluid after severe traumatic brain injury by reducing fluid requirements and eliminating the need for mannitol without affecting the coagulation profile [48].

Hypothermia prevention

Hypothermia is a significant problem in the management of combat casualties. In a recent review of combat injuries, Arthurs and colleagues [49] showed that 18% of combat casualties presented to the 31st CSH hypothermic (temperature $< 36°C$). The presence of hypothermia was an independent predictor of operative management, damage control procedures, factor VIIa use, and mortality. Temperature less than 34°C was associated with nearly 100% mortality. It also was associated with longer operative times, larger blood loss, and an increase in blood product requirement. Prevention of hypothermia before arrival to the upper echelon of care is critical and is emphasized at every level of care. At the lowest echelons, medics are trained to treat and prevent hypothermia after addressing ongoing hemorrhage, airway, and breathing problems. This is performed initially by limiting exposure of the patient to areas being treated and then completely covering the patient with blankets or solar blankets. Permissive hypotension is integral in limiting the amounts of cold fluids given to a casualty. In patients who require resuscitation, fluid warming devices, such as the Thermal Angel (Estill Medical Technologies, Inc., Dallas, Texas), can be used. The Thermal Angel is a portable battery-operated fluid warmer. It is disposable and requires no additional parts except for a standard infusion set. The most effective use of this device would probably be during transportation between echelons of care. The battery makes the unit heavy and limits its ability to be carried by medics in the field. In testing, the Thermal Angel was more effective at warming Hextend than lactate Ringer and it was not able to fully rewarm refrigerated fluids [50]. It was able to raise the temperature of Hextend an average of 14.8°C when starting at room temperature. In fixed treatment facilities, larger more effective fluid warmers are used. Additional techniques that have been effective in preventing hypothermia are the use of damage control procedures at forward surgical units and rapid transportation of the patient to higher echelons of care. A body bag is an effective transportation enclosure for patients that can reduce the loss of heat. Casualties are placed in the bag and covered with blankets. A hole is cut for the patient's face and for fluid access. The bag is closed, leaving only the face of the patient exposed, and then placed on a stretcher for transportation.

Prehospital concepts

Prehospital provider triage guidelines

Triage is a dynamic process that occurs at many levels of care, including the battlefield, battalion aid station, and the level of initial surgical care. For prehospital providers, it is particularly important to have a quick and reliable means of establishing priority of casualties not only for field care but also for order of evacuation on helicopters or ambulances. For this purpose, the traditional categories of immediate, delayed, minimal, and expectant casualties still apply. The definitions of these categories are well established elsewhere [51]. More critical are the training and means by which prehospital providers sort patients into these categories. Recent data demonstrate that manual vital signs and verbal and motor scores of the Glasgow Coma Scale (GCS) are as reliable as more sophisticated monitoring at identifying the need for life-saving interventions [52]. Medics and other prehospital personal are taught to assess radial pulse character and the GCS motor score; those patients who have a strong radial pulse character and a GCS motor score of 6 are triaged to a lower category of urgency. Obviously, patients who have signs of impending or actual airway compromise, uncontrolled hemorrhage, weak radial pulse or decreased mental status without head injury; patients who have penetrating or blunt injuries of the trunk, neck, head, or pelvis; and patients who have multiple long bone fractures are assumed to be unstable and require triage into an immediate category [51].

Permissive hypotension (in prehospital setting)

In 2003, COL John B. Holcomb [53] described the evolution of the term "hypotensive resuscitation" in a paper entitled, "Fluid Resuscitation in Modern Combat Casualty Care: Lessons Learned from Somalia". The recommended consensus algorithm for resuscitation of combat casualties is one that all military medical personnel should familiarize themselves with before deployment into a combat theater. In 1994, Bickell and colleagues [54] described a no-fluid resuscitation protocol in hypotensive patients after penetrating truncal injuries and concluded that traditional rapid fluid resuscitation significantly decreased survival in these patients. This study was the impetus for a drastic change in philosophy regarding management of an injured soldier on the battlefield and has been adopted by American Military [53,55,56] and Israeli Defense Forces [57].

Small volume resuscitation helps compensate for logistic problems in providing enough fluid on the battlefield to resuscitate a casualty adequately. Combat medics can only carry so much weight and still be effective.

Hypertonic saline dextran or HSD (7.5% NaCl/6% dextran-70) is an effective resuscitation fluid when used in small volumes [58]. The combination of intraosseous infusion and small volume resuscitation in line with the theme of hypotensive resuscitation are attractive and synergistic concepts for arming military first responders with the tools they need to save lives. Studies evaluating the efficacy of these synergistic modalities are currently underway.

Much remains to be elucidated regarding the concept of permissive hypotension. It currently is not known whether permissive hypotension would increase the incidence of late complications resulting from incomplete resuscitation [58]. It must be remembered that permissive hypotension is absolutely contraindicated in the setting of traumatic brain injury because of a resultant severe cerebral hypoperfusion with a potentially catastrophic outcome [59].

Casualty evacuation

Because of tactical situations, the combat casualty often presents to a forward surgical team (FST) or CSH several hours after the injury occurred. Prolonged evacuation time has long been a criticism of casualty care within the combat zone. Incoming fire, the need for light discipline in darkness, and other environmental factors have a profound impact on evacuation times. Military objectives remain to treat casualties in the field, prevent additional casualties, and complete the intended mission. Other than well-planned and executed evacuation routes and mass casualty exercises, there is little that will effect an improvement on evacuation times in a combat zone. This remains a reason to train combat medics, who often accompany these casualties during evacuation, in advanced techniques of resuscitation to include proper control of exsanguinating hemorrhage from wounded extremities.

Casualty evacuation (CASEVAC) can apply to injured soldiers or civilians and is used to denote the emergency evacuation of injured people from a war zone. CASEVAC can be accomplished by ground or air, the latter being done almost exclusively by helicopter. CASEVAC aircraft are not equipped with specific life saving equipment or specially trained medical personnel. Their primary purpose is to ferry personnel from the battlefield to the nearest appropriate medical facility available as quickly as possible. They are permitted to be armed and the pilots and crews often assume much more risk to their plane and crew to evacuate wounded personnel.

Standards for intra-theater medical evacuation are well established and routinely proceed in a unidirectional fashion from point of injury to the third echelon of care, typically a CSH [60–62]. Success of this system depends in large part on the maturity of the combat theater. In the early phases of a conflict, evacuation patterns are not well established and the Army FSTs at level 2 play a crucial role [63]. In 1997, Mattox [64] stated that the success of any forward deployed combat casualty management system relied on "qualified first responders," continuing care during secondary transport, and optimization of practical tele-medical technology. In reality, a large proportion of casualties presenting to a CSH do not follow standard routes of evacuation. A large number of casualties may be brought in by unit members in armored vehicles or HUMVEES or on flatbed trucks by local nationals, or simply walk in with significant penetrating injury.

Some authors have identified current military en route care as "not ideal," especially in an immature theater where precious personnel and resources are consumed during transport [63]. The current authors express concern over the existing intra-theater medical evacuation system. Rotary wing transport is space constrained and allows limited capacity for en route management of the acutely injured patient. In the authors' experiences, incidences occurred in which a casualty was stabilized at level 2, transported to level 3 by rotary wing, and arrived either in extremis or dead. In-flight monitoring is available but limited because of light discipline and other factors in a typically hostile environment. After-action reviews involving helicopter crews and receiving medical personnel for the purpose of quality and performance improvement are nearly impossible because of the rapid pace and high demands helicopter crews face. Fixed-wing aircraft, although more cumbersome and resource intensive, offer the unique advantage of allowing for general anesthesia and open surgery in flight as described by Peoples and coworkers in 2005 [65]. The intra-theater medical evacuation system, although vastly improved from prior conflicts, is in need of essential improvements to maximize casualty care during secondary transport.

Hospital care: concepts

Triage and evaluation of casualties at the level of surgical care

The manner in which triage was performed at the level of surgical care depended on the physical layout of the treatment facility, the provision of adequate shelter for casualties, and the primary means by which casualties arrived to the facility. Several CSHs regularly received incoming rocket and mortar fire, which on several occasions impacted the structures or the immediate surrounding areas. Creating an unprotected triage area outside the emergency department bay thus was not feasible. In addition, the casualties rarely arrived in large groups, but instead trickled in off multiple helicopter or ground transport vehicles in groups of two to eight patients. Gaining an overview of the entire group of patients before engaging in treatment in a given mass casualty event was difficult.

A rapid assessment using simple manual physical examination parameters, such as GCS and radial pulse character, was again used to sort casualties into three general categories: emergent, non-emergent, and expectant. A single experienced surgeon was designated as the sole triage officer and directed casualties into the main trauma bay if deemed emergent and into a secondary bay if deemed non-emergent. The triage officer assigned a trauma team, lead by a staff general surgeon, to each emergent casualty. Remaining general surgeons and orthopaedic surgeons would evaluate the non-emergent casualties who had been directed to the secondary emergency bay. As predicted in the latest edition of the War Surgery Manual, only 10% to 20% of arriving casualties would require immediate life-saving interventions. Ambulatory patients who had minor injuries were directed out of the immediate emergency department area to an outpatient clinic area for further assessment.

Casualties were systematically evaluated by the trauma team leader. In the setting of multiple casualties, a portable ultrasound machine to perform focused abdominal sonography for trauma (FAST) was used as a triage and evaluation tool. In unstable patients who had multisystem injuries, a positive FAST directed the surgeon to the operating room for exploration of the abdomen. In stable patients, a positive FAST allowed prioritization of patients going for further imaging using a CT scan. In patients arriving to one CSH after being injured by enemy fire, 3% had a reported motor vehicle crash or other blunt mechanism (eg, fall) as a secondary mechanism after the attack. In at least four of these instances in the authors' experiences, the blunt injury was the one that required surgical intervention.

Negative FAST examination was demonstrated to be unreliable in the authors' experiences, and hence patients with penetrating abdominal, flank, back, and buttock wounds who were hemodynamically stable and had a negative FAST underwent CT scan of the abdomen and pelvis. The presence of intra-abdominal or retroperitoneal fragments generally prompted exploratory laparotomy. Patients without penetration of the peritoneum or retroperitoneum were successfully managed nonoperatively in most cases [66].

Treatment of truncal injuries: damage control

The use of damage control techniques is essential in the management of the combat casualty. Casualties of modern warfare suffer massive tissue injury created by high-velocity weapons and improvised explosive devices (IED). The IED commonly damages patients with a combination of burns, amputation, penetrating, blunt, and inhalation injuries. High-velocity bullets or fragments that penetrate and cross the abdomen or pelvis create devastating injuries involving fractures, bowel, urologic, neurologic, and vascular systems. Tactical situations may delay the treatment and transportation of the patients, resulting in additional blood and heat losses. The constellation of injuries, evacuation times, and limited resources in the face of multiple casualties made damage control techniques essential to avoid physiologic burnout in severely injured patients.

In the experience of one CSH, 92 damage control procedures were performed on patients of all ages. This figure represented nearly 30% of all initial laparotomies. Damage control was the default procedure for casualties who had multiple injuries, and only if the patient's physiologic status remained stable or improved during the procedure would definitive procedures be performed. The use of damage control surgery was based on the number and types of injuries per patient, the physiologic status of the patient (ie, pH, temperature, and base deficit), and the types and numbers of patients waiting for surgery. A patient who required multiple procedures, such as laparotomy followed by intracranial or major vascular procedures, would have damage control procedures to temporize the abdominal injuries to allow a more rapid intervention on the other wounds. Forward surgical units performed damage control procedures and then promptly evacuated patients to higher echelons, such as the CSH, where more robust treatment capabilities were available. Second-look procedures occurred between 12 and 24 hours but could be performed as soon as the patient's physiologic status had improved. Patients required an average of 3.4 procedures and 77% of those that survived had definitive treatment of their injuries and closure of the abdomen at the CSH. The ability to transport critically injured patients out of the theater, including patients who had open abdomens after the initial damage control procedures, was routinely available. This transportation before definitive repair may be associated with higher complication rates, including failure to close the abdomen. If the patient remained in-theater, the average time to closure was 3.3 days. The overall survival was 72.8% and patients who had damage-control surgery at forward surgical units had a similar outcome of 66.6% survival.

Treatment of vascular injury in the field: damage control

The phrase "damage control" implies a rescue situation in which prevention of further injury is achieved. When applied to extremity vascular injuries, damage control is defined as control of exsanguinating hemorrhage, rapid restoration of blood flow to an ischemic limb and prevention of compartment syndrome. When dealing with the multiply injured patient, limb salvage may be a secondary priority or not a priority at all, depending on the physiologic status of the patient [67]. Pneumatic tourniquets, mentioned previously in this article, have proven invaluable in the combat setting [68]. When appropriately applied, they may serve as a proximal vascular clamp until definitive repair, damage control with rapid placement of an indwelling shunt, or debridement amputation can be performed (Fig. 4).

Shunts

Temporary intraluminal shunts allow for rapid restoration of blood flow to an ischemic limb while other procedures to include wound debridement, external fixation of fractures, or more life saving procedures such as trauma laparotomy or thoracotomy can be accomplished [69–71]. Shunts may be placed easily and rapidly after proximal vascular control with either

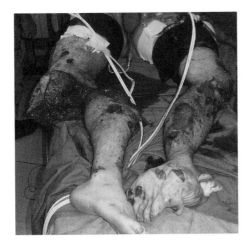

Fig. 4. Pneumatic tourniquets placed in emergency room for patient who had bilateral mangled lower extremities and traumatic amputations.

a pneumatic tourniquet or vascular clamp, and secured in place with Rummel tourniquets or simple silk ties to prevent dislodgement. After placement, patency should be confirmed with intraoperative continuous wave Doppler of the shunt. The authors recommend the specific use of Sundt shunts because their design minimizes risk for dislodgement when appropriately inserted. The Sundt shunt (Integra Lifesciences Corp., Plainsboro, New Jersey) is lined with an inner coil to prevent kinking or collapse. There is one small area within the shunt of discontinuous coils that should be used for clamping if needed. Clamping the shunt in any other location will crush the coil and occlude the shunt.

In a damage control setting in the far forward arena, an appropriately placed shunt can provide enough distal blood flow to perfuse a severely injured extremity until definitive repair can be performed at the CSH or, in some special situations, after strategic evacuation out-of-theater. We emphasize that most casualties who have shunts in place should be evacuated over short distances between facilities in-theater only, such as from the site of injury to an FST or CSH, or from FST to CSH. Casualties may have multiple injuries with associated coagulopathy, thus reducing the need for systemic heparinization [70]. The use of heparin in this setting is controversial, however, as some early reports from Operation Iraqi Freedom report that shunts that were inserted on the battlefield had clotted during tactical evacuation back to the CSH (47th CSH personal communication from MAJ Jerome McDonald, 2005). We emphasize the use of systemic heparinization in stable patients. Once the patient is evacuated to a facility where definitive repair can be performed, wound debridement and orthopedic repair is initiated first followed by vascular reconstruction.

Fasciotomy

One of the most important factors in managing the acutely injured extremity on the battlefield is the liberal use of fasciotomy to avoid or treat compartment syndrome [72]. A thorough understanding of the technique of fasciotomy for upper and lower extremities along with feet and hands must be possessed by a member of the surgical team. Principles for performance of fasciotomy in the lower extremity include two long skin incisions; at least 15 cm, on the medial and lateral aspect of each wounded extremity. Indications for fasciotomy in a combat zone are listed in Box 1.

Note the absence of compartment pressure measurement as an indication. As a routine, compartment pressures are not measured in a combat setting. Because of evacuation times and distance and discontinuous care by multiple providers, the mere thought of measuring compartment pressures should elicit fasciotomy. Regional pain management, such as CPNB, may cloud the examination of a casualty and the decision for fasciotomy should be dictated by the surgeon's experience and index of suspicion for development of compartment syndrome.

Massive transfusion, use of fresh whole blood, and hemostatic resuscitation

Multiple logistic hurdles to maintaining a robust blood bank exist in deployed settings. These hurdles include long transport times, limited number of temperature-controlled storage containers and vehicles, and rapid degradation or use of products. In particular, stored platelets were not readily available to CSHs until late December 2004, when a platelet apheresis machine capable of producing fresh platelets was brought into theater to the 86th CSH (personal communication, Kenneth Azarow, MD, COL, US Army Medical Corps, 2005). In addition, because of the aforementioned logistic problems, the storage age of red blood cells (RBC) in-theater was higher than in stateside trauma centers. The 31st CSH was deployed in

---

Box 1. Indications for fasciotomy in the combat setting

Greater than 4- to 6-hr evacuation delay to revascularization
Combined arterial and venous injuries
Crush injuries
High kinetic energy mechanism
Vascular repair
Arterial or venous ligation
Comatose, closed head injury, or epidural analgesia
Tense compartments
Prophylactic

Iraq from January to December 2004; during that time, 5294 RBC units were transfused in 930 patients. The mean age of the RBC units on delivery to the CSH was 27 days, and the mean age of the RBC units on transfusion was 33 days [73,74]. Several studies have suggested a detrimental effect of transfusions of blood greater than 14 to 21 days old [75–78].

The frequency of massive transfusions, defined as greater than 10 units of RBC in 24 hours [79,80], was high during the time period the authors' CSH was in-theater. During this year, the first Marine assault into Fallujah in April 2004, the assault on An Najaf in August 2004, and the second Marine assault on Fallujah in November 2004 occurred. These months represent some of the highest number of casualties to date for the war [1]. During this time period, 201 patients received massive transfusions [81]. The frequency of these cases meant that the hospital's blood bank would frequently be outstripped of standard blood products. By necessity, the CSH instituted a fresh whole blood program that recruited donors from within the hospital and from other neighboring units in the area. A total of 545 units of fresh whole blood were transfused in 87 patients during the CSH's deployment [73].

This experience of surgeons resuscitating with fresh warm whole blood provided anecdotal impressions of a hemostatic and perhaps survival benefit of fresh whole blood. Few modern clinical studies have revealed a benefit of fresh whole blood, partially because of its relative lack of use in favor of component therapy, although Manno and colleagues [82] demonstrated that use of whole blood or stored blood less than 72 hours old reduced blood loss and blood use in neonates post cardiac surgery. The use of fresh whole blood was integrated into a massive transfusion protocol that favored the delivery of fresh frozen plasma (FFP) to RBC in a ratio of 1:1, with the addition of early use of cryoprecipitate and recombinant factor VIIa, until the first units of fresh whole blood were available (usually in about 60 minutes from initiation of the blood drive) (Fig. 5). Once fresh whole blood was available, this became the favored resuscitation product in casualties requiring massive transfusion. This topic is being studied intensely by investigators from the 31st CSH and US Army Institute of Surgical Research, and early reports identify a survival benefit in patients receiving fresh whole blood compared with component therapy alone (personal communications, Philip Spinella, MD, MAJ(P), US Army Medical Corps and Jeremy Perkins, MD, MAJ, US Army Medical Corps, 2006). The rapid evacuation of casualties out of theater and across multiple continents has made accurate tracking of outcomes and complications challenging.

Nevertheless, several findings from this research are available. First, Borgman and colleagues [81] demonstrated that increased number of stored RBC units transfused in the first 24 hours of admission was independently associated with decreased survival, whereas increased units of FFP transfused in the first 24 hours of admission was independently associated with improved survival. The median ratio of FFP:RBC was 1:1.7 in survivors

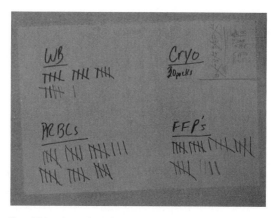

Fig. 5. Running tally of blood products hung on wall above casualty's bed. WB, fresh whole blood, 21 units; PRBCs, packed red blood cells, 33 units; Cryo, cryoprecipitate, 30 packs; FFP, fresh frozen plasma, 29 units. The casualty, treated by the authors (Beekley and Sebesta) and other members of a CSH, sustained the following injuries from multiple transabdominal gunshot wounds: Through-and-through perforation of distal esophagus, splenic rupture, splenic artery laceration, laceration to distal tail of pancreas, multiple perforations of stomach, left lobe of liver laceration, left diaphragm injury, multiple small bowel perforations, evisceration through left flank, right internal iliac artery and vein injury, intra- and extraperitoneal bladder perforations, extraperitoneal rectal injury, and open proximal left tibia/fibula fracture. He arrived somnolent with a blood pressure of approximately 50. As illustrated, the ratio of PRBC to FFP to cryoprecipitate packs he received was close to 1:1:1. The patient also received 21 units of fresh whole blood, which became his primary resuscitation modality once available. The patient received several doses of recombinant factor VIIa early in his course (drug was ordered in the emergency room). The patient survived his injuries and initial operations but ultimately succumbed to sepsis about 3 months later.

compared with 1:3 in nonsurvivors ($P < .001$). In addition, 30% of survivors received recombinant factor VIIa compared with 16% of nonsurvivors, although this did not reach significance ($P = .059$) [81]. The use of component therapy in a ratio of 1:1 for RBC, FFP, and platelets is becoming the standard resuscitation regimen in some trauma centers. Baltimore Shock Trauma Center currently thaws fresh frozen plasma each morning, allowing for the immediate transfusion of fresh thawed plasma once a trauma patient requiring transfusions arrives [83].

This early use of hemostatic products is based on data demonstrating that severely injured patients are suffering from a coagulopathy on arrival to hospital care, not just acquiring a coagulopathy from the resuscitation fluids [84,85]. In addition, hyperfibrinolysis may be more common in trauma patients than previously recognized. A recent study using rotational thromboelastography has shown that approximately 20% of multi-trauma patients suffering from massive bleeding have marked fibrinolysis [86]. Another recent large animal study demonstrated that fibrinogen replacement in a thrombocytopenic uncontrolled liver hemorrhage pig model provided improved median clot firmness, median blood loss, and survival time when compared with treatment with platelets or saline control [87]. Current military massive transfusion protocols feature early replacement of fibrinogen with FFP and cryoprecipitate, along with early use of recombinant factor VIIa, which reduces clot susceptibility to fibrinolysis [88]. Although no survival benefit favoring use of fresh whole blood was demonstrated in this analysis, the use of fresh whole blood as part of a comprehensive approach to resuscitation began in the second half of the 31st CSH's deployment. Earlier in the year, fresh whole blood at the 31st CSH was used as a therapy of last resort or after standard component resuscitation had failed or exhausted the blood bank's supply, rather than a central part of the resuscitation strategy. A comparison of its use and related clinical outcomes before and after its institution into a massive transfusion protocol is ongoing. In addition, accurate injury scoring for casualties is just now being completed for 31st CSH data to allow meaningful subgroup analysis (personal communication, Philip Spinella, MD, MAJ[P], US Army Medical Corps, 2006).

The other obvious issue with the use of fresh whole blood is the safety of its use from an infectious disease standpoint and from transfusion-related adverse events. The 31st CSH used a rapid immunochromatographic test (Biokit, Spain) for HIV 1 and 2, hepatitis B surface antigen (HBsAg), and hepatitis C virus (HCV). This test is not currently FDA approved. Manufacturer-reported sensitivities and specificities are shown in Table 1. The results of donors screened with this test are shown in Table 2. The two units contaminated with HCV were not transfused [89].

These results demonstrate that a fresh whole blood program can and should be integrated into deploying military medical units' blood bank plans. This program can provide an appropriately low risk for viral transmission as long as accurate point-of-care tests are available. The use of fresh whole blood is being reevaluated in civilian settings. For example, the Israeli medical system's blood banks now keep several of the daily collected units temporarily available as whole blood for use in patients who have severe hemorrhage, coagulopathy, or those that need massive transfusion. Unused units are separated and stored as components after 24 hours [90].

Recently, a clinical practice guideline was published governing the use of some of these controversial products and practices. Patients who have the following characteristics on arrival are candidates for early (as close to

Table 1
Manufacturer-reported sensitivities and specificities for rapid immunochromatographic test (Biokit, Spain) for HIV 1 and 2, HBsAg, and hepatitis C virus

Test	Specificity (%)	Sensitivity (%)
HIV 1, 2	98.2	98.5
HCV	98.7	99.4
HBsAg	>98	Not reported

Abbreviations: HBsAg, hepatitis B surface antigen; HCV, hepatitis C virus.

Table 2
The results of donors screened with rapid immunochromatographic test (Biokit, Spain) for HIV
1 and 2, HBsAg, and hepatitis C virus

Test	Positive results of rapid screening
HIV 1, 2	0/460
HCV	2/406
HBsAg	0/406

Abbreviations: HBsAg, hepatitis B surface antigen; HCV, hepatitis C virus.

casualty arrival as possible) use of hemostatic products, such as recombinant factor VIIa, cryoprecipitate, and FFP, and initiation of a fresh whole
blood drive: international normalized ration greater than or equal to 1.5;
base deficit (BD) greater than 6; temperature less than 96°F; hemoglobin
less than 11; and systolic blood pressure (SBP) less than 90 on arrival in
the setting of military trauma. This approach currently is being studied
in-theater (personal communication, John B. Holcomb, MD, COL, US
Army Medical Corps, 2006). Use of recombinant Factor VIIa has been
shown in ex vivo studies to function in the setting of hypothermia but not
in the setting of profound acidosis [91].

Critical care aeromedical transport

The US Air Force Critical Care Aeromedical Transport (CCAT) provides long-range transportation of critically injured patients while continuing sophisticated medical care. The CCAT program was developed after
Operation Just Cause when aeromedical evacuation systems designed to
transport stable patients found themselves transporting and treating fresh
casualties. In addition, the change in United States military doctrine from
large forward-based infrastructure of the Cold War era to today's light ex-
peditionary forces required the development of a method to transport all patients to higher echelons of care. This change resulted in the inclusion of
physicians on aeromedical flights to provide and direct treatment. CCAT
teams have transported thousands of injured troops from Iraq and Afghanistan to Germany and the United States. The CCAT team consists of a physician who has significant intensive care background, a critical care nurse,
and a respiratory therapist. Each CCAT team is capable of treating six
low-acuity patients or three high-acuity patients. In addition to their normal
training, each member completes additional training in aerospace physiology, equipment training, and medical care in austere environments. Teams
also can complete additional training and sustainment of trauma skills by
rotating at a stateside level one trauma center. CCAT team's equipment
has been designed and tested for use at various altitudes and cabin pressures.
The portable nature of this equipment makes it ideal for transporting patients by way of different modes of transportation including fixed-wing
and rotary-winged aircraft. CCAT teams must be able to function in low-
light and high-noise areas with limited access to the patients.

Training

The rapid expansion of knowledge regarding care of the combat casualty since the start of the Global War on Terror has required constant updating of training regimens and courses for prehospital providers, physicians, surgeons, and deploying units.

Currently, prehospital providers, in particular combat medics from line units, receive at least a 3-day training course called Combat Medic Advanced Skills Training, and many receive a 4- or 5-day Tactical Combat Casualty Care course that is enhanced with simulator mannequin (SimMAN, Laerdal Corporation) and controlled live-tissue training models. This training is administered as close to a unit's deployment as possible but at least within 6 months of a unit's upcoming deployment. The Pre-Hospital Trauma Life Support manual now has a chapter specifically dealing with prehospital care of the combat casualty, and provides a recommended equipment list for combat medics to carry.

In an effort to maintain trauma skills in military physicians and forward surgical teams who normally may not have any exposure to trauma on a day-to-day basis, the military uses stateside level 1 trauma centers for training. Teams rotate for 2- to 3-week long training at centers such as Ryder trauma center in Miami and Los Angeles County Hospital. The training includes didactic and laboratory sessions, animal and tissue models, simulators, and then training in an area of interest, such as the ICU, operating room, or the trauma bay as part of the resuscitation team. Additional instruction and exercises develop plans for mass casualty situations, triage scenarios, teamwork, and team building. After completing the initial training period, teams then take over the role as the trauma team and respond and treat all trauma patients for a given period of time. This practice allows teams to use all areas of training, practice sleep/rest cycles, and identify areas required for additional training. These training centers play an integral part in the preparation of teams and team members to prevent poor outcomes during the steep learning curve of treating combat casualties.

A 3-day Emergency War Surgery Course involving didactic sessions and practical exercises in cadavers or live-tissue models exists and was designed specifically for deploying surgeons. This course currently is being evaluated as a refresher for deploying surgeons (personal communication, David Burris, MD, COL, US Army Medical Corps, 2006). Another similar multidisciplinary course that involves training for surgeons and other trauma team members also has been created recently, and is being used as a combat casualty care preparation course by some deploying combat support hospitals. The Madigan Army Medical Center (MAMC) general surgery residency provides a twice-yearly live animal lab for residents to learn advanced laparoscopic skills. MAMC staff surgeons returning from combat-zone deployments (including the authors of this chapter) have since insisted on adding an afternoon session to this lab that focuses on identification and treatment of less common intraabdominal injuries, rapid mobilization of organs for various anatomic exposures, and damage control techniques. In addition, the MAMC vascular surgery service has hosted a Combat Extremity Trauma course, which is a didactic, saw-bones, and cadaver limb-based course that provides training in vascular exposures, vascular anastomoses, shunt placement, fasciotomies, and placement of external fixators.

Summary

The era of global terrorism and asymmetric warfare heralded by the September 11, 2001 attacks on the United States has continued with the Bali bombings and the Madrid and London train bombings (and other smaller terrorist events too numerous to list here). These types of incidents blur the traditional lines between civilian and military trauma victims. In addition, national and international natural disasters, such as Hurricane Katrina and the Asian tsunami in December 2004, have created intense focus on the medical community's preparation for such events. The lessons learned by physicians in the theaters of war, particularly regarding the response to mass casualties, blast and fragmentation injuries, and resuscitation of casualties in austere environments, likely resonate more strongly with our civilian counterparts in this current era. It is critical that we continue to share these valuable lessons with our civilian colleagues and in turn get critiques, guidance, and constructive feedback from these civilian trauma experts.

References

[1] US Department of Defense website. Operations Iraqi and Enduring Freedom US casualty status. http://www.defenselink.mil/news/casualty.pdf. Accessed June 27, 2006.
[2] Beekley AC. United States military surgical response to modern large-scale conflicts: the ongoing evolution of a trauma system. Surg Clin North Am 2006;86(3):689–709.
[3] Fox CJ, Gillespie DL, O'Donnell SD, et al. Contemporary management of wartime vascular trauma. J Vasc Surg 2005;41(4):638–44.
[4] Peleg K, Rivkind A, Aharonson-Daniel L. Does body armor protect from firearm injuries? J Am Coll Surg 2006;202(4):643–8
[5] Xydakis MS, Fravell MD, Nasser KE, et al. Analysis of battlefield head and neck injuries in Iraq and Afghanistan. Otolaryngol Head Neck Surg 2005;133(4):497–504.
[6] Helling E, McKinlay AJ. Considerations for the head-injured air-evacuated patient: a case report of frontal sinus fracture and review of the literature. Mil Med 2005;170(7):577–9.
[7] Gondusky JS, Reiter MP. Protecting military convoys in Iraq: an examination of battle injuries sustained by a mechanized battalion during Operation Iraqi Freedom II. Mil Med 2005;170(6):546–9.
[8] Harcke HT, Schauer DA, Harris RM, et al. Imaging body armor. Mil Med 2002;167(4): 267–71.
[9] Husum H, Gilbert M, Wisborg T, et al. Prehospital tourniquets: there should be no controversy. J Trauma 2004;56(1):214–5.
[10] Navein J, Coupland R, Dunn R. The tourniquet controversy. J Trauma 2003;54(5 Suppl): S219–20.

[11] Bellamy RF. The causes of death in conventional land warfare: implications for combat casualty care research. Mil Med 1984;149(2):55–62.

[12] Cuadrado D, Arthurs Z, Sebesta J, et al. Cause of death analysis at the 31st combat support hospital during Operation Iraqi Freedom. Presented at the 28th Annual Gary P. Wratten Army Surgical Symposium. Walter Reed Army Institute of Research, Silver Spring, Maryland. May 2006.

[13] Beekley A, Sebesta J, Blackbourne L, et al. Pre-hospital tourniquet use in Operation Iraqi Freedom: effect on hemorrhage control and outcomes. Presented at the 36th Annual Scientific Meeting of the Western Trauma Association. Big Sky, Montana. March 2006.

[14] Little R. Modern combat lacking in old medical supply. Baltimore Sun. March 6, 2005.

[15] Mabry RL. Tourniquet use on the battlefield. Mil Med 2006;171(5):352–6.

[16] Lakstein D, Blumenfeld A, Sokolov T, et al. Tourniquets for hemorrhage control on the battlefield: a 4-year accumulated experience. J Trauma 2003;54(Suppl 5):S221–5.

[17] Rhee P, Koustova E, Alam HB. Searching for the optimal resuscitation method: recommendations for the initial fluid resuscitation of combat casualties. J Trauma 2003;54(Suppl 5): S52–62.

[18] Alam HB, Burris D, DaCorta JA, et al. Hemorrhage control in the battlefield: role of new hemostatic agents. Mil Med 2005;170(1):63–9.

[19] Pusateri AE, Holcomb JB, Kheirabadi BS, et al. Making sense of the preclinical literature on advanced hemostatic products. J Trauma 2006;60(3):674–82.

[20] Pusateri AE, Delgado AV, Dick EJ Jr, et al. Application of a granular mineral-based hemostatic agent (QuikClot) to reduce blood loss after grade V liver injury in swine. J Trauma 2004;57(3):555–62.

[21] Alam HB, Chen Z, Jaskille A, et al. Application of a zeolite hemostatic agent achieves 100% survival in a lethal model of complex groin injury in Swine. J Trauma 2004;56(5): 974–83.

[22] Wright JK, Kalns J, Wolf EA, et al. Thermal injury resulting from application of a granular mineral hemostatic agent. J Trauma 2004;57(2):224–30.

[23] Arnaud F, Tomori T, Saito R, et al. Efficacy of Zeolite in groin injury: comparison of granular and bagged QuikClot. Abstract obtained at 1st International Miltranet Symposium. Koblenz, Germany. May 2006.

[24] McKeague A, Arnaud F, Tomori T, et al. Evaluation of bagged and powdered formulations of Zeolite hemostatic agent (QuikClot). Abstract obtained at 1st International Miltranet Symposium. Koblenz, Germany. May 2006.

[25] Pusateri AE, McCarthy SJ, Gregory KW, et al. Effect of a chitosan-based hemostatic dressing on blood loss and survival in a model of severe venous hemorrhage and hepatic injury in swine. J Trauma 2003;54(1):177–82.

[26] Fukasawa M, Abe H, Masaoka T, et al. The hemostatic effect of deacetylated chitin membrane on peritoneal injury in rabbit model. Surg Today 1992;22(4):333–8.

[27] Klokkevold PR, Subar P, Fukayama H, et al. Effect of chitosan on lingual hemostasis in rabbits with platelet dysfunction induced by epoprostenol. J Oral Maxillofac Surg 1992;50(1): 41–5.

[28] Klokkevold PR, Fukayama H, Sung EC, et al. The effect of chitosan (poly-N-acetyl glucosamine) on lingual hemostasis in heparinized rabbits. J Oral Maxillofac Surg 1999;57(1): 49–52.

[29] Wedmore I, McManus JG, Pusateri AE, et al. A special report on the chitosan-based hemostatic dressing: experience in current combat operations. J Trauma 2006;60(3):655–8.

[30] McPherson JJ, Feigin DS, Bellamy RF. Prevalence of tension pneumothorax in fatally wounded combat casualties. J Trauma 2006;60(3):573–8.

[31] Cullinane DC, Morris JA Jr, Bass JG, et al. Needle thoracostomy may not be indicated in the trauma patient. Injury 2001;32(10):749–52.

[32] Jenkins C, Sudheer PS. Needle thoracocentesis fails to diagnose a large pneumothorax Anaesthesia 2000;55(9):925–6.

[33] Jones R, Hollingsworth J. Tension pneumothoraces not responding to needle thoracocentesis. Emerg Med J 2002;19(2):176–7.

[34] Mines D, Abbuhl S. Needle thoracostomy fails to detect a fatal tension pneumothorax. Ann Emerg Med 1993;22(5):863–6.

[35] Lewis FR Jr. Prehospital intravenous fluid therapy: physiologic computer modelling J Trauma 1986;26(9):804–11.

[36] Drinker CK, Drinker KR, Lund CC. The circulation in the mammalian bone marrow. Am J Physiol 1922;62:1–92.

[37] Dubick MA, Holcomb JB. A review of intraosseous vascular access: current status and military application. Mil Med 2000;165(7):552–9.

[38] Johnson DL, Findlay J, Macnab AJ, et al. Cadaver testing to validate design criteria of an adult intraosseous infusion system. Mil Med 2005;170(3):251–7.

[39] Calkins MD, Fitzgerald G, Bentley TB, et al. Intraosseous infusion devices: a comparison for potential use in special operations. J Trauma 2000;48(6):1068–74.

[40] Butler F, O'Connor K. Antibiotics in tactical combat casualty care 2002. Mil Med 2003; 168(11):911–4.

[41] Hocking G, De Mello WF. Battlefield analgesia: an advanced approach. J R Army Med Corps 1999;145(3):116–8.

[42] Kotwal RS, O'Connor KC, Johnson TR, et al. A novel pain management strategy for combat casualty care. Ann Emerg Med 2004;44(2):121–7.

[43] Buckenmaier CC, McKnight GM, Winkley JV, et al. Continuous peripheral nerve block for battlefield anesthesia and evacuation. Reg Anesth Pain Med 2005;30(2):202–5.

[44] Dougherty PJ. Wartime amputations. Mil Med 1993;158(12):755–63.

[45] Hell K. Characteristics of the ideal antibiotic for prevention of wound sepsis among military forces in the field. Rev Infect Dis 1991;13(Suppl 2):S164–9.

[46] Davis KA, Moran KA, McAllister CK, et al. Multidrug-resistant Acinetobacter extremity infections in soldiers. Emerg Infect Dis 2005;11(8):1218–24.

[47] Handrigan MT, Bentley TB, Oliver JD, et al. Choice of fluid influences outcome in prolonged hypotensive resuscitation after hemorrhage in awake rats. Shock 2005;23(4):337–43.

[48] King DR, Cohn SM, Proctor KG. Changes in intracranial pressure, coagulation, and neurologic outcome after resuscitation from experimental traumatic brain injury with hetastarch. Surgery 2004;136(2):355–63.

[49] Arthurs Z, Cuadrado D, Beekley A, et al. The impact of hypothermia on trauma care at the 31st combat support hospital. Am J Surg 2006;191(5):610–4.

[50] Dubick MA, Brooks DE, Macaitis JM, et al. Evaluation of commercially available fluid-warming devices for use in forward surgical and combat areas. Mil Med 2005;170(1): 76–82.

[51] Emergency War Surgery. In: Burris DG, Fitzharris JB, Holcomb JB, Hetz SP, Jenkins DH, Muskat P, Roberts LH, Uhorchak JM, Venticinque S, Wedmore I, editors. 3rd United States Revision. Washington, DC: Borden Institute; 2004.

[52] Holcomb JB, Salinas J, McManus JM, et al. Manual vital signs reliably predict need for life-saving interventions in trauma patients. J Trauma 2005;59(4):821–8.

[53] Holcomb JB. Fluid resuscitation in modern combat casualty care: lessons learned from Somalia. J Trauma 2003;54(5 Suppl):S46–51.

[54] Bickell WH, Wall MJ Jr, Pepe PE, et al. Immediate versus delayed fluid resuscitation for hypotensive patients with penetrating torso injuries. N Engl J Med 1994;331(17):1105–9.

[55] Champion HR. Combat fluid resuscitation: introduction and overview of conferences J Trauma 2003;54(Suppl 5):S7–12.

[56] Butler FK Jr, Hagmann JH, Richards DT. Tactical management of urban warfare casualties in special operations. Mil Med 2000;165(Suppl 4):1–48.

[57] Krausz MM. Fluid resuscitation strategies in the Israeli army. J Trauma 2003;54(Suppl 5): S39–42.

[58] Dubick MA, Atkins JL. Small-volume fluid resuscitation for the far-forward combat environment: current concepts. J Trauma 2003;54(Suppl 5):S43–5.

[59] Sumann G, Kampfl A, Wenzel V, et al. Early intensive care unit intervention for trauma care: what alters the outcome? Curr Opin Crit Care 2002;8(6):587–92.

[60] Bricknell MC. The evolution of casualty evacuation in the 20th Century (Part 5)—Into the future. J R Army Med Corps 2003;149(4):357–63.

[61] Heaton LD. Emergency war surgery. Am J Surg 1965;110:358–9.

[62] Marshall TJ Jr. Combat casualty care: the Alpha Surgical Company experience during Operation Iraqi Freedom. Mil Med 2005;170(6):469–72.

[63] Bilski TR, Baker BC, Grove JR, et al. Battlefield casualties treated at Camp Rhino, Afghanistan: lessons learned. J Trauma 2003;54(5):814–21.

[64] Mattox KL. Introduction, background, and future projections of damage control surgery. Surg Clin North Am 1997;77(4):753–9.

[65] Peoples GE, Gerlinger T, Craig R, et al. The 274th Forward Surgical Team experience during Operation Enduring Freedom. Mil Med 2005;170(6):451–9.

[66] Beekley A, Blackbourne L, Sebesta J, et al. Evaluation for intra-abdominal injury from combat fragmentation wounds. Poster presentation at the American Association for the Surgery of Trauma meeting, Atlanta, Georgia, September 2005.

[67] Beekley AC, Watts DM. Combat trauma experience with the United States Army 102nd Forward Surgical Team in Afghanistan. Am J Surg 2004;187(5):652–4.

[68] Lovric Z, Lehner V, Wertheimer B, et al. Tourniquet occlusion technique for lower extremity artery reconstruction in war wound. J Cardiovasc Surg (Torino) 1997;38(2): 153–5.

[69] Johansen K, Bandyk D, Thiele B, et al. Temporary intraluminal shunts: resolution of a management dilemma in complex vascular injuries. J Trauma 1982;22(5):395–402.

[70] Granchi T, Schmittling Z, Vasquez J, et al. Prolonged use of intraluminal arterial shunts without systemic anticoagulation. Am J Surg 2000;180(6):493–6.

[71] Eger M, Golcman L, Goldstein A, et al. The use of a temporary shunt in the management of arterial vascular injuries. Surg Gynecol Obstet 1971;132(1):67–70.

[72] Jacob JE. Compartment syndrome. A potential cause of amputation in battlefield vascular injuries. Int Surg 1974;59(10):542–8.

[73] Spinella PC, Perkins J, Grathwohl K, Repine T, Sebesta J, Beekley A, et al. The Use and Risks of Warm Whole Blood to Manage Life Threatening Hemorrhage from Combat Injuries. Poster presentation at the 1st International Miltranet Symposium, Koblenz, Germany, May 2006. Ref Type: Generic.

[74] Spinella PC, Grathwohl K, Holcomb JB, et al. Fresh warm whole blood use during combat. Presented at the Society of Critical Care Meeting, January 2006. Crit Care Med 2005; 33(Suppl 12):A39, 146–S.

[75] Basran S, Frumento RJ, Cohen A, et al. The association between duration of storage of transfused red blood cells and morbidity and mortality after reoperative cardiac surgery. Anesth Analg 2006;103(1):15–20.

[76] Fitzgerald RD, Martin CM, Dietz GE, et al. Transfusing red blood cells stored in citrate phosphate dextrose adenine-1 for 28 days fails to improve tissue oxygenation in rats. Crit Care Med 1997;25(5):726–32.

[77] Purdy FR, Tweeddale MG, Merrick PM. Association of mortality with age of blood transfused in septic ICU patients. Can J Anaesth 1997;44(12):1256–61.

[78] Martin CM, Sibbald WJ, Lu X, et al. Age of transfused red blood cells is associated with ICU length of stay [Abstract]. Clin Invest Med 1994;17:124.

[79] Erber WN. Massive blood transfusion in the elective surgical setting. Transfus Apher Sci 2002;27(1):83–92.

[80] Stainsby D, MacLennan S, Hamilton PJ. Management of massive blood loss: a template guideline. Br J Anaesth 2000;85(3):487–91.

[81] Borgman M, Spinella PC, Perkins J, et al. Blood product replacement affects survival in patients receiving massive transfusions at a combat support hospital. Poster presentation at the 1st International Miltranet Symposium. Koblenz, Germany May 2006.

[82] Manno CS, Hedberg KW, Kim HC, et al. Comparison of the hemostatic effects of fresh whole blood, stored whole blood, and components after open heart surgery in children. Blood 1991;77(5):930–6.

[83] Dutton RP. Haemorrhage control in US trauma care. Presented at the 1st International Miltranet Symposium. Koblenz, Germany. May 2006.

[84] Brohi K, Singh J, Heron M, et al. Acute traumatic coagulopathy. J Trauma 2003;54(6): 1127–30.

[85] MacLeod JB, Lynn M, McKenney MG, et al. Early coagulopathy predicts mortality in trauma. J Trauma 2003;55(1):39–44.

[86] Martinowitz U, Michaelson M. Guidelines for the use of recombinant activated factor VII (rFVIIa) in uncontrolled bleeding: a report by the Israeli Multidisciplinary Task Force J Thromb Haemost 2005;3(4):640–8.

[87] Fries D, Velik-Salchner C, Haas T, et al. The effect of fibrinogen on thrombocytopenia. Poster presentation at the 1st International Miltranet Symposium. Koblenz, Germany. May 2006.

[88] Veldman A, Hoffman M, Ehrenforth S. New insights into the coagulation system and implications for new therapeutic options with recombinant factor VIIa. Curr Med Chem 2003; 10(10):797–811.

[89] Spinella PC, Grathwohl K, Holcomb JB, et al. Risks associated with fresh warm whole blood compared to PRBC transfusions during combat. Presented at the Society of Critical Care meeting, January 2006. Crit Care Med 2005;33[Suppl 12]:A44, 165-S.

[90] Martinowitz U. Recombinant Factor VIIa and Hemostatic Resuscitation. Invited address to 1st International Miltranet Symposium. Koblenz, Germany. May 2006.

[91] Schreiber MA, Holcomb JB, Rojkjaer R. Preclinical trauma studies of recombinant factor VIIa. Crit Care 2005;9(Suppl 5):S25–8.

ELSEVIER
SAUNDERS

SURGICAL
CLINICS OF
NORTH AMERICA

Surg Clin N Am 87 (2007) 185–206

Thermal and Electrical Injuries

Tam N. Pham, MD, Nicole S. Gibran, MD*

*University of Washington Burn Center, Department of Surgery, Harborview Medical Center,
Box 359796, 325 Ninth Avenue, Seattle, WA 98104, USA*

Modern burn care has been characterized by substantial increases in survival and improvements in functional outcomes for burn patients over the past 30 years. Twenty-first century optimal burn care consists of a specialized treatment scheme that incorporates early surgical wound closure, critical care management, and rehabilitation efforts. The success of burn treatment as a multidisciplinary model has fostered the organization of burn centers as regional resources for severely injured patients, including individuals with large open wounds.

The review in this article and the Burn Care Guidelines published by the American Burn Association both illustrate the need for Class I evidence to support standards of burn care [1]. In many cases, our practices are based on years of Class II evidence from small clinical trials. Multicenter research collaborations, such as the National Institutes of Health–funded genomics project "Inflammation and the Host Response" (http://www.gluegrant.org), have begun to codify standards of practice that should pave the way for improved future multicenter clinical trials [2,3].

Acute burn care

Burn wound management

Early eschar excision for massive burn injuries has had the greatest impact on burn patient survival by reducing the incidence of wound sepsis, hypercatabolism, numbers of operations, and hospital lengths of stay [4–6]. Wounds that take longer than 3 weeks to epithelialize typically heal with excessive scarring and contractures that produce aesthetic and functional impairment. Clinicians must be able to anticipate the healing potential of

---

* Corresponding author.

E-mail address: nicoleg@u.washington.edu (N.S. Gibran).

0039-6109/07/$ - see front matter © 2006 Elsevier Inc. All rights reserved.
doi:10.1016/j.suc.2006.09.013

a fresh wound to weigh the relative risks and benefits of excision and grafting of the burn wound. An accurate estimation of burn depth is paramount to proper wound management. An experienced burn provider usually can identify shallow or full-thickness wounds based on clinical grounds alone. Intermediate dermal injury ("indeterminate" burn) poses the greatest challenge. Unfortunately, several studies indicate that initial evaluation even by an experienced surgeon may be only 50% to 70% accurate as to whether an indeterminate dermal burn will heal within 3 weeks [7–9].

Investigators have searched for an objective adjunct to clinical judgment so that patients with indeterminate burns with poor healing potential also may benefit from early excision. Various techniques attempt to quantify physical changes associated with skin injury, such as the presence of denatured collagen, wound edema, and an altered blood flow pattern [10–13]. The most recent development in this field is noncontact laser Doppler imaging, which records the reflectance shift of moving red blood cells in the dermal capillary plexus to provide a color perfusion map of the wound [14]. Theoretically, reduced dermal blood flow portends a low likelihood of healing and could prompt a clinician to operate sooner. This technique is well tolerated by patients and avoids the artifact of pressure on the wound with the scanning device held at a distance. Noncontact laser Doppler imaging examinations can be repeated serially over the first several days after burn as wound bed perfusion evolves throughout the resuscitation phase. Indeterminate dermal burns may become progressively deeper several days after injury (a process termed "wound conversion") as healing potential is affected by perfusion, edema, and infection [15]. Wound conversion, however, is minimized when a patient receives adequate fluid resuscitation and proper wound management [16]. Although promising, noncontact laser Doppler imaging has not yet demonstrated consistent reproducibility and has been no more reliable than experienced burn surgeons [17–19]. It has not been incorporated into the mainstream of burn care.

Although full-thickness and deep dermal burns are best excised within the first week after injury, more superficial wounds may be treated with topical agents until they heal or have demonstrated that they will not heal within 3 weeks. An ideal dressing should be comfortable for the patient, easy to apply and remove, conform to the wound, be relatively cheap, and require infrequent changes. Biologically, it must provide a moist wound environment, limit growth of micro-organisms with good eschar penetration, have no or minimal systemic effect, and débride devitalized tissue as needed. Currently, such universal dressing does not exist; however, not all wounds require these features. Small shallow burns, for example, do not require dressings with antimicrobial activity. Greasy gauze is appropriate for shallow dermal burns. A recently marketed ointment containing β-glucan (Glucan-Pro, Brennan Medical, St Paul, Minnesota), a carbohydrate derived from oat, may be appropriate for shallow wounds because it is soothing and mitigates itching. β-glucan may have an immunomodulatory effect by stimulating macrophage activity [20,21]. β-glucan is also available as a dressing (Glucan II, Brennan Medical, St Paul, Minnesota) and is a favored dressing for donor sites at many centers across the United States [22,23].

Biologic dressings may enhance partial-thickness injury healing. Their proposed benefits stem from infrequent dressing reapplication, improved patient comfort, and topical administration of growth factors. A growing list of biologic dressings has been approved by the US Food and Drug Administration, with several more undergoing clinical trial. In larger burns in which cost is a limiting factor and outpatient therapy is not feasible, human cadaver skin and porcine skin remain good choices for temporary biologic dressings. Table 1 lists frequently used biologic and nonbiologic dressings for burn wounds.

Antibiotic activity becomes more relevant in dressings for deeper wounds, because they are more prone to infection. The most common

Table 1
Commonly used dressings for burn wounds, skin grafts, and donor sites

Dressings	Category	Examples	Appropriate indications
Nonbiologic			
	Petrolatum	Xeroform, Xeroflo, Adaptic, Aquaphor gauze	Partial-thickness burns, skin grafts, donor sites
	Silver	Acticoat, Acticoat-7, Aquacel-Ag, Silvasorb	Partial-thickness burns, skin grafts, donor sites
	Polyurethane	OpSite, Tegaderm	Partial-thickness burns, donor sites
	Foam	Lyofoam	Partial-thickness burns
	Silicone	Mepitel	Partial-thickness burns, skin grafts, donor sites
	Negative pressure therapy	Wound VAC system	Skin grafts
Biosynthetic and biologic	Oat	Glucan II	Partial-thickness burns, skin grafts, donor sites
	Collagen and fibroblasts	Transcyte, Apligraf	Partial-thickness burns
	Collagen, fibroblasts, and keratinocytes	OrCel	Partial-thickness burns
	Allograft (cadaver)	Fresh or cryopreserved	Partial-thickness burns
	Xenograft	Porcine skin, porcine intestinal submucosa (Oasis)	Partial-thickness burns

topical antimicrobial agent for deeper dermal burns is silver sulfadiazine (Thermazine, King Pharmaceuticals, Bristol, Tennessee). Silver is effective against a broad spectrum of gram-positive and gram-negative organisms, including most types of *Staphylococcus aureus* and *Pseudomonas aeruginosa* [24]. It has been incorporated in commercially available dressings, such as Acticoat (Smith and Nephew, Largo, Florida) and Aquacel-Ag (ConvaTec, Princeton, New Jersey) [25,26]. Both products can be used to cover partial-thickness burns, meshed skin grafts, and donor sites.

Ideally, when a burn wound is excised, the wound bed should be replaced with full-thickness autograft skin; unfortunately, full-thickness skin availability is limited by the number and size of full-thickness donor sites that can be primarily closed [27]. Whenever possible, split-thickness sheet grafts should be applied as sheet grafts to maximize function and aesthetics [28]. The standard practice of expanded meshed split-thickness skin autograft achieves wound closure over larger areas, but its disadvantages include fragile wound beds, suboptimal appearance, reduced pliability, and scarring. In patients with large burns, serial harvesting ("recropping") of donor sites may be necessary with larger body surface injuries; one must wait for donor sites to heal, and subsequent skin grafts are thinner and of lesser quality. In the meantime, fresh or cryopreserved cadaver (allograft) skin can be used as a temporary biologic dressing over the excised burn wound bed. Taken together, the current process of partial-thickness autografting for large burns yields suboptimal results for burn wounds covered with widely expanded skin grafts and the reharvested donor sites. The recognition of current limitations has created an impetus for research on commercially available skin substitutes.

There are two general classifications of skin substitutes: cultured epidermal grafts and dermal substitutes. Several caveats exist regarding use of skin substitutes for permanent wound coverage. Cultured epithelial autografts have limited use as a stand-alone replacement because they provide a thin and fragile sheet of keratinocytes that frequently sheer and offer little durability [29–31]. Although epithelial allografts may be suitable as biologic dressings, they cannot be used as skin substitutes because they are ultimately rejected by the recipient's immune system. The dermis determines optimal engraftment and graft durability. In vitro autologous dermal regeneration has not been achieved with current available technology. Providing a dermal layer for wounds requires an exogenous matrix template. Integra (Integra LifeSciences Corp., Plainsboro, New Jersey) is a dermal replacement template comprised of an inner matrix layer of bovine collagen and shark glycosaminoglycan, adhered to a silicone outer layer [32–34]. The inner layer forms a scaffold for in situ dermal regeneration while the outer layer contains water vapors and provides a physical barrier to the outside environment. After approximately 2 weeks, the neodermis is sufficiently vascularized to accept a thin partial-thickness autograft (0.06 in thick) [35]. Although Integra is relatively fragile and susceptible to infection, sufficient longitudinal experience in several centers suggests that consistently good results with this product are possible [32,36–38]. An acellular cryopreserved cadaver dermis (AlloDerm, LifeCell Corporation, Branchburg, New Jersey) also has been marketed as a dermal replacement, but clinical endorsement for this product as an acute burn wound replacement remains limited [39,40]. Boyce and colleagues [41] reported on a promising new approach of maturing the epidermal-dermal skin substitute in vitro by culturing autologous keratinocytes on a collagen matrix. The composite skin replacement is applied to the wound 2 to 3 weeks after harvesting autologous skin; in the meantime, the wound bed can be prepared with another layer of dermal substitute. If successful, this strategy could reduce the problem of shearing seen with application of cultured cells directly onto a wound bed and increase the elasticity, pliability, and function of the wound bed.

Fluid resuscitation

Judicious fluid resuscitation is one the greatest challenges in the care of acutely burned victims. Burn injuries over more than 20% of surface area result in increased capillary permeability and edema in burned and nonburned tissues. Vasoactive mediators from injured skin, such as histamine, prostaglandins, and oxygen-free radicals, mediate a massive capillary leak syndrome that typically lasts for 24 hours after injury [42]. Burn shock is characterized by persistent hypovolemia that demands continuous intravenous fluid rate modification over the first 24 to 48 hours of hospitalization. Several formulas developed over the past 50 years to estimate patient fluid needs have been based on body weight and burn surface area. Each formula differs on the amount and type of crystalloid and the necessity for colloid infusion during resuscitation. The most widely used formula in adults is the Parkland (or Baxter) formula [43], which calls for the infusion of 4 mL/kg/% total body surface area (TBSA) burn lactated Ringer's solution for 24 hours. Half of the volume should be administered over the first 8 hours and the other half during the next 16 hours. Throughout this period, the clinician must continuously re-evaluate patient response to resuscitation and titrate the fluids to achieve a mean arterial pressure of more than 60 mm Hg and urine output of more than 30 mL/h. In children, low glycogen stores and maintenance fluid needs should be addressed by augmenting the resuscitation fluid with an isotonic maintenance solution that contains dextrose. Controversy persists among burn specialists over the use and timing of colloids. Animal studies suggest that capillary permeability is maximal within the first 8 to 12 hours and may be exacerbated by colloid administration [42,44]. Centers that routinely use colloids generally administer them later in the resuscitation phase.

Deep burns, inhalation injury, comorbid illnesses, associated injuries, and delay in resuscitation are recognized to increase fluid requirements [45]. Formulas only serve as initial guidelines, and maintenance of urine output (0.5 mL/kg/h in adults and 1 mL/kg/h in children) is the best surrogate marker of adequate end-organ perfusion. Not satisfied with crude reliance on urine output, many investigators have sought to improve goal-directed therapy during resuscitation. Despite the appeal of invasive hemodynamic monitoring and the natural desire to augment oxygen delivery, a well-designed prospective randomized trial failed to show any advantages to preload-driven resuscitation [46]. Patients who were given preload-driven resuscitation had equally low central filling pressures and intrathoracic blood volumes compared with patients on the Parkland formula. The authors concluded that the additional fluid volume (60% over initial calculations) administered to the "preload" group leaked out of the intravascular space and contributed to peripheral edema.

Although Dr. Baxter repeatedly stressed that most patients could be resuscitated with 3.7 to 4.3 mL/kg/% TBSA burn, recent reports describe average resuscitation volumes significantly exceeding predicted needs, as high as 8 mL/kg/% TBSA [47,48]. This phenomenon has been termed "fluid creep." Proposed explanations for this discrepancy include not reducing fluid rates when urine outputs exceed 0.5 mL/kg/h, relying on invasive monitors to guide resuscitation, and administering larger doses of opioids to control burn pain (termed "opioid creep") [49]. It may be possible that the nature of burn injuries and inhalation injuries has evolved; patients who have been in methamphetamine explosions may exemplify this evolution, because they typically require large resuscitation volumes [50]. Whether higher fluid administration correlates with improved survival is unclear. Compared with the mid-twentieth century, acute renal failure, a common sequela of underresuscitation, is uncommon when resuscitation is initiated early and death because of failed resuscitation is even rarer. Excessive volume resuscitation generates its own complications. Edema may become severe enough in unburned extremities that escharotomies and, occasionally, fasciotomies become necessary [51]. Lung tissue edema may lead to acute respiratory failure [52]. Gut and mesenteric edema manifests as intra-abdominal hypertension; fascial release may be required to treat abdominal compartment syndrome [53,54]. Edema also may become symptomatic in the orbits, as evidenced by elevated intraocular pressures and need for lateral canthotomies [55].

Several strategies to mitigate "fluid creep" are currently being investigated. For instance, hourly urine output measurements have been criticized because hourly intervals are arbitrarily chosen for convenience. A recent animal study suggested that an automated closed-loop system that adjusts fluid administration to continuous urine output measurement may decrease fluctuations based on human interventions [56]. Such systems could be adapted with additional inputs, such as blood pressure or base deficit measurements, to guide resuscitation needs. Considerable interest also exists in antioxidant therapy, because membrane lipid peroxidation and oxygen-free radicals are major components of burn shock physiology [57]. Animal and clinical studies suggest that antioxidants reduce fluid requirements and burn wound edema during resuscitation [58,59]. Early administration of tocopherol and ascorbate in critically ill surgical trauma patients also shortens the duration of mechanical ventilation and decreases the incidence of multiorgan failure [60]. Antioxidant therapy as an adjunct to burn resuscitation mandates large-scale multicenter prospective validation before it should be accepted as standard of care. Another interesting strategy is plasma exchange, which theoretically removes inflammatory mediators circulating in the systemic circulation. Although Warden and colleagues [61] described the use of plasma exchange to salvage patients who were failing resuscitation more than 20 years ago, confirmatory studies to explain its salutary mechanisms or clinical benefits are still lacking.

Inhalation injury and intensive care management

Airway burn injuries can be divided into two types: upper airway thermal injury and lower airway chemical injury. Carbon monoxide poisoning is more accurately categorized as a systemic intoxication with the lung as a portal of entry. Clinicians often group all three into "inhalation injury" because all three insults may coexist, for example, in a patient who has been in a closed-space fire. The diagnosis of an upper airway burn can be made readily by assessment of hoarseness or stridor and examination of the posterior pharynx for edema or mucosal slough. Injuries to the lower airways can be diagnosed by direct visualization (fiberoptic bronchoscopy), suggestion of a ventilation/perfusion mismatch (xenon scan), or radiographic evidence of small airway inflammation and obstruction (CT scan) [62–64]. Xenon scanning is mostly of historical interest, and additional information obtained via CT scan is of questionable clinical value. The transport of patients to the radiology suite with ongoing resuscitation is cumbersome and at times hazardous. Although bronchoscopy confirms a clinical diagnosis of inhalation injury, it rarely alters clinical management.

The diagnosis of carbon monoxide poisoning can be measured easily with a serum carboxyhemoglobin level. Administration of 100% oxygen reduces the half-life of carboxyhemoglobin from 4 hours (on 21% O_2) to approximately 45 minutes. In practice, many patients with carbon monoxide poisoning have normalized values upon arrival to the burn center. Proponents of hyperbaric oxygen (HBO) therapy have argued that hyperbaric chamber treatment lessens long-term neurologic sequelae, even with normal pretreatment carbon monoxide levels. Two prospective randomized trials of HBO therapy have yielded conflicting results [65,66]. Scheinkestel and colleagues [65] described sequential chamber treatments over 3 to 6 days, with hyperbaric-treated individuals performing worse on neuropsychological testing compared with normobaric treatment. Conversely, Weaver and colleagues [66] used a treatment algorithm consisting of three HBO treatments within 24 hours of enrollment and reported that cognitive impairments were less frequent at 6 weeks in the HBO group and persisted at 1-year follow-up. The first study specifically excluded burn patients, whereas the second report apparently did not include major burn injuries, as evidenced by few being patients hospitalized (14%) or requiring mechanical ventilation (8%). The presence of a major burn requires careful fluid resuscitation, whereas mechanical ventilation imposes an additional logistical challenge for patients placed in HBO chambers. In our own experience, severely burned victims with concomitant carbon monoxide poisoning experience high complication rates when HBO therapy is attempted [67]. HBO treatment for carbon monoxide poisoning in patients probably should be limited to patients with burn injuries smaller than 15% TBSA.

Patients with lower airway inhalation injury are at risk for developing acute respiratory distress syndrome because of direct airway injury coupled with increased volume resuscitation requirements. Although an optimal ventilation strategy for inhalation injury remains to be defined, many burn centers have adopted the use of lower tidal volumes and reduced airway plateau pressures to treat acute respiratory distress syndrome based on compelling data from the Acute Respiratory Distress Syndrome Network group [68]. Although "prophylactic" use of a lung protective ventilation strategy in inhalation injury is an appealing concept, previous efforts have failed to show clinical benefits in patients at risk for acute respiratory distress syndrome [69]. For the small number of patients who oxygenate poorly on conventional settings, high-frequency oscillatory ventilation can improve oxygenation dramatically while acute respiratory distress syndrome resolves [70,71]. Several pharmacologic means to minimize airway narrowing, prevent airway obstruction, and improve clearance of debris have been shown to have variable success in animal models of lower airway inhalation injury. These strategies include mucus fragmentation (N-acetylcysteine), bronchodilation (β2 agonists, nitric oxide), clot dissolution (antithrombins, tissue plasminogen activator, and heparin), flow turbulence reduction (partial liquid ventilation), and inhibition of inflammation (steroidal and nonsteroidal anti-inflammatory agents) [72–77]. Widespread adoption of any of these agents awaits confirmation with level I evidence.

Prolonged mechanical ventilation often complicates the care of large burns, with or without inhalation injury. The debate over tracheostomy compared with translaryngeal intubation remains unresolved, because there are no prospective studies with appropriate side-by-side comparison [78–81]. For any benefit of tracheostomy to be realized, this procedure should be performed early in the patient's course. Predictors of successful ventilator weaning are often inaccurate, however, and tracheostomy can be a morbid procedure. Outcome comparison is also difficult because all patients with tracheostomy are cross-over from the translaryngeal intubation, and an accurate assessment of long-term tracheal complications can be made only by fiberoptic laryngoscopy on all patients studied. It is likely that individual burn centers will remain entrenched either on the conservative or aggressive side of the tracheostomy debate. Given the absence of Class I evidence, recommendations for airway management must include options rather than standards of clinical care.

Anemia

Hospitalized burn victims become anemic because of hemodilution, relative bone marrow suppression, and frequent laboratory draws. Early eschar excision, currently widely accepted as a standard of burn care in North America, traditionally has been associated with significant operative blood loss [82]. Blood transfusion is a life-saving treatment in some circumstances but has potential drawbacks, such as viral transmission, transfusion reactions, and immunosuppressive effects. "Passenger" leukocytes present in transfused packed red blood cell units are critical components of immune modulation [83]. Transfusion of leukocyte-depleted blood reduces the incidence of infection in postoperative cardiac and noncardiac surgery patients [84,85]; however, the validity of this approach in the injured patient remains to be established. In a multicenter retrospective study on blood use in burn centers, Palmieri and colleagues [86] reported that patients with burns over 20% received on average 14 units of packed red blood cells over the course of their hospitalization, and they suggested that transfusion requirements independently increased the risk of infections and mortality. Methods developed to reduce intraoperative blood loss include use of tourniquets, compression wrappings and elevation for extremities, application of hemostatic agents and epinephrine-soaked pads to excised wounds, and subcutaneous infusion of dilute epinephrine under the eschar and donor sites [82,87]. With accumulating data underscoring the safety of relative anemia (hemoglobin of 7 g/dL) in critically ill patients [88,89], burn centers are gradually accepting lower steady-state hemoglobin levels outside the operating room. The current trend is to adopt a restrictive transfusion policy based on individual patients' demonstrated needs.

The necessity for prophylaxis of deep venous thromboses and pulmonary emboli in burn patients remains unresolved. Although thromboembolic disease was historically viewed as a rare occurrence in burn patients, recent reports document a varying incidence of deep venous thromboses/pulmonary emboli in this patient population proportional to the frequency of duplex ultrasound examinations, whether performed as a serial screening tool or selectively based on symptomatology [90–92]. Compression devices are of unproven value, and their application is poorly tolerated in individuals with lower extremity open wounds. Administration of heparin and related compounds must be weighed against their side-effects. Most notably, heparin-induced thrombocytopenia has emerged as a recognized complication in the burn unit [93,94]. Heparin-induced thrombocytopenia is a severe prothrombotic state that is associated with dreaded complications, such as digit necrosis, limb loss, and even death. The efficacy of alternative anticoagulation agents, such as low molecular weight heparin compounds and pentasaccharides, has not yet been evaluated. Large-scale prospective studies are needed before we are able to define the indications and the most efficacious agents for deep venous thromboses/pulmonary emboli prophylaxis in burn patients.

Modulation of post-burn hypermetabolism

Burn injuries over more than 25% TBSA are associated with a hypermetabolic state that develops over the first 5 days and persists until the wounds are completely healed. Sometimes it lasts up to a year after injury [95]. Protein catabolism is a particularly deleterious feature of this response: the loss of lean body mass is a barrier to rehabilitation for all patients and retards normal growth in burned children. Early surgical wound excision and skin grafting remains the most expeditious way to reduce the inflammatory burden posed by the wound. Routine care in the burn intensive care unit also should include specific daily management strategies to manage hypermetabolism. Maintenance of warm ambient temperatures (33°C) partially reduces the obligatory heat loss created by fever [96]. Nutritional supplementation must be instituted early in the patient's course, ideally during the resuscitation phase and before ileus develops. Enteral feedings initially can be based on estimated needs and subsequently adjusted by indirect calorimetry. The prevention, prompt diagnosis, and treatment of infections represent a daily challenge in burn patients. Control of infection also significantly reduces energy expenditure over a patient's hospitalization. Hyperglycemia is another marker of severe metabolic derangement and has been associated with worse outcomes in burn patients [97,98]. Two recent prospective, randomized evaluations by Van den Berghe and colleagues [99,100] have established that maintenance of euglycemia via continuous insulin infusion is desirable in critically ill patients because it decreases the incidence of infections and reduces mortality.

During the recovery phase, a rehabilitation program that includes exercise against resistance builds not only lean body mass but also muscle strength [101,102]. Pharmacologic agents that help preserve and restore lean body mass represent adjuncts in modulating post-burn hypermetabolism. Recombinant growth hormone (administered over 1 year) prospectively evaluated in a double-blind trial in children with severe burns suggested that children on growth hormone gained more lean body mass, height, and bone-mineral content than control subjects [103]. The benefits of growth hormone are not applicable to adults, because hyperglycemia is a common side effect in this group [104]. Oxandrolone, a testosterone analog, is an anabolic steroid with reduced virilizing potential [105,106]. A prospective trial of oxandrolone in children demonstrated improvement in net protein balance after 1 week of administration [107]. In a recently completed randomized, placebo-controlled trial, adults who received oxandrolone had reduced lengths of hospital stay compared with patients on placebo [108]. Although many factors potentially impact length of stay, the study suggests a benefit to oxandrolone. Propranolol, a nonselective beta-blocker, reduces tachycardia, energy expenditure, and substrate cycling and prevents fatty infiltration of the liver [95,109]. In a randomized study of 25 children, Herndon and colleagues [110] demonstrated that propranolol attenuated the effect of hypermetabolism by reversing muscle protein catabolism. Beta-blockade also constitutes an attractive strategy for adults in which tachycardia is undesirable and less well tolerated in patients with pre-existing heart disease. Ongoing trials are indicated to evaluate the efficacy and safety of propranolol in adults.

Electrical injuries

Electrical burns represent a minority of admissions at major burn units but often cause severe morbidity beyond obvious skin injuries. In particular, high-voltage injuries (arbitrarily defined as >1000 V) may lead to temporary dysrhythmias in survivors, be associated with major blunt trauma, and cause deep tissue destruction. Other deficits may manifest themselves in a delayed fashion: two commonly described long-term sequelae are peripheral motor or sensory neuropathy and the appearance of cataracts [111,112]. Most patients with electrical burns are young men injured at work (eg, construction workers, electricians, and linemen). Injury and disability in this demographic group result in major loss of wages and significant medical costs [113,114]. No Class I evidence exists to support standardized management of electrical burns. Available guidelines recommend 24-hour telemetry monitoring for all patients with high-voltage injuries and for patients with low-voltage injuries who have an abnormal initial EKG [115]. Some data, however, suggest that monitoring high-voltage injuries with an initial normal EKG may be superfluous [116]. Deep electrical injuries generate rhabdomyolysis and myoglobinuria. In this setting, fluid resuscitation should be titrated to maintain a urine output of 100 mL/h until the urine clinically appears clear. Acute renal failure from myoglobinuria is rare unless resuscitation is delayed. Several methods have been proposed to enhance renal clearance of myoglobin, including alkalinization of urine and osmotic diuresis with mannitol [117]. These adjunct measures are of unproven value and represent individual centers' practices and will remain so until prospective evidence validates their benefit over simple isotonic crystalloid resuscitation.

Early fasciotomy or surgical débridement of necrotic muscle may be warranted when severe acidosis and myoglobinuria do not rapidly improve with aggressive resuscitation; management in a burn center in which these injuries can be monitored closely by a burn surgeon is optimal. Although most limbs can be salvaged with early diagnosis of compartment syndrome and compartment fasciotomies, major débridement and early amputation occasionally may be necessary [118]. Although routine fasciotomy has been advocated, a review of national trends in management of patients with electrical burns supports selective decompression [119]. Mann and colleagues [113] reported that most patients with high-voltage injuries (70%) did not require emergent operation and no amputations were required in patients who were monitored. Monitoring consists of serial clinical assessments of tissue perfusion and peripheral nerve function in at-risk extremities. The use of technetium scan has not gained wide acceptance for it is overly sensitive in detecting deep tissue damage [120]. Fibrosis is the end of result of limited deep-tissue necrosis, whereas overly aggressive débridement may introduce infection and increase the risk of amputation.

Rehabilitation and reconstruction

With an increasing number of survivors of major burn injuries, successful re-entry into society becomes the next major challenge. A coordinated burn center program that includes surgeons, physiatrists, pediatricians, occupational and physical therapists, vocational rehabilitation specialists, and psychologists is essential to successful rehabilitation. Perhaps because of their resilience and adaptive ability, children recover well even after major burn injury. Sheridan and colleagues [121] reported that most children treated at Shriners Burn Institute (Boston) who survived massive burns ($\geq 70\%$ TBSA) became productive members of society. In their series however, 20% of patients had physical scores below norm; indicating that this subgroup had persistent sequelae. In adults, an important benchmark may be return to work. There is little information reported in the literature on this subject, however. A recent two-center review reported that median time off work approximated 12 weeks, and 90% of patients had regained employment by 2 years [122]. It is noteworthy that only 37% of patients returned to their preinjury job without accommodations. Several factors contributed to this finding: burn size, location of burns, and psychiatric history. A related but seldom reported outcome is impairment. Standard methods to calculate physical impairment are not widely used in burn care because they require either tedious calculations (whole person impairment rating) or initial investment in costly equipment ($27,000 for the Dexter Evaluation system) [123,124]. Psychological assessment is another important component of impairment rating. Efforts are underway in this arena to develop tools that are appropriate gauges of the quality of life in burn survivors. The ongoing multicenter collaborative Burn Injury Rehabilitation Model System Program funded by the National Institute of Disability and Rehabilitation Research has increased awareness among burn providers and patients about burn survivor needs; despite progress since its inception, much more can be done to improve our patients' return to function.

Reconstructive surgery is essential to the rehabilitation process because it helps restore function and body image. The problems of hypertrophic scarring and contracture remain enormous challenges for reconstructive burn surgeons. Hypertrophic scars may develop in healed burn areas, grafted sites, and even donor sites. Commonly used preventive strategies aimed at reducing raised scars include pressure therapy, topical silicone gel application, and massage [125–127]. Well-designed prospective studies to support use of these modalities are lacking. Patients with large burns can expect to undergo several scar revisions over their lifetime, because each procedure results in small incremental gains in function and appearance. Current understanding of the pathophysiology of hypertrophic scarring unfortunately remains limited, because many previous studies have studied mature scars and not scars in evolution. A standard animal model for hypertrophic scarring does not yet exist. Recent laboratory efforts have focused on the female red Duroc pig as multiple laboratories attempt to validate similarities in skin healing between this model and humans [128–130].

Access to burn care

The success of modern burn care, characterized by improved survival rates and return to preinjury function, is closely associated with the development of specialized burn centers. The burn center is not just "an area of the hospital" but a system of care that includes a specialized infrastructure, highly trained providers, and treatment algorithms that serve the unique needs of the burn victim. The burn center must be equipped to deliver all aspects of burn care, from initial management and acute surgical wound coverage, through rehabilitation and long-term reconstruction. Akin to other areas of medicine in which a relationship between volume and outcome has been established, the same appears true for burn centers. This process has driven regionalization of burn care in the past two decades, with many low-volume centers closing and seriously injured patients being referred to regional burn centers for definitive care. The American Burn Association has participated actively in this transformation by generating criteria for burn center referral (Box 1). The American Burn Association in association with the American College of Surgeons also has established a burn center verification program for approximately two decades. So far, 43 of the 139 listed burn centers in the United States have been certified by this process, and it is likely that they will continue to serve as centers of excellence for the foreseeable future.

Specialized burn care has created a demand for highly trained providers, including surgeons, nurses, therapists, psychologists, pharmacists, and rehabilitation physiatrists to form a multidisciplinary care team. The ranks of burn surgeons are usually filled with individuals having completed training in general surgery or plastic surgery. Their scope of practice, however, also includes components of pediatric and surgical critical care. Surgeons interested in burn care often seek additional training through burn fellowships. Whereas these individuals only number five to seven per year,

---

Box 1. American Burn Association burn unit referral criteria

1. Partial thickness burns >10% TBSA
2. Burns that involve the hands, face, feet, genitalia, perineum, or major joints
3. Third-degree (full-thickness) burns in any age group
4. Electrical burns, including lightning injury
5. Chemical burns
6. Inhalation injury
7. Burn injury in patients with pre-existing medical disorder that could complicate management or recovery or affect mortality
8. Patients with concomitant burn and trauma in which the burn injury poses the greatest risk of morbidity or mortality
9. Burned children in hospitals without qualified personnel or equipment for the care of children
10. Burn injury in patients who require special social, emotional, or long-term rehabilitative intervention

-----

Adapted from the American Burn Association. Burn unit referral criteria. Available at http://www.ameriburn.org. Accessed June 30, 2006.

---

many fellowship positions remained unfilled. A similar situation exists for other burn team specialists. Experienced burn therapists are in short supply because proficiency requires many months of on-the-job training, and advertised positions may stay unfilled for indefinite periods of time. Whether this reality will result in a workforce shortage or create additional impetus for regionalization remains an unanswered question.

The large-scale use of air transport for burn patients started during the Vietnam War, during which field burn casualties were flown to the Brooke Army Medical Center in San Antonio, TX. Since that time, transport of burn patients has become more sophisticated, especially with the addition of respirators that were not available in the Vietnam Era. Successful transfer/transport over large distances requires good communication and coordination between referring and receiving facilities and highly trained personnel in the prehospital phase of care. Although our regional burn center covers an area one-fourth the land mass of the United States, outcomes for long-distance transfer patients are equivalent to that of patients directly admitted to the burn center [131].

Regionalization of care also creates two additional challenges: (1) proper patient triage and (2) coordination of transport, sometimes over great distances. It has been long recognized that referring physicians often under- or overestimate burn surface area, which leads to inappropriate initial care, increased morbidity and mortality, and unnecessary use of air transport systems. Initial burn triage appears well suited for televideoconference consultation because most injuries can be assessed rapidly by an experienced provider at a remote location. Several burn centers in the United States and abroad have gained experiences with the application of telemedicine to initial burn treatment and patient follow-up [132–134]. Its reported advantages include improved access to tertiary care in rural and medically underserved areas, cost savings with fewer air transports for minor burns, increased patient satisfaction thanks to reduced travel expenses, and more time spent with providers. Cost savings are mainly felt on the patient side, whereas the use of videoconference technology represents a major expenditure for health care systems because of investments in infrastructure, maintenance costs, and communication expenses. Others have reported on the use of e-mail, including pictures for patient data communication [135]. This method has the added benefit of minimal technologic investment. So far, regulations have lagged behind technology with many unresolved issues such as patient confidentiality, licensure and credentialing, malpractice liability for providers, and reimbursement agreements that could offset the cost of telemedicine. Clearly, this area represents a most exciting development in burn care and likely will mature over the next few years.

Burn disaster planning

Mass disasters caused by explosions or structure fires typically result in a large number of burn casualties. The Rhode Island Station nightclub fire on February 20, 2003 resulted in 100 deaths and 215 injured patients, more than 50 of them with serious burns [136]. The terrorist attacks on September 11, 2001 were so lethal that the number of injured survivors was actually small. Still, one third of injured patients in New York City needed treatment for severe burns [137]. One could imagine that had the World Trade Center towers not collapsed, the number of burn casualties would have been much higher. The optimal care for burn victims follows a sequence of rapid and proper field triage, followed by intensive care management, burn excision and wound coverage procedures, and finally rehabilitation. For all these reasons, early access to specialized burn care is of paramount importance.

The triage of casualties at the scene naturally involves the activation of state and local response systems. To augment local capacities, the federal government can deploy disaster medical assistance teams to the scene. Burn specialty teams are specialized disaster medical assistance teams that consist of burn-experienced personnel to provide assistance needed in the initial care of burn victims. Four regional burn specialty teams are currently available for federal deployment. Burn specialty teams were deployed after the World Trade Center attack on September 11 and to support local resources after the Rhode Island nightclub fire. The last layer of this tiered response system involves military support to civil authority via activation of US Army special medical augmentation response teams. Two burn-specialized special medical augmentation response teams are currently based in San Antonio, TX, but so far have never been used for US civilian mass casualties. Because special medical augmentation response teams possess long-range air evacuation capabilities, they could become invaluable in the secondary triage and transfer of victims outside the disaster area.

Recognizing that casualty numbers exceeding 50% of maximum capacity (surge capacity) would quickly exhaust resources of local burn centers, the American Burn Association has advocated for a triage system unique to mass casualty burn events [138]. Primary triage is handled according to state and local activation plans, with burn patients triaged to a burn center within 24 hours of injury. Secondary triage is the coordinated transfer of patients from one burn center to a verified burn center after surge capacity is reached. In the event that casualties overwhelm local and national resources, patients would be triaged according to a survival probability grid that prioritizes treatment for patients with the highest likelihood of survival.

Burn research

A central tenet of any burn center should be its commitment to education and research. The physiologic challenge caused by burn injury may be greater than any other type of insult on the human body. It is a model that lends itself to study and can be replicated in the laboratory. In 2006, the official publication of the American Burn Association was renamed the *Journal of Burn Care and Research*. This change underscores the need for additional research to validate current practices and test unanswered questions in our field. In the clinical arena, several projects are worthy of mention because they embrace the concept of economy of scale to patient-oriented research. First, the organization of the National Burn Repository has created a large patient database accessible for research. Second, many centers across the United States have organized into a burn multicenter trial group. Their efforts have resulted in noteworthy publications on transfusion practices [85], toxic epidermal necrolysis syndrome treatment [107], and validation of oxandrolone as anabolic agent [86,108,139]. "Inflammation and the Host Response to Injury" is a major National Institute of Health–funded multicenter program that includes trauma and burn patients. This ambitious translational project aims to correlate genomic and proteomic responses to physiologic perturbations observed at the bedside. Finally, the burn injury model system is a multi-institutional project funded by the National Institute of Disability and Rehabilitation Research (http:// bms-dcc.uchsc.edu) to evaluate longitudinal outcomes after major burns. Optimally, current efforts in bench research, translational science, and outcome analyses will generate the necessary Class I evidence to create standards in burn care for the next generation.

References

[1] Gibran NS. Committee on organization and delivery of burn care, American Burn Association. Practice guidelines for burn care, 2006. J Burn Care Res 2006;27(4):437–8.

[2] Klein MB, Silver G, Gamelli R, et al. Inflammation and the host response to injury: an overview of the multicenter study of the genomic and proteomic response to burn injury. J Burn Care Res 2006;27(4):448–51.

[3] Nathens AB, Johnson JL, Minei JP, et al. Inflammation and the host response to injury: a large-scale collaborative project. Patient-oriented research core: standard operating procedures for clinical care. I. Guidelines for mechanical ventilation of the trauma patient. J Trauma 2005;59(3):764–9.

[4] Janzekovic Z. A new concept in the early excision and immediate grafting of burns. J Trauma 1970;10(12):1103–8.

[5] Burke JF, Bondoc CC, Quinby WC. Primary burn excision and immediate grafting: a method shortening illness. J Trauma 1974;14(5):389–95.

[6] Engrav LH, Heimbach DM, Reus JL, et al. Early excision and grafting vs. nonoperative treatment of burns of indeterminate depth: a randomized prospective study. J Trauma 1983;23(11):1001–4.

[7] Niazi ZB, Essex TJ, Papini R, et al. New laser Doppler scanner, a valuable adjunct in burn depth assessment. Burns 1993;19(6):485–9.

[8] Hlava P, Moserova J, Konigova R. Validity of clinical assessment of the depth of a thermal injury. Acta Chir Plast 1983;25(4):202–8.

[9] Yeong EK, Mann R, Goldberg M, et al. Improved accuracy of burn wound assessment using laser Doppler. J Trauma 1996;40(6):956–61 [discussion: 961–2].

[10] Moserova J, Hlava P, Malinsky J. Scope for ultrasound diagnosis of the depth of thermal damage: preliminary report. Acta Chir Plast 1982;24(4):235–42.

[11] Kaufman T, Hurwitz DJ, Heggers JP. The india ink injection technique to assess the depth of experimental burn wounds. Burns Incl Therm Inj 1984;10(6):405–8.

[12] Heimbach DM, Afromowitz MA, Engrav LH, et al. Burn depth estimation: man or machine. J Trauma 1984;24(5):373–8.

[13] Pape SA, Skouras CA, Byrne PO. An audit of the use of laser Doppler imaging (LDI) in the assessment of burns of intermediate depth. Burns 2001;27(3):233–9.

[14] Kloppenberg FW, Beerthuizen GI, ten Duis HJ. Perfusion of burn wounds assessed by laser Doppler imaging is related to burn depth and healing time. Burns 2001;27(4): 359–63.

[15] Pham TN, Gibran NS, Heimbach DM. Evaluation of the burn wound: management decisions. In: Herndon DN, editor. Total burn care. 3rd edition. In press.

[16] Zawacki BE. Reversal of capillary stasis and prevention of necrosis in burns. Ann Surg 1974;180(1):98–102.

[17] Kim DE, Phillips TM, Jeng JC, et al. Microvascular assessment of burn depth conversion during varying resuscitation conditions. J Burn Care Rehabil 2001;22(6):406–16.

[18] Jeng JC, Bridgeman A, Shivnan L, et al. Laser Doppler imaging determines need for excision and grafting in advance of clinical judgment: a prospective blinded trial. Burns 2003; 29(7):665–70.

[19] Chatterjee JS. A critical evaluation of the clinimetrics of laser Doppler as a method of burn assessment in clinical practice. J Burn Care Res 2006;27(2):123–30.

[20] Estrada A, Yun CH, Van Kessel A, et al. Immunomodulatory activities of oat beta-glucan in vitro and in vivo. Microbiol Immunol 1997;41(12):991–8.

[21] Honari S. Topical therapies and antimicrobials in the management of burn wounds. Crit Care Nurs Clin North Am 2004;16(1):1–11.

[22] Ho WS, Ying SY, Choi PC, et al. A prospective controlled clinical study of skin donor sites treated with a 1-4,2-acetamide-deoxy-B-D-glucan polymer: a preliminary report. Burns 2001;27(7):759–61.

[23] Delatte SJ, Evans J, Hebra A, et al. Effectiveness of beta-glucan collagen for treatment of partial-thickness burns in children. J Pediatr Surg 2001;36(1):113–8.

[24] Atiyeh BS, Gunn SW, Hayek SN. State of the art in burn treatment. World J Surg 2005; 29(2):131–48.

[25] Tredget EE, Shankowsky HA, Groeneveld A, et al. A matched-pair, randomized study evaluating the efficacy and safety of Acticoat silver-coated dressing for the treatment of burn wounds. J Burn Care Rehabil 1998;19(6):531–7.

[26] Caruso DM, Foster KN, Hermans MH, et al. Aquacel Ag in the management of partial-thickness burns: results of a clinical trial. J Burn Care Rehabil 2004;25(1):89–97.

[27] Andreassi A, Bilenchi R, Biagioli M, et al. Classification and pathophysiology of skin grafts. Clin Dermatol 2005;23(4):332–7.

[28] Archer SB, Henke A, Greenhalgh DG, et al. The use of sheet autografts to cover extensive burns in patients. J Burn Care Rehabil 1998;19(1 Pt 1):33–8.

[29] Gallico GG III, O'Connor NE, Compton CC, et al. Permanent coverage of large burn wounds with autologous cultured human epithelium. N Engl J Med 1984;311(7):448–51.

[30] Desai MH, Mlakar JM, McCauley RL, et al. Lack of long-term durability of cultured keratinocyte burn-wound coverage: a case report. J Burn Care Rehabil 1991;12(6):540–5.

[31] Wood F, Liddiard K, Skinner A, et al. Scar management of cultured epithelial autograft. Burns 1996;22(6):451–4.

[32] Burke JF, Yannas IV, Quinby WC Jr, et al. Successful use of a physiologically acceptable artificial skin in the treatment of extensive burn injury. Ann Surg 1981;194(4):413–28.

[33] Yannas IV, Burke JF. Design of an artificial skin. I. Basic design principles. J Biomed Mater Res 1980;14(1):65–81.

[34] Yannas IV, Burke JF, Gordon PL, et al. Design of an artificial skin. II. Control of chemical composition. J Biomed Mater Res 1980;14(2):107–32.

[35] Fang P, Engrav LH, Gibran NS, et al. Dermatome setting for autografts to cover INTEGRA. J Burn Care Rehabil 2002;23(5):327–32.

[36] Heimbach D, Luterman A, Burke J, et al. Artificial dermis for major burns: a multi-center randomized clinical trial. Ann Surg 1988;208(3):313–20.

[37] Heitland A, Piatkowski A, Noah EM, et al. Update on the use of collagen/glycosaminoglycate skin substitute: six years of experiences with artificial skin in 15 German burn centers. Burns 2004;30(5):471–5.

[38] Klein MB, Engrav LH, Holmes JH, et al. Management of facial burns with a collagen/glycosaminoglycan skin substitute: prospective experience with 12 consecutive patients with large, deep facial burns. Burns 2005;31(3):257–61.

[39] Wainwright DJ. Use of an acellular allograft dermal matrix (AlloDerm) in the management of full-thickness burns. Burns 1995;21(4):243–8.

[40] Gore DC. Utility of acellular allograft dermis in the care of elderly burn patients. J Surg Res 2005;125(1):37–41.

[41] Boyce ST, Kagan RJ, Meyer NA, et al. The 1999 clinical research award. Cultured skin substitutes combined with Integra Artificial Skin to replace native skin autograft and allograft for the closure of excised full-thickness burns. J Burn Care Rehabil 1999;20(6):453–61.

[42] Warden GD. Burn shock resuscitation. World J Surg 1992;16(1):16–23.

[43] Baxter CR, Shires T. Physiological response to crystalloid resuscitation of severe burns. Ann N Y Acad Sci 1968;150(3):874–94.

[44] Demling RH. The burn edema process: current concepts. J Burn Care Rehabil 2005;26(3): 207–27.

[45] Shirani KZ, Vaughan GM, Mason AD Jr, et al. Update on current therapeutic approaches in burns. Shock 1996;5(1):4–16.

[46] Holm C, Mayr M, Tegeler J, et al. A clinical randomized study on the effects of invasive monitoring on burn shock resuscitation. Burns 2004;30(8):798–807.

[47] Engrav LH, Colescott PL, Kemalyan N, et al. A biopsy of the use of the Baxter formula to resuscitate burns or do we do it like Charlie did it? J Burn Care Rehabil 2000;21(2):91–5.

[48] Friedrich JB, Sullivan SR, Engrav LH, et al. Is supra-Baxter resuscitation in burn patients a new phenomenon? Burns 2004;30(5):464–6.

[49] Sullivan SR, Friedrich JB, Engrav LH, et al. "Opioid creep" is real and may be the cause of "fluid creep". Burns 2004;30(6):583–90.

[50] Warner P, Connolly JP, Gibran NS, et al. The methamphetamine burn patient. J Burn Care Rehabil 2003;24(5):275–8.

[51] Sheridan RL, Tompkins RG, McManus WF, et al. Intracompartmental sepsis in burn patients. J Trauma 1994;36(3):301–5.

[52] Pruitt BA Jr. Protection from excessive resuscitation: pushing the pendulum back. J Trauma 2000;49(3):567–8.

[53] Greenhalgh DG, Warden GD. The importance of intra-abdominal pressure measurements in burned children. J Trauma 1994;36(5):685–90.

[54] Hobson KG, Young KM, Ciraulo A, et al. Release of abdominal compartment syndrome improves survival in patients with burn injury. J Trauma 2002;53(6):1129–33 [discussion: 1133–4].

[55] Sullivan SR, Ahmadi AJ, Singh CN, et al. Elevated orbital pressure: another untoward effect of massive resuscitation after burn injury. J Trauma 2006;60(1):72–6.

[56] Hoskins SL, Elgjo GI, Lu J, et al. Closed-loop resuscitation of burn shock. J Burn Care Res 2006;27(3):377–85.

[57] Horton JW. Free radicals and lipid peroxidation mediated injury in burn trauma: the role of antioxidant therapy. Toxicology 2003;189(1–2):75–88.

[58] Matsuda T, Tanaka H, Williams S, et al. Reduced fluid volume requirement for resuscitation of third-degree burns with high-dose vitamin C. J Burn Care Rehabil 1991;12(6): 525–32.

[59] Tanaka H, Matsuda T, Miyagantani Y, et al. Reduction of resuscitation fluid volumes in severely burned patients using ascorbic acid administration: a randomized, prospective study. Arch Surg 2000;135(3):326–31.

[60] Nathens AB, Neff MJ, Jurkovich GJ, et al. Randomized, prospective trial of antioxidant supplementation in critically ill surgical patients. Ann Surg 2002;236(6):814–22.

[61] Warden GD, Stratta RJ, Saffle JR, et al. Plasma exchange therapy in patients failing to resuscitate from burn shock. J Trauma 1983;23(10):945–51.

[62] Masanes MJ, Legendre C, Lioret N, et al. Using bronchoscopy and biopsy to diagnose early inhalation injury: macroscopic and histologic findings. Chest 1995;107(5):1365–9.

[63] Moylan JA Jr, Wilmore DW, Mouton DE, et al. Early diagnosis of inhalation injury using 133 xenon lung scan. Ann Surg 1972;176(4):477–84.

[64] Park MS, Cancio LC, Batchinsky AI, et al. Assessment of severity of ovine smoke inhalation injury by analysis of computed tomographic scans. J Trauma 2003;55(3):417–27 [discussion: 427–9].

[65] Scheinkestel CD, Bailey M, Myles PS, et al. Hyperbaric or normobaric oxygen for acute carbon monoxide poisoning: a randomised controlled clinical trial. Med J Aust 1999; 170(5):203–10.

[66] Weaver LK, Hopkins RO, Chan KJ, et al. Hyperbaric oxygen for acute carbon monoxide poisoning. N Engl J Med 2002;347(14):1057–67.

[67] Grube BJ, Marvin JA, Heimbach DM. Therapeutic hyperbaric oxygen: help or hindrance in burn patients with carbon monoxide poisoning? J Burn Care Rehabil 1988;9(3):249–52.

[68] Acute Respiratory Distress Syndrome Network. Ventilation with lower tidal volumes as compared with traditional tidal volumes for acute lung injury and the acute respiratory distress syndrome. N Engl J Med 2000;342(18):1301–8.

[69] Stewart TE, Meade MO, Cook DJ, et al. Evaluation of a ventilation strategy to prevent barotrauma in patients at high risk for acute respiratory distress syndrome: Pressure- and Volume-Limited Ventilation Strategy Group. N Engl J Med 1998;338(6):355–61.

[70] Cioffi WG, Graves TA, McManus WF, et al. High-frequency percussive ventilation in patients with inhalation injury. J Trauma 1989;29(3):350–4.

[71] Cioffi WG, deLemos RA, Coalson JJ, et al. Decreased pulmonary damage in primates with inhalation injury treated with high-frequency ventilation. Ann Surg 1993;218(3):328–35 [discussion: 335–7].

[72] Suter PM, Domenighetti G, Schaller MD, et al. N-acetylcysteine enhances recovery from acute lung injury in man: a randomized, double-blind, placebo-controlled clinical study. Chest 1994;105(1):190–4.

[73] Palmieri TL, Enkhbaatar P, Bayliss R, et al. Continuous nebulized albuterol attenuates acute lung injury in an ovine model of combined burn and smoke inhalation. Crit Care Med 2006;34(6):1719–24.

[74] Enkhbaatar P, Murakami K, Shimoda K, et al. The inducible nitric oxide synthase inhibitor BBS-2 prevents acute lung injury in sheep after burn and smoke inhalation injury. Am J Respir Crit Care Med 2003;167(7):1021–6.

[75] Enkhbaatar P, Murakami K, Shimoda K, et al. Ketorolac attenuates cardiopulmonary derangements in sheep with combined burn and smoke inhalation injury. Clin Sci (Lond) 2003;105(5):621–8.

[76] Murakami K, Enkhbaatar P, Shimoda K, et al. High-dose heparin fails to improve acute lung injury following smoke inhalation in sheep. Clin Sci (Lond) 2003;104(4): 349–56.

[77] Nieman GF, Clark WR, Hakim T. Methylprednisolone does not protect the lung from inhalation injury. Burns 1991;17(5):384–90.

[78] Barret JP, Desai MH, Herndon DN. Effects of tracheostomies on infection and airway complications in pediatric burn patients. Burns 2000;26(2):190–3.

[79] Palmieri TL, Jackson W, Greenhalgh DG. Benefits of early tracheostomy in severely burned children. Crit Care Med 2002;30(4):922–4.

[80] Hunt JL, Purdue GF, Gunning T. Is tracheostomy warranted in the burn patient? Indications and complications. J Burn Care Rehabil 1986;7(6):492–5.

[81] Kadilak PR, Vanasse S, Sheridan RL. Favorable short- and long-term outcomes of prolonged translaryngeal intubation in critically ill children. J Burn Care Rehabil 2004; 25(3):262–5.

[82] Gomez M, Logsetty S, Fish JS. Reduced blood loss during burn surgery. J Burn Care Rehabil 2001;22(2):111–7.

[83] Bordin JO, Heddle NM, Blajchman MA. Biologic effects of leukocytes present in transfused cellular blood products. Blood 1994;84(6):1703–21.

[84] Bilgin YM, van de Watering LM, Eijsman L, et al. Double-blind, randomized controlled trial on the effect of leukocyte-depleted erythrocyte transfusions in cardiac valve surgery. Circulation 2004;109(22):2755–60.

[85] Jensen LS, Andersen AJ, Christiansen PM, et al. Postoperative infection and natural killer cell function following blood transfusion in patients undergoing elective colorectal surgery. Br J Surg 1992;79(6):513–6.

[86] Palmieri TL, Caruso DM, Foster KN, et al. Effect of blood transfusion on outcome after major burn injury: a multicenter study. Crit Care Med 2006;34(6):1602–7.

[87] Kahalley L, Dimick AR, Gillespie RW. Methods to diminish intraoperative blood loss. J Burn Care Rehabil 1991;12(2):160–1.

[88] Hebert PC, Wells G, Blajchman MA, et al. A multicenter, randomized, controlled clinical trial of transfusion requirements in critical care: Transfusion Requirements in Critical Care Investigators, Canadian Critical Care Trials Group. N Engl J Med 1999;340(6):409–17.

[89] Palmieri TL, Greenhalgh DG. Blood transfusion in burns: what do we do? J Burn Care Rehabil 2004;25(1):71–5.

[90] Wibbenmeyer LA, Hoballah JJ, Amelon MJ, et al. The prevalence of venous thromboembolism of the lower extremity among thermally injured patients determined by duplex sonography. J Trauma 2003;55(6):1162–7.

[91] Wahl WL, Brandt MM, Ahrns K, et al. The utility of D-dimer levels in screening for thromboembolic complications in burn patients. J Burn Care Rehabil 2002;23(6):439–43.

[92] Fecher AM, O'Mara MS, Goldfarb IW, et al. Analysis of deep vein thrombosis in burn patients. Burns 2004;30(6):591–3.

[93] Horner BM, Myers SR. Don't miss HIT (heparin induced thrombocytopenia). Burns 2004; 30(1):88–90.

[94] Scott JR, Klein MB, Gernsheimer T, et-al. Heparin-induced thrombocytopenia in burns: a retrospective review. J Burn Care Res, in press.

[95] Herndon DN, Tompkins RG. Support of the metabolic response to burn injury. Lancet 2004;363(9424):1895–902.

[96] Wilmore DW, Mason AD Jr, Johnson DW, et al. Effect of ambient temperature on heat production and heat loss in burn patients. J Appl Physiol 1975;38(4):593–7.

[97] Gore DC, Chinkes D, Heggers J, et al. Association of hyperglycemia with increased mortality after severe burn injury. J Trauma 2001;51(3):540–4.

[98] Pham TN, Warren AJ, Phan HH, et al. Impact of tight glycemic control in severely burned children. J Trauma 2005;59(5):1148–54.

[99] Van den Berghe G, Wouters P, Weekers F, et al. Intensive insulin therapy in the critically ill patients. N Engl J Med 2001;345(19):1359–67.

[100] Van den Berghe G, Wilmer A, Hermans G, et al. Intensive insulin therapy in the medical ICU. N Engl J Med 2006;354(5):449–61.

[101] Suman OE, Spies RJ, Celis MM, et al. Effects of a 12-wk resistance exercise program on skeletal muscle strength in children with burn injuries. J Appl Physiol 2001;91(3):1168–75.

[102] Suman OE, Thomas SJ, Wilkins JP, et al. Effect of exogenous growth hormone and exercise on lean mass and muscle function in children with burns. J Appl Physiol 2003;94(6):2273–81.

[103] Klein GL, Wolf SE, Langman CB, et al. Effects of therapy with recombinant human growth hormone on insulin-like growth factor system components and serum levels of biochemical markers of bone formation in children after severe burn injury. J Clin Endocrinol Metab 1998;83(1):21–4.

[104] Takala J, Ruokonen E, Webster, et al. Increased mortality associated with growth hormone treatment in critically ill adults. N Engl J Med 1999;341(11):785–92.

[105] Demling RH, DeSanti L. The rate of restoration of body weight after burn injury, using the anabolic agent oxandrolone, is not age dependent. Burns 2001;27(1):46–51.

[106] Demling RH, DeSanti L. Oxandrolone induced lean mass gain during recovery from severe burns is maintained after discontinuation of the anabolic steroid. Burns 2003;29(8):793–7.

[107] Hart DW, Wolf SE, Ramzy PI, et al. Anabolic effects of oxandrolone after severe burn. Ann Surg 2001;233(4):556–64.

[108] Wolf SE, Edelman LS, Kemalyan N, et al. Effects of oxandrolone on outcome measures in the severely burned: a multicenter prospective randomized double-blind trial. J Burn Care Res 2006;27(2):131–9 [discussion: 140–1].

[109] Wolfe RR, Herndon DN, Jahoor F, et al. Effect of severe burn injury on substrate cycling by glucose and fatty acids. N Engl J Med 1987;317(7):403–8.

[110] Herndon DN, Hart DW, Wolf SE, et al. Reversal of catabolism by beta-blockade after severe burns. N Engl J Med 2001;345(17):1223–9.

[111] Saffle JR, Crandall A, Warden GD. Cataracts: a long-term complication of electrical injury. J Trauma 1985;25(1):17–21.

[112] Luce EA. Electrical burns. Clin Plast Surg 2000;27(1):133–43.

[113] Mann R, Gibran N, Engrav L, et al. Is immediate decompression of high voltage electrical injuries to the upper extremity always necessary? J Trauma 1996;40(4):584–7 [discussion: 587–9].

[114] Arnoldo BD, Purdue GF, Kowalske K, et al. Electrical injuries: a 20-year review. J Burn Care Rehabil 2004;25(6):479–84.

[115] Arnoldo B, Klein M, Gibran NS. Practice guidelines for the management of electrical injuries. J Burn Care Res 2006;27(4):439–47.

[116] Purdue GF, Hunt JL. Electrocardiographic monitoring after electrical injury: necessity or luxury. J Trauma 1986;26(2):166–7.

[117] Yowler CJ, Fratianne RB. Current status of burn resuscitation. Clin Plast Surg 2000;27(1): 1–10.
[118] Yowler CJ, Mozingo DW, Ryan JB, et al. Factors contributing to delayed extremity amputation in burn patients. J Trauma 1998;45(3):522–6.
[119] Engrav LH, Gottlieb JR, Walkinshaw MD, et al. Outcome and treatment of electrical injury with immediate median and ulnar nerve palsy at the wrist: a retrospective review and a survey of members of the American Burn Association. Ann Plast Surg 1990;25(3):166–8.
[120] Hunt J, Lewis S, Parkey R, et al. The use of Technetium-99m stannous pyrophosphate scintigraphy to identify muscle damage in acute electric burns. J Trauma 1979;19(6):409–13.
[121] Sheridan RL, Hinson MI, Liang MH, et al. Long-term outcome of children surviving massive burns. JAMA 2000;283(1):69–73.
[122] Brych SB, Engrav LH, Rivara FP, et al. Time off work and return to work rates after burns: systematic review of the literature and a large two-center series. J Burn Care Rehabil 2001; 22(6):401–5.
[123] Costa BA, Engrav LH, Holavanahalli R, et al. Impairment after burns: a two-center, prospective report. Burns 2003;29(7):671–5.
[124] Moore ML, Engrav LH, Vedder NB, et al. Dexter: a tool to facilitate impairment ratings. J Burn Care Rehabil 2001;22(6):397–400.
[125] Chang P, Laubenthal KN, Lewis RW II, et al. Prospective, randomized study of the efficacy of pressure garment therapy in patients with burns. J Burn Care Rehabil 1995;16(5):473–5.
[126] Patino O, Novick C, Merlo A, et al. Massage in hypertrophic scars. J Burn Care Rehabil 1999;20(3):268–71 [discussion: 267].
[127] So K, Umraw N, Scott J, et al. Effects of enhanced patient education on compliance with silicone gel sheeting and burn scar outcome: a randomized prospective study. J Burn Care Rehabil 2003;24(6):411–7 [discussion: 410].
[128] Zhu KQ, Engrav LH, Gibran NS, et al. The female, red Duroc pig as an animal model of hypertrophic scarring and the potential role of the cones of skin. Burns 2003;29(7):649–64.
[129] Zhu KQ, Engrav LH, Tamura RN, et al. Further similarities between cutaneous scarring in the female, red Duroc pig and human hypertrophic scarring. Burns 2004;30(6):518–30.
[130] Gallant CL, Olson ME, Hart DA. Molecular, histologic, and gross phenotype of skin wound healing in red Duroc pigs reveals an abnormal healing phenotype of hypercontracted, hyperpigmented scarring. Wound Repair Regen 2004;12(3):305–19.
[131] Klein MB, Nathens AB, Emerson D, et al. An analysis of the long-distance transport of burn patients to a regional burn center. J Burn Care Res 2006;32(8):940–5.
[132] Saffle JR, Edelman L, Morris SE. Regional air transport of burn patients: a case for telemedicine? J Trauma 2004;57(1):57–64 [discussion: 64].
[133] Nguyen LT, Massman NJ, Franzen BJ, et al. Telemedicine follow-up of burns: lessons learned from the first thousand visits. J Burn Care Rehabil 2004;25(6):485–90.
[134] Massman NJ, Dodge JD, Fortman KK, et al. Burns follow-up: an innovative application of telemedicine. J Telemed Telecare 1999;5(Suppl 1):S52–4.
[135] Smith AC, Youngberry K, Mill J, et al. A review of three years experience using email and videoconferencing for the delivery of post-acute burns care to children in Queensland. Burns 2004;30(3):248–52.
[136] Harrington DT, Biffl WL, Cioffi WG. The station nightclub fire. J Burn Care Rehabil 2005; 26(2):141–3.
[137] Yurt RW, Bessey PQ, Bauer GJ, et al. A regional burn center's response to a disaster: September 11, 2001, and the days beyond. J Burn Care Rehabil 2005;26(2):117–24.
[138] ABA Board of Trustees; Committee on organization and delivery of burn care. Disaster management and the ABA Plan. J Burn Care Rehabil 2005;26(2):102–6.
[139] Palmieri TL, Greenhalgh DG, Saffle JR, et al. A multicenter review of toxic epidermal necrolysis treated in US burn centers at the end of the twentieth century. J Burn Care Rehabil 2002;23(2):87–96.

ELSEVIER
SAUNDERS

Surg Clin N Am 87 (2007) 207–228

SURGICAL
CLINICS OF
NORTH AMERICA

Pediatric Injuries: Prevention to Resolution

Kim G. Mendelson, MD, PhD, Mary E. Fallat, MD*

*Division of Pediatric Surgery, Department of Surgery, University of Louisville,
233 East Gray Street, Suite 708, Louisville, KY 40202, USA*

Despite improved education and prevention initiatives, trauma remains the leading cause of death in children over 1 year of age, and exceeds all other causes of death combined. In 2003, there were 14,110 deaths from injury in children less than 18 years old reported to the National Center for Injury Prevention and Control. Of these, deaths from motor vehicle and traffic-related incidents were responsible for 63%, followed distantly by homicide or suicide and drowning. The leading cause of nonfatal injuries was falls, and of the more than 8 million nonfatal injuries receiving medical attention, 151,319 required hospitalization [1].

Age and sex are factors in the type and severity of pediatric injuries. Male children overall have higher injury and mortality rates [2]. Falls are most common in younger children, bicycle and pedestrian collisions in elementary-aged children, and motor vehicle collisions in adolescents. In both sexes, motor vehicle collisions are the leading cause of deaths. In adolescent boys, however, homicide is the second leading cause, whereas in girls it is suicide [1]. Contributing factors include premorbid conditions, such as behavioral disorders. For example, children with attention-deficit disorders have a more than 1.5 times risk of sustaining a traumatic injury [3].

Most injuries in children are a result of blunt trauma. Traumatic brain injury (TBI) is the most common injury, and can result in long-term disability. Abdominal trauma is also a leading cause of morbidity and mortality and can be challenging to diagnose, especially in younger nonverbal patients. Children often sustain injuries to multiple systems, including the head, chest, abdomen, genitourinary, and musculoskeletal systems. In these polytrauma patients, there is a death rate of 3% to 27% that correlates with the degree of TBI [4–7].

---
* Corresponding author.
E-mail address: mefall01@louisville.edu (M.E. Fallat).

0039-6109/07/$ - see front matter © 2006 Elsevier Inc. All rights reserved.
doi:10.1016/j.suc.2006.09.016

A variety of trauma registries and databases have been developed as a means to document and follow trauma trends and outcomes. The data accumulated in these registries can then be analyzed and used to influence local prevention initiatives and legislation. Examples of national databases that have or can be used include the now retired National Pediatric Trauma Registry and the current National Trauma Data Bank. A Web-based Injury Statistics Query and Reporting System has been developed by the National Center for Injury Prevention and Control to provide customized reports of injury statistics. In addition, individual states and trauma centers maintain internal registries.

Clearly, the financial burden of trauma on the health care system is substantial. Injury prevention efforts both in existence and development have the common goal to decrease the morbidity and mortality rates from trauma and thereby lower health care costs. The most effective efforts focus on severe but preventable injuries, such as those involving the brain and spinal cord, which often result in extended hospital stays and long-term disabilities. Public education and regulatory legislation aimed at proper child safety seat, booster seat, seat belt, and helmet use act as measures potentially to decrease the number and severity of severe traumatic injuries in children.

Injury prevention

Effective strategies for injury prevention follow a stepwise approach. The target issue is identified, goals are specified, interventions are planned, and these interventions are then executed and evaluated. Methods can be either active or passive. Passive prevention strategies work automatically. Some examples of passive strategies include reducing speed limits and requiring smoke detectors. These methods tend to be more successful than active intervention, which requires a behavioral change, such as wearing a helmet.

Education and legislation are often used in conjunction to address injury prevention. All-terrain vehicles (ATVs) were introduced in the early 1970s as recreational vehicles capable of negotiating rough terrain and adverse conditions. These machines have motorcycle-styled handlebars, a high center of gravity, and large tires. The first ATV, a three-wheeled vehicle made by Honda, was featured in the James Bond movie "Diamonds are Forever." These soon became popular, and were more widely manufactured. In 1983, Suzuki presented the first four-wheeled ATV as a vehicle for beginners. Although appearing safe, the inherently unstable design of the three-wheeled variety caused increasing numbers of injuries and deaths [8,9]. This machine tended to roll over during sharp turns, and flip backward while going uphill. In 1988, the United States Consumer Product Safety Commission entered into a binding 10-year consensus decree with ATV manufacturers that banned the sale of three-wheeled vehicles, established an ATV training program, and improved warning labels [10]. In addition, the American Academy of Pediatrics issued a policy statement discouraging the use of ATVs among children under 16 years of age [11].

Injuries and deaths from ATV crashes continue, however, to rise. An analysis of the Kids' Inpatient Database revealed a 79.1% increase in ATV-related hospitalizations in children under 18 years of age between 1997 and 2000, with a mortality rate in both years of 0.9%. Most patients were boys, and the largest age group was children 10 to 14 years of age. The mean charge per hospitalization was $13,000 [12]. The Consumer Product Safety Commission estimated that 33,071 children were treated for ATV-related injuries in 2001, which represented a 64% increase from 1997 [13]. Disturbingly, despite increasing public awareness and education, sales have climbed 89% in the past 5 years, [14] and children under 16 years of age comprise 35% of ATV-related deaths, representing a risk of death 4.5 to 12 times that of adults [15,16].

Numerous injury prevention strategies have been attempted, including safety education courses and safety legislation. Private organizations and state agencies offer hands-on safety courses designed for new riders and families. Most states have some usage restrictions involving age of driver or weight of vehicle, and 25 states require helmet and safety equipment. The challenge is to enforce these regulations, because even in states requiring helmets, usage approaches only 35% [16]. In one study, when asked to discuss prevention issues in focus groups, children admitted to risk-taking behavior and were resistant to age-based restrictions. They were receptive, however, to mandatory licensing and public service announcements containing straight-forward graphic messages about consequences [17].

It is estimated that over 30,000 injuries occur each year to children living on farms and ranches. Prevention strategies include restricting access to worksites and increasing education [18]. Farm safety day-camps, which have been held since the early 1900s, are attended by thousands of children in rural areas. Pretesting and posttesting done 3 to 4 months following these camps have shown an increase in knowledge and safe behaviors, especially in the areas of animal, grain, power take-off, and tractor safety. For those using ATVs, there was increased use of protective gear including helmets [19]. A similar intervention called Agricultural Disability Awareness and Risk Education (AgDARE), performed in schools in Kentucky, Iowa, and Mississippi, showed increases in safety behavioral changes [20,21]. It has been suggested that such educational programs might be useful in farming communities, such as the Amish, in which common mechanisms of pediatric injuries are falls, buggy versus motor vehicles collisions, and animal injuries [22].

Educational and legislative initiatives are also in effect for safety seat and seat belt compliance in motor vehicles. These may be partially responsible for the decline in the annual rate of child fatalities during 1978 to 2004 from 31.8 to 22.3 deaths per million [23]. State laws require safety seats for children less than 4 years of age and 40 lb, and an increasing number are now requiring booster seats for children up to 8 years of age and 80 pounds. Data from the National Electronic Injury Surveillance System-All Injury Program during 2004, however, revealed that 45% of children aged 12 years and under injured in motor vehicle collisions were either not restrained or inappropriately restrained. Unrestrained children were three times more likely to be hospitalized. Most inappropriate restraint use occurred among children aged 4 to 8 years who were placed in seat belts instead of booster seats [23]. Increased education is necessary for this high-risk population.

Legislation has also been effective in decreasing alcohol-related fatal motor vehicle crashes during 1982 to 2001, especially among drivers under 21 years of age. Interventions, such as raising the minimum legal drinking age to 21 years and zero tolerance blood alcohol concentration standards for drivers under 21 years, have countered the increased likelihood of these drivers to be involved in fatal crashes [24].

Even in the setting of penetrating injury, there is evidence that legislation can have a positive effect. In 12 states between 1990 and 1994, individual laws making gun owners responsible for storing firearms in a manner that makes them inaccessible to children were in effect for at least 1 year. During this time, unintentional shooting deaths in these states were reduced by 23% among children younger than 15 years [25]. Community initiatives have also been used to achieve firearm injury prevention [26,27]. A combination of education and enforced legislation that reaches target groups may be more effective.

Prehospital care

Optimal care and transport of pediatric trauma patients requires well-trained and well-equipped medical personnel. Educational courses, such as Pediatric Advanced Life Support [28] and Pediatric Education for the Prehospital Professional [29], are available but many rural communities rely on volunteers to provide prehospital care. These individuals may not have the time or resources to participate in these educational offerings. For example, more than 65% of Washington's certified emergency medical technicians are volunteers who undergo a community-based training program [30].

Variability in training and experience with pediatric patients is a key issue in prehospital management. The ability to manage the pediatric airway and venous access requires adequate education, experience, and skill maintenance. Studies of intubation attempts in children reveal a significantly increased risk of intubation failure, and often multiple attempts, which then leads to complications. This suggests not only that further education is necessary, but that bag-valve mask ventilation may be the safest method of airway control under certain circumstances [31,32]. Ambulances responding to pediatric trauma, whether advanced life support or basic life support, should have the appropriate-sized equipment for their expertise, including bag-valve masks, endotracheal tubes, blood pressure cuffs, and venous access devices.

Under ideal circumstances, for all potential multisystem trauma victims, an adequate airway must be established, spinal precautions maintained, and venous access attained, especially for long transports. The most common pediatric traumatic injury is TBI, and appropriate attention to limiting hypoxia and hypotension minimizes the potential for secondary brain injury. The initial stabilization of the pediatric trauma patient in the prehospital setting is similar to that for adults. The ABCs (airway, breathing, circulation) of trauma management are assessed and stabilized, and the child is transported as quickly as possible to a trauma center.

Although there is some evidence that transport to pediatric trauma centers versus community hospitals may result in lower mortality, the geographic limitations may be difficult to overcome. Especially in rural areas, time and distance problems exist, and adverse weather conditions may contribute to a triage decision to take a child to a closer facility without a trauma designation [33].

Initial evaluation and resuscitation

The initial evaluation and resuscitation of the pediatric trauma patient is similar to that of adults, and follows the Advanced Trauma Life Support guidelines [34]. The primary survey ensures adequacy of airway, breathing, and circulation, whereas the secondary survey assesses additional injuries. In trauma centers, a team approach is often used to address these issues simultaneously and thereby achieve greater time efficiency.

The pediatric airway is best stabilized by maintaining the middle face in a sniffing position while keeping the cervical spine immobilized. A careful jaw thrust can be used and the airway cleared of particulate matter and blood. If the patient has a decreased Glasgow Coma Scale (GCS) score of ≤ 8, or is experiencing respiratory distress, immediate intubation is warranted. Drug-assisted intubation is preferred in semiconscious children in the controlled setting of an emergency department. Orotracheal intubation is preferred in children < 8 years of age because of the more anterior and cephalad positioned airway, large adenoids and tonsils, and short trachea. The endotracheal tube size can be estimated by using a length-based pediatric tape; gauging the diameter of the little finger or nares; or using an age-based formula, such as [(age in years $+ 16)/4$]. Proper placement is confirmed by a combination of auscultation, end-tidal carbon dioxide detection, pulse oximetry, and chest radiograph. If an airway is unable to be established by the most experienced personnel, a temporizing needle cricothyroidotomy can be performed.

Appropriate intravenous access sites include the back of the hand, antecubital fossa, or saphenous vein at the ankle. If no intravenous line can be established after two attempts, intraosseous access in an uninjured proximal tibia or percutaneous femoral venous access should be obtained. At the same time venous access is initiated, laboratory studies can be drawn. Representative baseline laboratory work can include a complete blood count, liver function tests, and amylase. Urine is dipped for blood, and sent for urinalysis if positive. Additional laboratory work can include a type and crossmatch, an arterial blood gas if the child has been intubated, and a coagulation panel if indicated by GCS less than 13, hypotension, open fractures, and major soft tissue wounds [35].

Fluid resuscitation should begin immediately on arrival, because initial signs of shock are subtle in children and can be limited to tachycardia and lethargy. Hypotension, which is commonly estimated as less than 70 mm Hg plus twice the age in years, is a late sign of shock because of increased physiologic reserve. Loss of blood from external wounds may have occurred before presentation, and the presence of hypotension indicates a loss of approximately 40% of circulating blood volume. The initial fluid bolus is generally 10 or 20 mL/kg, or 25% of the blood volume of a child. Transfusion of O Rh-negative packed red blood cells at 20 mL/kg is considered if the child does not respond to repeated crystalloid boluses. If this is necessary, sources of bleeding should be rapidly identified. If bleeding sites are external and visible, direct pressure should be held and pressure dressings applied. Unless the patient has an unstable pelvic fracture or blood at the meatus, a Foley catheter should be placed for continued resuscitation monitoring. Signs of adequate resuscitation include resolution of tachycardia, return of capillary refill, clearing of the sensorium, and a sustained urine output of 1 to 2 mL/kg/h. Hypothermia should also be rectified through the use of external warming devices and heated intravenous fluids.

Initial radiographic evaluation of the patient includes chest and pelvis films. Cervical spine immobilization is maintained, because the requisite three views can be obtained after resuscitation and stabilization. In addition, radiographs of obviously injured extremities can be performed using the contralateral limb as a control for comparison. Evaluation of the abdomen is performed by physical examination followed by appropriate studies as necessary. Positive predictors of intra-abdominal injury include abdominal tenderness, ecchymosis and abrasions [36], tenderness combined with abnormal urinalysis [37], low systolic blood pressure [38], and decreased mental status [38,39]. Children with femur fractures have also been found to have a slightly increased incidence of intra-abdominal injury [38]. Especially in young nonverbal children, physical examination findings or concerning mechanism of injury should lead to a heightened awareness of the possibility of injury.

Radiographic imaging of the abdomen can include CT scanning or ultrasound. The Focused Assessment for the Sonographic Examination of the Trauma patient (FAST) examination surveys for the presence or absence of blood in dependent regions of the abdomen including the right upper quadrant, left upper quadrant, and pelvis. This rapid ultrasound assessment can be performed in the trauma bay using mobile equipment. In unstable trauma patients, a positive FAST examination mandates surgical intervention to determine the source of bleeding. Although the FAST examination has been found to have a high specificity and positive predictive value in the pediatric patient, it is operator dependent, and is most accurate when done by experienced personnel. In addition, the FAST examination does not detect intraparenchymal or retroperitoneal blood, and cannot grade solid organ injuries. Its use remains controversial, and may be suited for situations requiring rapid surgical decisions, such as in the unstable patient [40–44].

Liberal CT scanning is supported in the adult literature because of its sensitivity and rapidity [45]. Increased imaging, however, adds to the medical radiation burden and the cancer induction risk. For example, a standard chest CT has the radiation dose of 250 chest radiographs. In the pediatric population, this is especially concerning, because children are more radiosensitive and have longer life spans during which to acquire tumors. In addition, many findings identified on CT scanning do not impact patient management or outcome. For these reasons, initial plain radiographs should be carefully evaluated with the injury mechanism taken into consideration, and further imaging by CT scanning performed in a focused manner [46–50].

Abdominal CT scanning is indicated in the stabilized trauma patient with abdominal tenderness or external signs of injury. An unexplained drop in hemoglobin, hematuria, lower rib or pelvic fractures, uncorrected acidosis, severe head injury, or positive FAST examination can also be indications for abdominal imaging. CT scanning is more time consuming than the FAST examination, but has the advantage of specifically identifying and grading injuries. Neither CT nor ultrasound reliably detects intestinal injury.

Head CT scans are commonly obtained in children with a history of loss of consciousness or significant mechanism of injury, although the additional presence of headache, emesis, intoxication, seizure, short-term memory deficits, or physical evidence of trauma above the clavicles make the scan more likely to show an intracranial abnormality [51–53]. Chest CT scans are helpful in patients with abnormal chest radiographs, obvious trauma to the chest wall, or high-force impact [46,54]. CT scans of the cervical spine may be useful in patients with head injuries, [55] but can usually be performed after identification of life-threatening injuries unless there is obvious neck trauma or neurologic disability.

Throughout the resuscitation and evaluation period, the presence of family members can be calming and reassuring to the frightened child. There is often a perception that family presence during trauma resuscitation is disruptive. Fear that a family member will hinder medical personnel, either through emotional outbursts or by making the providers uncomfortable, has often resulted in protocols mandating removal of family from the area. It is also conceivable, however, that the inclusion of family members in the resuscitation environment reduces their and their child's anxiety and allows for an improved flow of information. Several medical associations, including the American Academy of Pediatrics [56] and the American Heart Association [57], recommend allowing family members to be present during procedures and resuscitation under certain circumstances according to guidelines and protocols.

A survey of parents permitted to maintain a family presence during procedures and resuscitations indicated that it was a positive experience, their presence eased their fears, and it was beneficial to the child. Three months after the encounter, they still had a positive recollection and no traumatic memories. Most of the health care providers were also positive about the experience, commenting that the presence of family members did not disrupt patient care, and may have resulted in increased professionalism among the staff [58].

Management by systems

Traumatic brain injury

TBI, defined as a trauma-induced alteration in mental status that may or may not involve the loss of consciousness, is the leading cause of traumatic death and disability in children [5–7]. In infants and young children, falls are the most common cause, with falls from heights greater than 3 ft most likely to cause intracranial injury. Motor vehicle crashes are a common cause in older children, and often result in more significant intracranial pathology than falls. TBI can also result from sports trauma and child maltreatment. TBI is often associated with other injuries and has been reported in 17% of children with polytrauma [5].

Primary brain injury, which occurs immediately after the insult, is typically characterized by focal lesions that can lead to impaired autoregulation of cerebral blood flow and contribute to cerebral edema. Although the skulls of children have an "architectural advantage" because of the cranial sutures and the buttress support provided by the sphenoid and petrous bones [59], intracranial hemorrhage, intraparenchymal contusion, and skull fractures occur, with the parietal bone the most commonly fractured (60%–70%) [60]. Basilar skull fractures involving the temporal or parietal bone may lead to permanent hearing loss if the cochlear-vestibular apparatus is affected, or meningitis if a dural tear occurs [61,62].

Evaluation of injured children involves a complete neurologic examination, including assessment of the GCS score, which has been adapted for application in infants and young children [63]. Additional imaging can then be performed to assess the extent of intracranial injury. Studies to define better the group of children needing a head CT scan have not been definitive, with even a documented loss of consciousness lacking predictive value [64,65]. The presence of altered mental status, focal neurologic deficit, skull fracture, loss of consciousness, emesis, amnesia, headache, or drowsiness have all been suggested as indications for imaging [51,66]. In addition, scalp abnormalities [63,65,67,68] or facial fractures [69–71] have been correlated with injury. Because even neurologically intact children can have intracranial injury, and those with GCS scores of 13 to 15 have an incidence of intracranial pathology of up to 33% [63], a high index of suspicion is necessary. Nonverbal or poorly verbal children under 2 years of age have also been found to have a high incidence of skull fracture and intracranial injury. A management strategy that categorizes these patients into four subgroups based on risk of injury has been devised; in this scheme, only children in the lowest risk category (ie, falls less than 3 ft), no clinical signs or symptoms of TBI, and age >1 year, are not imaged and are treated only with observation [72].

A goal of clinical management is to minimize secondary brain injury by supporting oxygenation, ventilation, and perfusion, which minimizes or prevents hypoxemia and hypoperfusion. Neurosurgical intervention to evacuate intracranial blood is directed by imaging studies. Intracranial pressure monitoring may be needed in children with evidence of cerebral edema and a GCS of ≤8 to measure and maintain adequate cerebral perfusion pressure. There is variation in the use of paralytic agents, sedatives, seizure medications, and intracranial pressure monitoring across pediatric critical care units because of lack of evidence-based standards.

Despite aggressive therapy, the overall mortality rate from severe TBI is approximately 8%. Although this is less than in the adult population, children are more vulnerable to long-term disability. Speech and feeding difficulties are associated with increasing severity of head injury [73], whereas personality changes are found across the injury severity continuum [74,75]. Even children with mild head injury may have difficulties with behavior and cognition, although these are usually transient. These injuries may have a major impact on the lives of the children and their families long after the actual event.

Spine and spinal cord injury

Although the incidence in children is less than that in adults, pediatric spine injuries have been reported as 2% to 5% of all spine injuries [76]. The greater mobility and elasticity of the pediatric spine and the smaller body mass of a child offer some protection to injury. Certain anatomic features, however, predispose children to cervical spine injury. In children under 8 years of age, a heaver head and weak ligaments permit greater mobility of C-1 on C-2 compared with the lower spine. In addition, horizontally inclined facets, immature vertebral joints, growth centers susceptible to shear forces, and a higher fulcrum of flexion make injury from the occiput to the base of C-2 more likely. In older children, cervical spine fractures mainly occur at C-5 to C-6 [77,78].

Improper restraint of children in motor vehicles results in specific patterns of injury. Airbags deploy by releasing hot effluent at 300 km/h. If children are positioned close to the airbag, injury can result either from direct contact of hot gas or from energy transmission to the head and neck. TBI and spinal injuries including atlanto-occipital dislocation and cervical spinal cord transaction can occur [79–81]. Seat belt injuries are also common. The term "seat belt syndrome" was coined by Garrett and Braunstein [82] in 1962 to describe a distinctive pattern of injuries associated with lap seat belts, which ride across the abdomen rather than the bony prominences of the pelvis. These include hip and abdominal contusions, or the "seat belt sign"; pelvic fractures; lumbar spine injuries; and intra-abdominal injuries (Fig. 1). Both compression fractures and Chance fractures, or flexion-distraction injuries, of the lumbar spine have been described as part of seat belt syndrome. Children aged 3 to 9 years are at particular risk because of improper use of seat belt restraints riding above the iliac crests, although seat belt syndrome has been reported in children as young as 2 months of age [83–87].

Evaluation of the cervical spine typically begins with plain radiographs. The lateral view is sensitive for most injuries, but can miss pathology up to 25% of the time. Anatomic variables, such as pseudosubluxation, which occurs normally in up to 40% of children, physiologic increased distance between the dens and the anterior arch of C-1, and skeletal growth centers, may make interpretation challenging. In children under age 12, up to 5 mm at the atlanto-dens interval and 3 mm of C-2 on C-3 may be physiologic. CT scanning in these cases may be indicated but can be done at the discretion of a neurosurgeon given the radiation exposure involved. MRI is needed if spinal cord injury is suspected. Plain radiographs also serve as the initial evaluation of the thoracic and lumbar spines, with further imaging performed as indicated. A subtle indication of thoracic spine injury on the initial chest radiograph is widening of the paraspinal lines, which should lead to focused CT imaging [46].

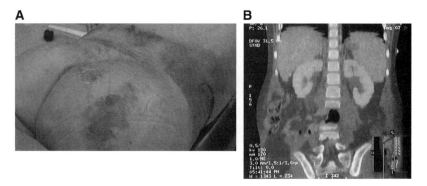

Fig. 1. (*A*) Circumferential seat-belt sign caused by lap belt. (*B*) L3 Chance fracture caused by lap belt trauma. The aorta was acutely occluded at this level. Additional injuries included degloving of the sigmoid colon and a transected right ureter.

A clinical entity specific to children is spinal cord injury without radiographic abnormality. It is thought that the increased elasticity of the pediatric spine predisposes it to injury from stretch, hyperflexion, or hyperextension. This results in neurologic deficits without radiographic evidence of bony injury. MRI scans are helpful in determining the level and extent of injury [78,88].

Once spinal injury is suspected, high-dose steroid therapy may be initiated. The National Acute Spinal Cord Injury Studies reported improvement in motor function and sensation when patients with complete or incomplete spinal cord injury from nonpenetrating mechanisms were treated with high doses of methylprednisolone within 8 hours [89–91]. The standard protocol is an initial loading dose of 30 mg/kg followed by a drip at 5.4 mg/kg/h. Patients treated earlier than 3 hours after injury are given methylprednisolone for 24 hours, whereas patients treated 3 to 8 hours after injury receive it for 48 hours. There is much controversy, however, concerning the positive effect of steroid administration. The American College of Surgeons has recently amended the Advanced Trauma Life Support guidelines to refer to steroids as "a recommended" rather than "the recommended" treatment. Although methylprednisolone possesses neuroprotective effects, the risks of steroid therapy include an increased incidence of infection and avascular necrosis [92–94]. High-dose steroids should not be used for patients with spinal cord injury from penetrating trauma [95].

Unstable fractures and those associated with spinal cord injury should be treated with early operative intervention. Generally, management includes posterior fusion with internal fixation.

Orthopedic injury

Orthopedic injuries are often seen in combination with other organ system injuries, and affect long-term morbidity after polytrauma. Up to 76% of children with multiple injuries have extremity fractures [6]. Evaluation of the musculoskeletal system begins with a complete physical examination. A neurovascular examination is essential to document distal perfusion and neurologic status. Radiographic evaluation begins with plain films of suspicious areas. Adjacent joints and bones should also be radiographed, because there are often fractures at multiple levels, especially in association with calcaneal fractures and cervical spine injuries. Children with femur fractures have a high incidence of concomitant injury, and should be thoroughly evaluated. Pelvic fractures are often associated with high-energy mechanisms, and with multiple organ system involvement. If an unstable pelvic fracture is suspected, stabilization of the pelvis is essential to prevent excessive blood loss, and this may require the urgent placement of an external fixator. In addition, because 9% to 24% of children with pelvic fractures have genitourinary injuries [4], caution is advised in placing urinary catheters.

Initial care consists of immobilizing and splinting. Although most orthopedic injuries do not require emergent surgical intervention, there is evidence that early fracture stabilization may decrease complications and
allow for early mobilization. Most patients with multiple injuries undergo
fixation within 24 to 72 hours. Stable pelvic fractures are treated nonoperatively, whereas unstable pelvic fractures and acetabular fractures usually
require surgical stabilization. Open fractures, which occur when the broken
bone penetrates the skin, are initially treated with Betadine dressing and
limb alignment and splinting. These require thorough operative debridement, preferably within 6 hours. Tetanus prophylaxis should be given depending on the child's immunization history. Because the infection rate
approaches 50% in contaminated wounds, intravenous antibiotics should
be started [4]. Guidelines developed by the Eastern Association for the Advancement of Trauma suggest the use of gram-positive coverage for grade I
and II fractures with the addition of gram-negative coverage for grade III
fractures. The length of treatment is controversial, especially for more extensive injuries. Antibiotic coverage for 24 hours postinjury is probably adequate for primarily closed grade I and II injuries [96].

Thoracic injury

Thoracic injury has been reported in 8% to 62% of children with multiple
system injuries, and has a 25% mortality rate in association with TBI or abdominal trauma [4]. The most common thoracic injuries in children are pulmonary contusions, hemothorax, and pneumothorax. Rib fractures are
uncommon because of the greater pliability of the bones and cartilage of
children, but if present can be an indicator of more severe injuries. Similarly,
injuries to the heart and great vessels are less common than in adults because
of greater elasticity and mobility, and imply high-energy mechanisms
[4,46,97].

The initial radiograph is an anteroposterior chest film. Although the
supine film obtained in the trauma bay may be affected by technical factors
and artifact, life-threatening conditions, such as a tension pneumothorax,
can be diagnosed and treated. Pulmonary contusions may be evident on
plain film or be seen on CT scan as peripheral areas of consolidation without air bronchograms. If great vessel injury is suspected, CT angiography or
arch angiography should be performed [46].

Pulmonary contusions lead to focal edema and hemorrhage. The radiographic appearance typically worsens over the first few days because of secondary edema from disruption of the alveolar-capillary interface. This is
treated with oxygen or mechanical ventilatory support. Pneumothoraces
and hemothoraces are typically treated with chest tubes on initial evaluation. The persistence of pneumothorax and pneumomediastinum can indicate tracheobronchial injury, which can be further delineated with
thoracic CT scan and bronchoscopy. Injury to the tracheobronchial tree

in children typically occurs within 2 cm of the carina in the right mainstem bronchus and requires surgical repair. Benign pneumomediastinum can also occur as a result of blunt abdominal trauma against a closed glottis, and generally does not cause pneumothorax and is self-limiting [46].

Other less common injuries include blunt cardiac injuries, great vessel injuries, esophageal injuries, and diaphragmatic ruptures. Each of these should be suspected on the basis of mechanism, initial radiographs, clinical appearance, and associated injuries. Additional studies and interventions should then be performed.

Abdominal injury

Motor vehicle collisions, pedestrian trauma, and falls are the most common causes of intra-abdominal injury. Children injured by mechanisms resulting in direct force applied to the abdomen, such as with lap belts, vehicle handlebars, sports, or direct blows, should also have careful evaluation [98]. Lap belt injuries with seat belt signs frequently result in small bowel mesenteric tears and perforations [82–87]. Handlebar blows to the abdomen can cause small bowel and pancreatic injury (Fig. 2) [99]. Solid organ injury to the kidney, spleen, and liver can be seen in sports-related trauma [100].

Useful laboratory tests include the complete blood count, liver function tests, and urinalysis. An initial hematocrit of less than 30 could indicate an intra-abdominal injury but is not specific for injury [38]. More usefully, serial hematocrits are used to follow the progress of solid organ injuries. Similarly, serial pancreatic enzymes may be useful in diagnosing intestinal injury, but the initial value is less helpful [101]. Liver transaminases have been shown to be predictors of hepatic injury, and can direct CT scanning [102]. Gross and microscopic hematuria has also been described as a marker of renal injuries in children, although asymptomatic hematuria is of low yield in the absence of physical findings [37,38,103–105].

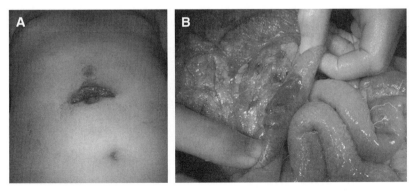

Fig. 2. (*A*) Bicycle handlebar trauma. The handlebar entered the peritoneal cavity inferiorly. (*B*) Transverse colon and jejunum injury caused by handlebar trauma.

Solid organ injuries are common in children sustaining blunt trauma. The liver is the most commonly injured, and may result in most fatalities directly related to abdominal injury. Hepatic injury can be staged using CT scanning with intravenous contrast. The American Association for the Surgery of Trauma has developed a grading scale for liver injury ranging from subcapsular hematoma to global destruction (Table 1) [106]. Hemodynamically stable children with hepatic injury are managed nonoperatively with resuscitation and serial examinations and laboratory studies. Hemodynamic instability may necessitate emergent operative intervention. Arterial embolization, either alone or in combination with operative management, has also been described [107,108]. Nonoperative management is successful in 85% to 90% [98,109]. Follow-up CT scans are routinely not necessary unless new symptoms arise [110].

The spleen is also commonly injured by blunt traumatic mechanisms, and has a similar grading system (Table 2) [106]. Most injured spleens in children can be salvaged, with a success rate of 90% to 98% [98]. This may be partially caused by the favorable anatomy of the pediatric spleen, which has a thicker capsule and tends to fracture along avascular horizontal planes. Even if a contrast blush is evident on CT scanning, splenic preservation can be achieved, although in these patients eventual operative intervention is more likely [111,112]. In children with concurrent mononucleosis, in which spontaneous splenic rupture occurs in 0.6% to 0.7% of patients between 14 and 28 days of infection, splenic salvage may also be successful [113,114]. Children with splenic injuries are closely observed with bed rest

Table 1
Liver injury grading scale

I	Hematoma	Subcapsular, <10% surface area
	Laceration	Capsular tear, <1 cm parenchymal depth
II	Hematoma	Subcapsular, 0%–50% surface area; intraparenchymal, <10 cm in diameter
	Laceration	1–3 cm parenchymal depth, <10 cm in length
III	Hematoma	Subcapsular, >50% surface area or expanding; ruptured subcapsular or parenchymal hematoma. Intraparenchymal hematoma >10 cm or expanding
IV	Laceration	Parenchymal disruption involving 25%–75% of hepatic lobe or 1–3 Couinaud's segments within a single lobe
V	Laceration	Parenchymal disruption involving >75% of hepatic lobe or >3 Couinaud's segments within a single lobe
	Vascular	Juxtahepatic venous injuries (ie, retrohepatic vena cava or central major hepatic veins)
VI	Vascular	Hepatic avulsion

Adapted from Moore EE, Cogbill TH, Jurkovich GJ, et al. Organ injury scaling: spleen and liver (1994 revision). J Trauma 1995;38:323–4; with permission.

Table 2
Spleen injury grading scale

I	Hematoma	Subscapular, <10% surface area
	Laceration	Capsular tear, <1 cm parenchymal depth
II	Hematoma	Subscapular, 10%–50% surface area; intraparenchymal, 5 cm in diameter
	Laceration	1–3cm parenchymal depth, which does not involve a trabecular vessel
III	Hematoma	Subscapular, >50% surface area or expanding; ruptured subscapular or parenchymal hematoma. Intraparenchymal hematoma >5 cm or expanding
IV	Laceration	Laceration involving segmental or hilar vessels producing major devascularization (>25% of spleen)
V	Laceration	Completely shattered spleen
	Vascular	Hilar vascular injury, which devascularizes spleen

Adapted from Moore EE, Cogbill TH, Jurkovich GJ, et al. Organ injury scaling: spleen and liver (1994 revision). J Trauma 1995;38:323–4; with permission.

and monitoring. In cases of hemodynamic instability or continually decreasing hematocrit, splenectomy, splenorrhaphy, or arterial embolization is indicated.

For both liver and spleen injuries, a standardized approach to hospital management has been suggested. This includes recommendations for hospital stay and activity restriction for each grade of injury (Table 3) [115].

Other intra-abdominal injuries include those involving the kidneys, intestines, and pancreas. Similar to injuries of the liver and spleen, most renal injuries are treated nonoperatively. Absolute indications for operative intervention and reconstruction are an expanding or pulsatile hematoma, and relative indications include arterial injury or urinary extravasation. The success rate of renal preservation is greater than 98% [116,117]. Intestinal injuries commonly occur in association with direct blunt force or seat belt trauma during deceleration [82–87]. A high index of suspicion is necessary to diagnose these injuries, because the initial clinical presentation may be benign and CT scans equivocal. Worsening of abdominal pain and

Table 3
Proposed guidelines for resource use in children with isolated spleen or liver injury

	CT grade			
	I	II	III	IV
ICU stay (d)	None	None	None	1
Hospital stay (d)	2	3	4	5
Predischarge imaging	None	None	None	None
Postdischarge imaging	None	None	None	None
Activity restriction (wk)	3	4	5	6

From Stylianos S, APSA trauma committee. Evidence-based guidelines for resource utilization in children with isolated spleen or liver injury. J Pediatr Surg 2000;35:164–9; with permission.

feeding intolerance should lead to further studies or intervention. Direct force, such as from handlebars, may also lead to pancreatic injury, which is more common in children because of the underdeveloped abdominal musculature and horizontally oriented costal margins, which allow the body of the pancreas to be compressed against the vertebral column [118]. Pancreatic injury can be suggested from pancreatic enzyme levels, although these are relatively insensitive and nonspecific [101]. CT scanning can be diagnostic, or endoscopic retrograde cholangiopancreatography may be done in difficult cases to delineate ductal injury. Pancreatic injury without ductal involvement may be managed nonoperatively, but major ductal disruption requires resection. Spleen-preserving distal pancreatectomy is the preferred operation if no injury to the spleen has occurred.

Child maltreatment

The four defined types of child maltreatment are neglect, physical abuse, sexual abuse, and emotional abuse. The Centers for Disease Control and Prevention estimates that 906,000 children in the United States in 2002 were maltreated, and 1500 children died from maltreatment, as confirmed by child protective service agencies. The direct costs to the judicial, law enforcement, and health care systems are estimated at $24 billion per year, whereas the indirect long-term economic costs are more than $69 billion annually [119]. The societal consequences of child maltreatment are significant, because physical abuse during infancy or early childhood has effects on brain development, and children who experience maltreatment are at increased risk for adverse health effects and behaviors as adults [120–122].

Because children are often brought to the emergency department repetitively with nonspecific complaints, there are opportunities to intervene before a fatal outcome [123]. Discrepancies in the history or inconsistency between the history and anatomic injury should act as red flags to all health care providers. Common injuries associated with maltreatment include acute or chronic subdural hematomas, genital or perianal injuries, burn scars, bruises, multiple healed fractures with callus, and multiple aligned posterior rib fractures that may result from anteroposterior chest compression [46,123,124]. Characteristics helpful in distinguishing abusive head injury from other trauma include retinal hemorrhages, especially if they are bilateral; abnormal mental status; and seizures at initial presentation [125]. If maltreatment is suspected, the involvement of child protective services is mandatory, and most states require a formal report.

Recovery phase

Discharge from the hospital is only the start of a long recovery phase. Children may need inpatient or outpatient rehabilitation services, and close follow-up with medical specialists, and may experience long-term physical and psychologic problems as a result of trauma. Acute stress disorder is common within the month following the trauma, and risk factors include family stress, caregiver stress, child's experience of pain, and child's age. There is also an increased incidence of longer-term posttraumatic stress disorder in children initially diagnosed with acute stress disorder, with over 30% of children involved in trauma found to have posttraumatic stress symptoms [126]. Interventional programs that target acute stress disorder and posttraumatic stress disorder may provide an opportunity to improve functional recovery after injury in children.

References

[1] Centers for Disease Control and Prevention, National Centers for Injury Prevention and Control. Web-based injury statistics query and reporting system (WISQARS). Available at: www.cdc.gov/ncipc/wisqars. Accessed June 18, 2006.

[2] Dandrinos-Smith S. The epidemiology of pediatric trauma. Crit Care Nurs Clin North Am 1991;3:387–9.

[3] Brehaut JC, Miller A, Raina P, et al. Childhood behavior disorders and injuries among children and youth: a population based study. Pediatrics 2003;111:262–9.

[4] Kay RM, Skaggs DL. Pediatric polytrauma management. J Pediatr Orthop 2006;26: 268–77.

[5] Letts M, Davidson D, Lapner P. Multiple trauma in children: predicting outcome and long-term results. Can J Surg 2002;45:126–31.

[6] Schalamon J, von Bismarck S, Schober PH, et al. Multiple trauma in pediatric patients. Pediatr Surg Int 2003;19:417–23.

[7] van der Sluis CK, Kingma J, Eisma WH, et al. Pediatric polytrauma: short-term and long-term outcomes. J Trauma 1997;43:501–6.

[8] Smith LM, Pittman MA, Marr AB, et al. Unsafe at any age: a retrospective review of all-terrain vehicle injuries in two level I trauma centers from 1995 to 2003. J Trauma 2005;58: 783–7.

[9] Moroney P, Doyle M, Mealy K. All-terrain vehicles – unstable, unsafe, and unregulated: a prospective study of ATV-related trauma in rural Ireland. Injury 2003;34:203–5.

[10] US District Court for the District of Columbia. United States of America versus American Honda Motor Co., Inc., et al: Final Consent Decree: Civil Action 87–3525. March 14, 1988.

[11] American Academy of Pediatrics, Committee on Injury and Poison Prevention. All-terrain vehicle injury prevention: two-, three-, and four-wheeled unlicensed motor vehicles. Pediatrics 2000;105:1352–4.

[12] Killingsworth JB, Tilford JM, Parker JG, et al. National hospitalization impact of pediatric all-terrain vehicle injuries. Pediatrics 2005;115:316–21.

[13] Levenson MS. All-terrain vehicle 2001 injury and exposure studies. Washington: US Consumer Product Safety Commission; 2003.

[14] Fialka JJ. As ATVs take off in sales, deaths and injuries mount. Wall Street Journal, February 10, 2004. p. A-1.

[15] Brown RL, Koepplinger ME, Mehlman CT, et al. All-terrain vehicle and bicycle crashes in children: epidemiology and comparison of injury severity. J Pediatr Surg 2002;37:375–80.

[16] Kelleher CM, Metze SL, Dillon PA, et al. Unsafe at any speed: kids riding all-terrain vehicles. J Pediatr Surg 2005;40:929–35.

[17] Aitken ME, Graham CJ, Killingworth JB, et al. All-terrain vehicle injury in children: strategies for prevention. Inj Prev 2004;10:303–7.

[18] Brison RJ, Pickett W, Berg RL, et al. Fatal agricultural injuries in preschool children: risks, injury patterns and strategies for prevention. CMAJ 2006;174:1723–6.

[19] McCallum DM, Conaway MB, Drury S, et al. Safety-related knowledge and behavior changes in participants of farm safety day camps. J Agric Saf Health 2005;11:35–50.

[20] Reed DB, Westneat SC, Kidd P. Observation study of students who completed a high school agricultural safety education program. J Agric Saf Health 2003;9:275–83.

[21] Reed DB, Kidd P, Westneat S, et al. Agricultural Disability Awareness and Risk Education (AgDARE) for high school students. Inj Prev 2001;7(Suppl 1) i59–63.

[22] Vitale MA, Rzucidlo S, Shaffer ML, et al. The impact of pediatric trauma in the Amish community. J Pediatr 2006;148:359–65.

[23] Centers for Disease Control and Prevention (CDC). Nonfatal injuries and restraint use among child passengers— United States, 2004. MMWR Morb Mortal Wkly Rep 2006; 55:624–7.

[24] Elder RW, Shults RA. Involvement by young drivers in fatal alcohol-related motor-vehicle crashes—United States, 1982–2001. MMWR 2002;519480:1089–91.

[25] Cummings P, Grossman DC, Rivara FP, et al. State gun safe storage laws and child mortality due to firearms. JAMA 1997;278:1084–6.

[26] Kallenborn JC, Gonzales K, Crane NB, et al. Cease Fire Tampa Bay: a three-tiered approach to firearm injury prevention. J Trauma Nurs 2004;11:6–11.

[27] Hardy MS. Behavior-oriented approaches to reducing youth gun violence. Dallas (TX): Future Child 2002;12:100–17.

[28] Pediatric advanced life support. American Heart Association: 2002.

[29] Pediatric education for the prehospital professional. Elk Grove Village (IL): American Academy of Pediatrics: 2001.

[30] Washington State Department of Health. Available at: http://www.doh.wa.gov. Accessed June 19, 2006.

[31] Garza AG, Algren DA, Gratton MC, et al. Populations at risk for intubation nonattempt and failure in the prehospital setting. Prehosp Emerg Care 2005;9:163–6.

[32] Ehrlich PF, Seidman PS, Atallah O, et al. Endotracheal intubations in rural pediatric trauma patients. J Pediatr Surg 2004;39:1376–80.

[33] Poltavski D, Muus K. Factors associated with incidence of inappropriate ambulance transport in rural areas in cases of moderate to severe head injury in children. J Rural Health 2005;21:272–7.

[34] Advanced trauma life support. Chicago: American College of Surgeons: 2006.

[35] Holmes JF, Goodwin HC, Land C, et al. Coagulation testing in pediatric blunt trauma patients. Pediatr Emerg Care 2001;17:324–8.

[36] Cotton BA, Beckert BW, Smith MK, et al. The utility of clinical and laboratory data for predicting intraabdominal injury among children. J Trauma 2004;56:1068–74 [discussion: 1074–5].

[37] Isaacman DJ, Scarfone RJ, Kost SI, et al. Utility of routine laboratory testing for detecting intra-abdominal injury in the pediatric trauma patient. Pediatrics 1993;92:691–4.

[38] Holmes JF, Sokolove PE, Brant WE, et al. Identification of children with intra-abdominal injuries after blunt trauma. Ann Emerg Med 2002;39:500–9.

[39] Beaver BL, Colombani PM, Fal A, et al. The efficacy of computed tomography in evaluating abdominal injuries in children with major head trauma. J Pediatr Surg 1987;22: 1117–22.

[40] Suthers SE, Albrecht R, Foley D, et al. Surgeon-directed ultrasound for trauma is a predictor of intra-abdominal injury in children. Am Surg 2004;70:164–7.

[41] Ballard RB, Rozycki GS, Newman PG, et al. An algorithm to reduce the incidence of false-negative FAST examinations in patients at high risk for occult injury. Focused Assessment for the Sonographic Examination of the Trauma patient. J Am Coll Surg 1999;189:145–50.

[42] Soudack M, Epelman M, Maor R, et al. Experience with focused abdominal sonography for trauma (FAST) in 313 pediatric patients. J Clin Ultrasound 2004;32:53–61.

[43] Thourani VH, Pettitt BJ, Schmidt JA, et al. Validation of surgeon-performed emergency abdominal ultrasonography in pediatric patients. J Pediatr Surg 1998;33:322–8.

[44] Coley BD, Mutabagani KH, Martin LC, et al. Focused abdominal sonography for trauma (FAST) in children with blunt abdominal trauma. J Trauma 2000;48:902–6.

[45] Salim A, Sangthong B, Martin M, et al. Whole body imaging in blunt multisystem trauma patients without obvious signs of injury: results of a prospective study. Arch Surg 2006;141: 468–73.

[46] Westra SJ, Wallace EC. Imaging evaluation of pediatric chest trauma. Radiol Clin North Am 2005;43:267–81.

[47] Frush DP. Review of radiation issues for computed tomography. Semin Ultrasound CT MR 2004;25:17–24.

[48] Frush DP, Donnelly LF, Rosen NS. Computed tomography and radiation risks: what pediatric health care providers should know. Pediatrics 2003;112:951–7.

[49] Berrington de Gonzalez A, Darby S. Risk of cancer from diagnostic x-rays: estimates for the UK and 14 other countries. Lancet 2004;363:345–51.

[50] Brenner D, Elliston C, Hall E, et al. Estimated risks of radiation-induced fatal cancer from pediatric CT. AJR Am J Roentgenol 2001;176:289–96.

[51] Haydel MJ, Shembekar AD. Prediction of intracranial injury in children aged five years and older with loss of consciousness after minor head injury to nontrivial mechanisms. Ann Emerg Med 2003;42:515–8.

[52] Munson S, Schroth E, Ernst M. The role of functional neuroimaging in pediatric brain injury. Pediatrics 2006;117:1372–81.

[53] Simon B, Letourneau P, Vitorino E, et al. Pediatric minor head trauma: indications for computed tomographic scanning revisited. J Trauma 2001;51:231–7.

[54] Renton J, Kincaid S, Ehrlich PF. Should helical CT scanning of the thoracic cavity replace the conventional chest x-ray as a primary assessment tool in pediatric trauma? An efficacy and cost analysis. J Pediatr Surg 2003;38:793–7.

[55] Keenan HT, Hollingshead MC, Chung CJ, et al. Using CT of the cervical spine for early evaluation of pediatric patients with head trauma. AJR Am J Roentgenol 2002; 179:533.

[56] Henderson DP, Knapp JF. Report of the national consensus conference on family presence during pediatric cardiopulmonary resuscitation and procedures. J Emerg Nurs 2006;32: 23–9.

[57] American Heart Association. 2005 American Heart Association guidelines for cardiopulmonary resuscitation and emergency cardiovascular care. Circulation 2005;112(24 Suppl) IV-1–211.

[58] Mangurten J, Scott SH, Guzzeta CE, et al. Effects of family presence during resuscitation and invasive procedures in a pediatric emergency department. J Emerg Nurs 2006;32: 225–33.

[59] Ghajar J, Hariri RJ. Management of pediatric head injury. Pediatr Clin North Am 1992;39: 1093–125.

[60] Schutzman SA, Greenes DS. Pediatric minor head trauma. Ann Emerg Med 2001;37:65–74.

[61] Woestman R, Perkin R, Serna T, et al. Mild head injury in children: identification, clinical evaluation, neuroimaging, and disposition. J Pediatr Health Care 1999;5(6 Pt 1): 288–98.

[62] Thiessen ML, Woolridge DP. Pediatric minor closed head injury. Pediatr Clin North Am 2006;53:1–26.

[63] Holmes JF, Palchak MK, MacFarlane T, et al. Performance of the pediatric Glasgow coma scale in children with blunt head trauma. Acad Emerg Med 2005;12:814–9.

[64] Davis RL, Mullen N, Makela M, et al. Cranial computed tomography scans in children after minimal head injury with loss of consciousness. Ann Emerg Med 1994;24:713–4.

[65] Mitchell KA, Fallat ME, Raque GH, et al. Evaluation of minor head injury in children. J Pediatr Surg 1994;29:851–4.

[66] Quayle KS, Jaffe DM, Kuppermann N, et al. Diagnostic testing for acute head injury in children: when are head computed tomography and skull radiographs indicated? Pediatrics 1997;99:E11.

[67] Greenes DS, Schutzman SA. Clinical indicators of intracranial injury in head-injured infants. Pediatrics 1999;104(4 Pt 1):861–7.

[68] Gruskin KD, Schutzman SA. Head trauma in children younger than 2 years: are there predictors for complications? Arch Pediatr Adolesc Med 1999;153:15–20.

[69] Holmgren EP, Dierks EJ, Homer LD, et al. Facial computed tomography use in trauma patients who require a head computed tomogram. J Oral Maxillofac Surg 2004;62:911–2.

[70] Alvi A, Doherty T, Lewen G. Facial fractures and concomitant injuries in trauma patients. Laryngoscope 2003;113:102–6.

[71] Keenan HT, Brundage SI, Thompson DC, et al. Does the face protect the brain? A case-control study of traumatic brain injury and facial fractures. Arch Surg 1999;134:14–7.

[72] Schutzman SA, Barnes P, Duhaime AC, et al. Evaluation and management of children younger than two years old with apparently minor head trauma: proposed guidelines. Pediatrics 2001;107:983–93.

[73] Pavlovitch C, DiRusso SM, Risucci D, et al. Mortality and functional outcome in pediatric trauma patients with and without head injuries. Acad Emerg Med 2003;10:495–6.

[74] Hawley CA, Ward AB, Magnay AR, et al. Outcomes following head injury: a population study. J Neurol Neurosurg Psychiatry 2004;75:737–42.

[75] Hawley CA. Behaviour and school performance after brain injury. Brain Inj 2004;18:645–59.

[76] Parisini P, DiSilvestre M, Greggi T. Treatment of spinal fractures in children and adolescents: long-term results in 44 patients. Spine 2002;27:1989–94.

[77] Orenstein JB, Klien BL, Gotschall CS, et al. Age and outcome in pediatric cervical spine injury: 11-year experience. Pediatr Emerg Care 1994;10:132–7.

[78] Hayes JS, Arriola T. Pediatric spinal injuries. Pediatr Nurs 2005;31:464–7.

[79] Quinones-Hinojosa A, Jun P, Manley GT, et al. Airbag deployment and improperly restrained children: a lethal combination. J Trauma 2005;59:729–33.

[80] Giguere JF, St-Vil D, Turmel A, et al. Airbags and children: a spectrum of C-spine injuries. J Pediatr Surg 1998;33:811–6.

[81] Morrison AL, Chute D, Radentz S, et al. Air bag-associated injury to a child in the front passenger seat. Am J Forensic Med Pathol 1998;19:218–22.

[82] Garrett JW, Braunstein PW. The seat belt syndrome. J Trauma 1962;2:220–38.

[83] Durbin DR, Arbogast KB, Moll EK. Seat belt syndrome in children: a case report and review of the literature. Pediatr Emerg Care 2001;17:474–7.

[84] Walsh A, Sheehan E, Walsh MG. Lumbar Chance fracture associated with use of the lap belt restraint in an adolescent. Ir Med J 2003;96:148–9.

[85] Jordan B. Lap belt complex: recognition and assessment of seatbelt injuries in pediatric trauma patients. JEMS 2001;26:36–43.

[86] Santschi M, Echave V, Laflamme S, et al. Seat-belt injuries in children involved in motor vehicle crashes. Can J Surg 2005;48:373–6.

[87] Davies KL. Buckled-up children: understanding the mechanism, injuries, management, and prevention of seat belt related injuries. J Trauma Nurs 2004;11:16–24.

[88] Betz RR, Mulcahey MJ, D'Andrea LP, et al. Acute evaluation and management of pediatric spinal cord injury. J Spinal Cord Med 2004;27(Suppl 1):S11–5.

[89] Bracken MB, Collins WF, Freeman DF, et al. Efficacy of methylprednisolone in acute spinal cord injury. JAMA 1984;251:45–52.

[90] Bracken MB, Shepard MJ, Hellenbrand KG, et al. Methylprednisolone and neurological function 1 year after spinal cord injury. Results of the National Acute Spinal Cord Injury Study. J Neurosurg 1985;63:704–13.

[91] Bracken MB. Treatment of acute spinal cord injury with methylprednisolone: results of a multicenter, randomized clinical trial. J Neurotrauma 1991;8(Suppl 1):S47–50.

[92] Gerndt SJ, Rodriguez JL, Pawlik JW, et al. Consequences of high-dose steroid therapy for acute spinal cord injury. J Trauma 1997;42:279–84.

[93] Pointillart V, Petitjean ME, Wiart L, et al. Pharmacological therapy of spinal cord injury during the acute phase. Spinal Cord 2000;38:71–6.

[94] Matsumoto T, Tamaki T, Kawakami M, et al. Early complications of high-dose methyl-prednisolone sodium succinate treatment in the follow-up of acute cervical spinal cord injury. Spine 2001;26:426–30.

[95] Heary RF, Vaccaro AR, Mesa JJ, et al. Steroids and gunshot wounds to the spine. Neurosurgery 1997;41:576–83 [discussion: 583–4].

[96] Luchette FA, Bone LB, Born CT, et al. EAST practice management guidelines work group: practice management guidelines for prophylactic antibiotic use in open fractures. Available at: http://www.east.org/tpg/openfrac.pdf. Accessed June 20, 2006.

[97] Bliss D, Silen M. Pediatric thoracic trauma. Crit Care Med 2002;30(11 Suppl):S409–15.

[98] Wegner S, Colletti JE, Van Wie D. Pediatric blunt abdominal trauma. Pediatr Clin North Am 2006;53:243–56.

[99] Nadler EP, Potoka DA, Shultz BL, et al. The high morbidity associated with handlebar injuries in children. J Trauma 2005;58:1171–4.

[100] Wan J, Corvino TF, Greenfield SP, et al. The incidence of recreational genitourinary and abdominal injuries in the Western New York pediatric population. J Urol 2003;170(4 Pt 2): 1525–7 [discussion: 1527].

[101] Adamson WT, Hebra A, Thomas PB, et al. Serum amylase and lipase alone are not cost-effective screening methods for pediatric pancreatic trauma. J Pediatr Surg 2003;38: 354–7 [discussion: 354–7].

[102] Puranik SR, Hayes JS, Long J, et al. Liver enzymes as predictors of liver damage due to blunt abdominal trauma in children. South Med J 2002;95:203–6.

[103] Stalker HP, Kaufman RA, Stedje K. The significance of hematuria in children after blunt abdominal trauma. AJR Am J Roentgenol 1990;154:569–71.

[104] Stein JP, Kaji DM, Eastham J, et al. Blunt renal trauma in the pediatric population: indications for radiographic evaluation. Urology 1994;44:406–10.

[105] Taylor GA, Eichelberger MR, Potter BM. Hematuria: a marker of abdominal injury in children after blunt trauma. Ann Surg 1988;208:688–93.

[106] Moore EE, Cogbill TH, Jurkovich GJ, et al. Organ injury scaling: spleen and liver (1994 revision). J Trauma 1995;38:323–4.

[107] Kushimoto S, Koido Y, Omoto K, et al. Immediate postoperative angiographic embolization after damage control surgery for liver injury: report of a case. Surg Today 2006;36: 566–9.

[108] Mohr AM, Lavery RF, Barone A, et al. Angiographic embolization for liver injuries: low mortality, high morbidity. J Trauma 2003;55:1077–81.

[109] Kozar RA, Moore JB, Niles SE, et al. Complications of nonoperative management of high-grade blunt hepatic injuries. J Trauma 2005;59:1066–71.

[110] Cox JC, Fabian TC, Maish GO III, et al. Routine follow-up imaging is unnecessary in the management of blunt hepatic injury. J Trauma 2005;59:1175–8.

[111] Cloutier DR, Baird TB, Gormley P, et al. Pediatric splenic injuries with a contrast blush: successful nonoperative management without angiography and embolization. J Pediatr Surg 2004;39:969–71.

[112] Nwomeh BC, Nadler EP, Meza MP, et al. Contrast extravasation predicts the need for operative intervention in children with blunt splenic injuries. J Trauma 2004;56:537–41.

[113] Meguid AA, Ivascu FA, Bair HA, et al. Management of blunt splenic injury in patient with concurrent infectious mononucleosis. Am Surg 2004;70:801–4.

[114] Statter MB, Liu DC. Nonoperative management of blunt splenic injury in infection mononucleosis. Am Surg 2005;71:376–8.

[115] Stylianos S, APSA Trauma Committee. Evidence-based guidelines for resource utilization in children with isolated spleen or liver injury. J Pediatr Surg 2000;35:164–9.

[116] Broghammer JA, Langenburg SE, Smith SJ, et al. Pediatric blunt renal trauma: its conservative management and patterns of associated injuries. Urology 2006;67:823–7.

[117] Buckley JC, McAninch JW. The diagnosis, management, and outcomes of pediatric renal injuries. Urol Clin North Am 2006;33:33–40.

[118] Fanta K, Cook BS, Schweer L. Traumatic injury to the pancreas: the challenges of care in the pediatric patient. J Trauma Nurs 2003;10:72–8.

[119] Centers for Disease Control and Prevention. Child maltreatment fact sheet. Available at: http://www.cdc.gov/ncipc/factsheets/cmfacts.htm. Accessed June 20, 2006.

[120] Barlow KM, Thomson E, Johnson D, et al. Late neurologic and cognitive sequelae of inflicted traumatic brain injury in infancy. Pediatrics 2005;116 e174–85.

[121] Gushurst CA. Child abuse: behavioral aspects and other associated problems. Pediatr Clin North Am 2003;50:919–38.

[122] Nemeroff CB. Neurobiological consequences of childhood trauma. J Clin Psychiatry 2004; 65(Suppl 1):18–28.

[123] King WK, Kiesel EL, Simon HK. Child abuse fatalities: are we missing opportunities for intervention? Pediatr Emerg Care 2006;22:211–4.

[124] Kleinman PK, Schlesinger AE. Mechanical factors associated with posterior rib fractures: laboratory and case studies. Pediatr Radiol 1997;27:87–91.

[125] Bechtel K, Stoessel K, Leventhal JM, et al. Characteristics that distinguish accidental from abusive injury in hospitalized young children with head trauma. Pediatrics 2004;114:165–8.

[126] Saxe GN, Miller A, Bartholomew D, et al. Incidence of and risk factors for acute stress disorder in children with injuries. J Trauma 2005;59:946–53.

ELSEVIER
SAUNDERS

SURGICAL
CLINICS OF
NORTH AMERICA

Surg Clin N Am 87 (2007) 229–245

Injury in the Elderly and End-of-Life Decisions

Tammy T. Chang, MD, PhD[a],
William P. Schecter, MD[a,b],*

[a]Department of Surgery, University of California, San Francisco, San Francisco, CA, USA
[b]San Francisco General Hospital, San Francisco, CA, USA

Case presentation

A 65-year-old woman struck by an automobile at 30 miles per hour presented to the emergency department with a systolic blood pressure (BP) of 110 mm Hg, a heart rate of 84, a respiratory rate of 18, and a Glasgow Coma Scale score (GCS) of 15. Her only initial complaint was right upper extremity pain. During the secondary survey, her BP fell to 60/30 mm Hg and her GCS decreased to 12. The initial Focused Abdominal Sonogram for Trauma (FAST) examination was negative, but a repeat FAST examination demonstrated fluid in Morison's pouch. Other pertinent positive physical findings included pain on palpation of the pelvis and the presence of blood at the introitus. The patient was intubated and a large-bore femoral venous catheter placed for fluid resuscitation. Type-specific blood was transfused when her BP failed to improve after infusion of 2 L of crystalloid and she was transported directly to the operating room for abdominal exploration. A family member reported that the patient's underlying medical problems included hypertension, diabetes, atrial fibrillation, osteoporosis, and hypothyroidism. Her daily medications included metoprolol and warfarin.

Epidemiology of aging

The population of the United States is aging. Individuals ages 65 and older made up 12% of the population in the year 2000 and are expected

* Corresponding author. Department of Surgery, University of California, San Francisco, San Francisco General Hospital, 1001 Potrero Avenue, Ward 3A17, San Francisco, CA 94110.
E-mail address: bschect@sfghsurg.ucsf.edu (W.P. Schecter).

0039-6109/07/$ - see front matter © 2006 Elsevier Inc. All rights reserved.
doi:10.1016/j.suc.2006.09.010
surgical.theclinics.com

to be 20% of the population by 2030. The elderly will be the most rapidly growing sector of the population, increasing from 35 million people to 72 million people between 2000 and 2030 [1]. Today's senior citizens have fewer disabilities and more active lifestyles than those of previous generations, which increase their risk of injury. One study estimates that 40% of all trauma patients will be 65 or older by 2050 [2].

Definition of geriatric trauma

Geriatric trauma usually is defined as injury in people ages 65 and older. Some published studies, however, include people older than 55, or even 45, in their analysis of geriatric trauma outcomes. The mortality rate from minor injury (Injury Severity Score [ISS] <9) is increased in people older than 65, and the mortality rate from moderate injury (ISS 9–24) begins to increase at age 45 [3]. The risk of death from major trauma rises sharply after age 45 and doubles by age 75 [4].

Other studies stratify the elderly population into two groups: patients between ages 65 and 80 and the very elderly, who are older than 80. Octogenarian trauma patients have an overall higher mortality rate (10%) compared with those between ages 65 and 80 (6.6%). They also have worse functional outcomes if they survive their injuries and are more likely to lose the ability to walk and transfer independently [5].

Mechanism of injury

Falls are the most common mechanism of injury in the elderly population [6] and are responsible for significant morbidity, mortality, and medical cost [7]. Motor vehicle collisions are the second most common mechanism of injury followed by pedestrian–motor vehicle accidents. Pedestrian–motor vehicle injuries affect children and the elderly disproportionately and result in a higher mortality rate in elderly patients compared with other age groups [8].

Predictors of morbidity and mortality

Age

There may be many reasons why elderly patients have increased morbidity and mortality rates after trauma. They are more likely to have underlying medical conditions that limit their physiologic response to injury. Eighty percent of the population over age 65 has at least one chronic medical condition and 50% has at least two [1]. In addition, elderly patients tend to sustain more severe injuries [9], and ISS is one of the strongest predictors of mortality [10]. Age in and of itself, however, is an independent predictor of poor outcome even when controlled for comorbidities and ISS. In a retrospective analysis of 22,571 patients who had blunt trauma, of whom 7117

(32%) were older than 65, elderly patients had almost twice the mortality rate when stratified for ISS and pre-existing medical conditions [11]. Age, injury severity, and pre-existing medical conditions all were independent predictors of death as determined by a logistic regression analysis of 5139 patients, including 448 (9%) patients older than 65. After controlling for ISS and pre-existing medical conditions, trauma patients older than 65 still were 4.6 times more likely to die than younger patients (P < .001) [12]. These results indicate that age alone is a powerful predictor of mortality in trauma patients.

Comorbidities

Other factors contribute to the morbidity and mortality of elderly trauma patients. Certain pre-existing medical conditions increase the risk of death after trauma significantly. Cirrhosis increases the relative mortality risk by 4.5, coagulopathy by 3.2, ischemic heart disease by 1.8, chronic obstructive pulmonary disease by 1.8, and diabetes by 1.2 [13]. Other conditions found to increase the risk of death significantly include renal disease and malignancy [14,15]. In addition, not only are comorbidities more prevalent in the elderly population, but also cardiovascular disease and diabetes are associated with significantly higher mortality rates in patients over 65 than in younger patients who have these conditions [12].

Severity of injury

The severity of injury tends to increase in older patients. In a study of 1039 trauma patients, the average ISS of 45 patients ages 75 and older was 18 compared with an ISS of 11–12 in the remaining 994 patients (P < .0005). Less than 20% of the younger patients had an ISS greater than 20 compared with almost 50% of the patients older than 75 [9]. The mortality rate was 40% in patients who had severe injury (ISS > 25) in a study of 852 trauma patients older than 65. The ISS was the variable that correlated most significantly with the risk of death. Other physiologic factors associated with poor prognosis (mortality rate > 80%) were hypoventilation (respiratory rate < 10), hypotension (systolic BP < 90), and GCS less than 3 on admission [10].

Age as a trauma center triage criterion

Evidence indicates that many injured elderly patients are undertriaged to trauma centers despite the increased risk of death and complications. The mean age of severely injured patients (ISS > 16) admitted to level I trauma centers was 33 compared with 56 at nontrauma hospitals in Portland, Oregon. Patients over age 65 were 5 times more likely to be undertriaged to a nontrauma hospital (P < .0001) [16]. Another study based on statewide data from Maryland demonstrated that significantly fewer elderly patients meeting physiologic and mechanism criteria were transported to trauma centers than with younger patients [17]. Appropriate triage is important, because very elderly patients who have severe injury have better outcomes when treated at a trauma center. In a study of 455 severely injured octogenarians (ISS 21–45), inhospital survival was 56% in trauma centers but only 8% in hospitals without a trauma program [18].

One possible cause of the undertriage of elderly trauma patients is the late presentation of physical findings indicating hypovolemia. Sixty-three percent of patients 70 years old and older who had severe injuries (ISS > 15) did not meet the standard hemodynamic criteria for trauma team activation at one trauma center [19]. There was a trend toward a decreased mortality rate once age greater than 70 was added as a criterion for trauma team activation [20].

Special physiologic and medical considerations

Physiologic reserve

Why does age in itself increase the risk of morbidity and mortality in trauma patients? The elderly have decreased reserve, limiting the physiologic response to hypovolemia. Cardiac index decreases 1% per year with age whereas systemic vascular resistance rises 1% per year. Maximal heart rate and the effect of adrenergic stimulation are reduced with age [21]. Trauma patients over age 65 demonstrate significantly lower measured cardiac index, oxygen delivery, and oxygen consumption compared with younger trauma patients [22]. Not only are elderly patients less able to compensate for the physiologic demands of hypovolemia, they suffer more adverse consequences from hypoperfusion than do younger patients. In one study of 264 patients, prolonged lactic acidosis was associated with an increased risk of death in patients older than 55 but not in younger patients [23].

β-Blockers

In addition to diminished physiologic reserve, many elderly patients take medications that alter their response to stress. Approximately 20% of the elderly who have coronary artery disease and 10% of those who have hypertension take β-blockers [24]. Tachycardia is an important sign of hypovolemia and may be masked in elderly patients taking β-blocker medications. Thus, elderly patients often may not exhibit the hemodynamic indications for trauma team activation despite severe injury [19]. Interpretation of hemodynamic parameters in elderly trauma patients is difficult, especially in the presence of beta-blockade.

Anticoagulation

Warfarin is a common anticoagulant used in the management of elderly patients who have a variety of medical conditions, including atrial fibrillation, deep vein thrombosis, and prosthetic heart valves. Chronic oral anticoagulation carries a 1% per year risk of spontaneous intracranial hemorrhage [25]. Head trauma in elderly patients on oral anticoagulation can be deadly. The mortality rate of 25 elderly patients on warfarin (international normalized ratio [INR] 3.2 ± 1.9) with traumatic intracranial hemorrhage was 48% compared with a mortality rate of 10% in age-matched controls who were not taking warfarin (INR 1.0 ± 0.1) [26]. A more recent study showed even worse outcomes when anticoagulation was supratherapeutic. In 49 anticoagulated patients who had severe brain injury (GCS ≤8) and an average INR of 6.5, the mortality rate was 87.8%. The mortality rate for 77 anticoagulated patients who had minor brain injury (initial GCS 13–15) and an average INR of 4.4 was similarly high at 80.6%. Fifty-four of the 77 patients who had minor brain injury were admitted for observation. Nearly 70% of these patients had an initial normal head CT scan. Eighty percent of the patients deteriorated within 12 hours to a GCS less than or equal to 10 with significant intracranial hemorrhage. The mortality rate was 84% [27]. One large retrospective study did not demonstrate a difference in mortality between head and nonhead injury patients on anticoagulation versus matching controls. The INR data of the study population, however, were not reported and the degree of anticoagulation could not be assessed [28].

Rapid reversal of anticoagulation with fresh frozen plasma (FFP) transfusion is beneficial. Compared with a mortality rate of 48% reported in a previous study [26], the mortality rate was decreased to 10% with FFP reversal in 19 patients on warfarin (average initial INR 2.7) who had documented intracranial hemorrhage and GCS less than or equal to 14. The INR was normalized to an average of 1.5 within 2 hours with up to 4 units of FFP transfusion and intravenous vitamin K [29].

There is increasing evidence that factor VIIa reverses the coagulopathy associated with prolonged shock and massive transfusion in selected trauma patients [30,31]. Factor VIIa also is effective in reversing the anticoagulation effects of warfarin in patients who have intracranial hemorrhage [32]. The precise indications for factor VIIa administration remain to be determined.

Antiplatelet agents, aspirin and clopidogrel, frequently are used for treatment and prophylaxis of cardiovascular disease. In a study of 110 elderly head injury patients (ages 60 and older), there was no significant difference in the frequency of intracranial hemorrhage between the patients who had and who did not have preinjury low-dose aspirin therapy [33]. Two other studies, however, indicated that antiplatelet drugs increased mortality in elderly patients who had head trauma. Forty-seven percent of elderly intracranial hemorrhage patients receiving aspirin died compared with 8% of case-matched controls not receiving aspirin [34]. A more recent retrospective report studied the effect of aspirin and clopidogrel in elderly patients who had head injury. Fifty of 90 intracranial hemorrhage patients 50 and older were treated with antiplatelet agents before injury; 58 received aspirin;

12 received clopidogrel; and 20 received aspirin and clopidogrel. The mortality rate was 23% in patients taking antiplatelet drugs and 8% in case-matched control patients not taking any antiplatelet drugs ($P = .016$). There was no difference in mortality between patients taking aspirin or clopidogrel as single agents. There also was no difference in mortality between patients taking only one drug compared with those taking aspirin and clopidogrel. Platelet transfusions were given to 24 patients who had received antiplatelet drugs, although the impact of platelet therapy on survival was unclear [35].

Elderly patients on oral anticoagulation with signs of head trauma require closer monitoring even without depressed GCS or overt neurologic symptoms. One retrospective study of 144 asymptomatic elderly patients who had mild head trauma and were taking warfarin showed that 7% had clinically important intracranial injury [36]. Given the high mortality rate and the subtle presentation of significant intracranial hemorrhage in anticoagulated patients, head CT scan and close neurologic monitoring are warranted on all head trauma patients receiving oral anticoagulation.

> An intracranial bolt was placed during surgery because of a decline in GCS to 12 during resuscitation. The initial intracranial pressure was 15 mm Hg. Exploratory laparotomy revealed a grade II splenic laceration and a large retroperitoneal hematoma. She was resuscitated aggressively with 14 units of packed red blood cells. Her coagulopathy was corrected with 13 units of FFP, two units of cryoglobulin, and two six-packs of platelets. She continued to bleed from the open pelvic fracture, however, which was packed. After surgery, the patient was transferred to the interventional radiology suite for an angiogram, which demonstrated active extravasation from the left and the right internal iliac and the right L4 lumbar arteries. These arteries were embolized, resulting in hemostasis.
>
> After stabilization in an ICU, the patient underwent CT imaging of the head and abdomen in addition to standard roentgenograms of the upper and lower extremities demonstrating the following injuries:
>
> 1. Extensive bilateral subarachnoid hemorrhage with blood in the left lateral ventricle
> 2. A grade II splenic lacerations
> 3. Bilateral superior and inferior pubic rami fractures
> 4. A right sacral fracture
> 5. A comminuted fracture of the right proximal humeral head
> 6. A right tibial plateau fracture

Head injury

Head injury in the elderly most often is caused by falls and pedestrian–motor vehicle collisions [37]. Subdural hematomas are common in the elderly population because of the fragile bridging veins and increased distance between the dura and brain parenchyma. In contrast, epidural hematomas are relatively uncommon because the dura tends to adhere to the skull with increasing age. The initial clinical presentation of an intracranial space-occupying lesion may be subtle in elderly patients because of the presence of cerebral atrophy [6].

The mortality rate and functional outcome is poorer in elderly as compared with younger patients. In a study of 661 patients from the Traumatic Coma Data Bank, the overall mortality rate was 38% compared with 80% for patients older than 55. Age was an independent predictor of death starting at age 45 [37]. There seems to be a linear relationship between age and worsening outcome after severe traumatic brain injury (GCS 3 to 8). The odds of death, vegetative state, or severe disability increases by 50% with every 10-year increase in age [38]. Patients older than 65 demonstrated larger subdural hematoma volumes, greater midline shifts, and a mortality rate 4 times greater than younger patients in a study of traumatic subdural hematomas [39]. Elderly trauma patients who present with a GCS of 8 or lower have an extremely poor prognosis. In an analysis of 136 head injury patients older than 70 who had GCS less than or equal to 8, the mortality rate was nearly 100% for those who had significant space-occupying lesions and 80% for those who had nonsurgical lesions [40]. In another study of 40 patients 65 or older with GCS less than or equal to 8, only 13 patients survived to be discharged from the hospital (survival rate 32%); all patients who had an initial GCS of 3 died. After hospital discharge, 85% had long-term survival up to 3 years. Only three patients who had an initial GCS of 8, however, lived with functional independence; all patients who had GCS between 4 and 7 were in a persistent vegetative state or required intensive supportive care [41].

Some investigators suggest that elderly patients who have head trauma should be re-evaluated after 72 hours of aggressive treatment because the functional outcome is so poor. These investigators suggest that further aggressive therapy is unlikely to benefit these patients if significant improvement is not seen within this period [21].

Abdominal injury

Nonoperative management of blunt abdominal solid organ injury in hemodynamically stable patients now is standard care [42]. Nonoperative management of splenic injury in the elderly, however, must be approached with particular caution. Although the spleen tends to be more fragile in elderly patients, their diminished physiologic reserve makes them less tolerant of hypovolemia because of hemorrhage. Some studies report success rates of nonoperative management of splenic trauma in patients over 55 comparable to the results achieved in younger adults (success rates 83%–100%) [43–47]. In a series of 23 hemodynamically stable patients over age 55 who had nonoperative management of splenic trauma, only four required splenectomy because of clinical decompensation [43]. In another series of 18 patients older than 55 who met hemodynamic criteria for nonoperative management, three patients failed conservative management and required splenectomy or splenorrhaphy; two of these three patients died [44]. All these studies suffer from small sample size and many do not include the grade of splenic injury in the analysis, making comparison between the elderly and younger cohorts impossible.

In a retrospective study of 1485 patients, 1261 patients (85%) were younger than 55, and 224 patients (15%) were 55 or older. The proportion of patients requiring immediate surgical exploration was similar between the two groups (38% and 41%, respectively). The mortality rate in the elderly group was 43%, significantly higher than the 23% mortality rate in the younger group ($P < .05$). Only 24 of the 132 elderly patients who underwent nonoperative management required subsequent surgical exploration. This 80% success rate for nonoperative management in patients older than 55 is comparable to the reported rates of previous studies. The mortality rate was significantly higher in elderly patients, however, for either successful nonoperative management (8% versus 4%, $P < .05$) or failed nonoperative management (29% versus 12%, $P = .054$). There was a trend toward an increased failure rate for nonoperative management in the elderly with increasing grade of splenic injury. The success rates for nonoperative management were comparable, between less than 55 and greater than or equal to 55 age groups for grade I splenic injury (74% versus 84%). Success rates, however, were lower in the elderly patients for grade II injury (73% versus 54%) and grade III injury (52% versus 28%). Although 17% of patients younger than 55 who had grade IV-V splenic injury still were managed successfully without an operation, all patients in the elderly group who had grade IV-V injury either went directly to the operating room or failed nonoperative management [48].

These results highlight the vulnerability of elderly patients who have blunt splenic trauma. The data suggest that nonoperative management of splenic trauma in the elderly should be undertaken with caution because older patients have an increased risk of death after failed nonoperative management compared with younger patients. Age greater than 55 is not an absolute contraindication to nonoperative management; in fact, the majority of elderly patients (approximately 80%) who have blunt splenic trauma can be managed successfully nonoperatively. The success of nonoperative management likely is lower in elderly who have higher grades of splenic injury. A prerequisite for nonoperative management for blunt splenic injury for any patients is hemodynamic stability. Regardless of age, signs of hemodynamic compromise in patients who have splenic injury mandate prompt exploration in the operating room.

Pelvic and extremity fractures

Osteoporosis is common in elderly women. Fractures of the spine, hip, and distal forearm frequently are associated with osteoporotic bone, but all types of fractures are increased in patients who have low bone density [49]. Pelvic fracture is the most serious skeletal injury in the elderly. The overall mortality rate from acute or delayed complications of pelvic fracture is up to 81% in elderly patients who have open pelvic fracture [50]. The pattern of pelvic fracture is different in elderly compared with younger patients. The elderly were 4.6 times more likely to have lateral compression fractures than anterior-posterior compression fractures in a study of 234 patients who had pelvic fracture, 39 of whom were above age 55. Although 98% of the fractures were minor (lateral compression types I and II), elderly patients were nearly 3 times more likely to receive blood transfusions than younger patients. Elderly patients also were more likely to require angiographic intervention. Despite aggressive therapy, the 21% mortality rate for patients 55 or older was significantly higher than the 6% mortality rate in the younger group ($P < .005$) [51]. Another study of 350 patients, including 57 patients over age 55, corroborated the finding that elderly patients who had pelvic fractures have a higher mortality rate (12.3% versus 2.3%, $P < .05$) [52]. Despite less severe pelvic fractures, blood loss and the risk of death are higher in elderly compared with younger patients.

Elderly patients are more likely to have unsatisfactory functional outcomes regardless of the type of extremity fracture treatment. In a study of 40 patients who had tibial plateau fractures and were 50 or older, 23 (72%) of 32 patients treated operatively and three (38%) of eight patients treated nonoperatively believed that their outcomes were unsatisfactory based on a self-assessment questionnaire [53]. Elderly patients who have periarticular fractures may require primary prosthetic replacement to avoid complications of delayed union, nonunion, loss of fixation, or osteonecrosis. Prosthetic replacement may be a particularly attractive surgical option for displaced or comminuted fractures of the femoral neck, proximal humerus, and elbow. Osteopenic bones in the elderly usually require intramedullary devices for optimal fixation. Other materials, such as polymethylmetharcylate, calcium phosphate, and calcium sulfate cements, are used to enhance hardware fixation in elderly osteoporotic patients [54].

Timing orthopedic surgery in geriatric trauma patients depends on the nature and severity of the visceral, neurologic, and orthopedic injuries and on the physiologic status of patients. In a series of 367 elderly patients who had hip fractures, a delay in surgical treatment for more than 2 days was associated with more than double the risk of death within the first postoperative year [55]. Another study of hip fractures demonstrated that patients who had three or more comorbidities had a poorer survival rate if they had their operation within 24 hours of admission compared with more than 24 hours after admission [56]. Surgical correction of most orthopedic injuries in the elderly should occur as soon as possible after treatment of shock and life-threatening injuries and optimization of comorbid conditions.

The patient was brought to the ICU where resuscitation efforts continued. Her BP remained marginal and required vasopressor support. A pulmonary artery catheter (PAC) was placed to help guide fluid resuscitation. Although the initial chest radiograph did not show any evidence of chest trauma, the following day the patient developed bilateral pulmonary infiltrates consistent with the acute respiratory distress syndrome. She became increasingly difficult to oxygenate, requiring a high inspired oxygen concentration and positive end-expiratory pressure. A repeat head CT scan 48 hours later demonstrated increasing subarachnoid hemorrhage and massive cerebral edema. Further aggressive therapy was deemed futile. After discussion with the patient's family, aggressive support was withdrawn and the patient expired.

Intensive care of geriatric trauma patients

A study of 26,237 trauma patients, of whom 7117 (27%) were 65 or older, demonstrated that age was an independent risk factor for morbidity and mortality. Elderly patients have longer hospital lengths of stay (mean 9.2 ± 9.6 days) compared with younger patients between ages 18 and 65 (mean 8.3 ± 10.0 days, $P < .001$). Although elderly patients have a lower ICU admission rate (36.7%) compared with younger patients (45.5%), presumably because of death of more elderly patients before ICU admission, once admitted they have a longer period of ICU stay compared with younger patients (mean 6.7 ± 9.2 versus 5.4 ± 8.7, $P < .001$) [11].

Not surprisingly, preventable complications are associated with 32% of all deaths and 62% of deaths caused by multiple organ failure or sepsis in patients 65 or older [57]. The risk of death increases significantly with the number of complications [58].

Elderly patients are at particular risk for nosocomial infections. Thirty-nine percent of patients 65 or older, compared with 17% of younger patients ($P < .005$), developed nosocomial infection in a study of 3254 patients. The mortality rate for elderly patients who had nosocomial infection in this study was 28% compared with 5% for younger patients ($P < .005$). The presence of chronic obstructive pulmonary disease was an independent risk factor for nosocomial infection [59]. Prevention and early aggressive treatment of nosocomial infection is essential to improve outcome of geriatric trauma patients requiring intensive care [21].

The optimal method of hemodynamic monitoring in ICUs is unclear. Arterial and central venous pressure (CVP) catheters are routine monitors for critically injured patients. A prospective randomized study of 70 elderly hip fracture patients in 1985 suggested that the mortality rate could be significantly reduced by use of PACs [60]. PAC monitoring has been recommended for optimal management of critically ill geriatric trauma patients [21]. No clinical benefit, however, from PAC monitoring was demonstrated in large prospective studies of either ICU patients or high-risk geriatric surgical patients. PAC monitoring was associated with an increase in risk of death in the ICU study [61] and pulmonary embolism in the geriatric surgery study [62]. CVP and PAC have risks of technical complications and nosocomial infection.

Transthoracic echocardiography (TTE) and transesophageal echocardiography (TEE) can provide information on cardiac anatomy, ventricular wall motion and filling, and ejection fraction. They can be used to supplement or replace the information derived from the CVP and PAC as a guide to hemodynamic management of geriatric trauma patients. TTE and TEE have the disadvantages of requiring interval examinations to answer volume status and cardiac function questions at different points in time. Both require extensive training for the technical examination and correct interpretation of images [63–65].

Long-term functional outcome

Long-term functional outcomes of elderly trauma patients who survive their injuries can be good. In a large-scale retrospective study of 38,707 patients, ages 65 and older, 50% of the survivors were discharged to home and 25% of the survivors were transferred to a skilled nursing facility [66]. In another study, 48 of 495 geriatric trauma patients (9.7%) survived for 3 years after injury. Eight of the 48 survivors (16.6%) returned to their preinjury level of function and 32 survivors (67%) were able to live independently [67]. In another study of 279 patients, ages 75 and older, 77 of 93 patients (83%) who survived for 4 years after injury were living in an independent setting [68]. The available data indicate that age alone is not an indication to withhold aggressive therapy [21].

Advance directives and health care proxies

There are two basic types of advance directives: the living will and the health care proxy. Elderly patients should have the opportunity to execute a living will to guide physicians and family members in the event of devastating injury. A living will is a legal document in which a mentally competent person expresses wishes regarding continued medical care in the event of incompetence resulting from injury or illness. Unfortunately, living wills require patients to predict specific circumstances of future injury accurately. Trauma surgeons, who usually have not met the patients before a severe injury, therefore must be guided by a document sometimes written years before an injury instead of by an in-depth discussion with the patients.

A heath care proxy is an individual appointed by a mentally competent adult to make health care decisions in the event of catastrophic injury or illness resulting in incompetence. Patients and the general public desire advance directives [69,70]. The lack of physician initiative in raising the issue is the barrier to advance directives perceived most frequently by patients.

Withholding and withdrawing life support

Withholding and withdrawing life support is a common occurrence in ICUs in the United States. Support was withheld or withdrawn in 57% of the ICU patients who died in a prospective study of two ICUs at the University of California, San Francisco (UCSF). The reasons cited by health care providers for limiting care in the UCSF study included brain death, futility, patient suffering, and anticipated poor quality of life [71].

The concept of brain death was introduced to meet the challenges and requirements of organ transplantation. The initial diagnostic criteria for brain death were published by Beecher in 1968 [72] and since have been modified to include complete cessation of brain and brainstem function as evidenced by (1) irreversible coma, (2) absent brainstem reflexes, (3) apnea, (4) serial observations separated by 6 hours in adults over age 18, and (5) confirmatory tests documenting absence of cerebral blood flow if the diagnosis is in doubt [73].

Physicians, nurses, and medical ethicists use the word futile to describe continued intensive care without hope of survival. Unfortunately, the futility of continued care not always is obvious. Opinions about the futility of care can be influenced by the skill and experience of surgeons, the discipline of clinicians, and personal and cultural values [74]. The key is to focus on the principles of beneficence and autonomy for individual patients [75].

Perceived suffering of geriatric trauma patients is a frequent cause of emotional distress for ICU staff [76]. Nurses frequently are the first members of the team to raise the question of limiting care because of futility and patient suffering. The routine use of continuous analgesics and sedatives in ventilated patients is an essential part of management, but the science of analgesia and sedation remains imperfect [77]. Most surgical ICU patients who survive, however, indicate that they would repeat the experience again if necessary [78]. Withdrawal of support based solely on the criterion of patient suffering is not indicated.

The use of poor anticipated quality of life as a sole indication for withdrawal of support in incompetent patients is dangerous. Members of a health care team may substitute their own concept of poor quality of life for a patient's and deny a patient a chance for survival. All trauma patients may struggle with psychologic and physical challenges after injury [79,80]. Most ICU survivors studied indicate, however, that they have an "acceptable" quality of life and would undergo treatment again [81]. Data related specifically to quality of life in geriatric trauma survivors are sparse.

Competition for ICU beds is a fact of life. Appropriate allocation of limited health care resources often is an unarticulated influence on these fateful decisions. Balancing the interests of society and patients can be a challenging experience for trauma surgeons [82]. The authors believe firmly that poor clinical decisions are made by surgeons acting as health economists at the bedside. In the absence of a mass casualty event, individual patients' best interests always must guide clinicians' actions. The body politic must set the rules after open public debate and the medical profession must provide the best possible care given those rules. Poorly understood personal, professional, and cultural values no doubt influence these decisions. Surgeons are shown to be less likely than other intensivists to be influenced by factors, such as scarcity of resources and anticipated quality of life, when considering limiting care [83].

Withholding and withdrawing life support in hopelessly ill geriatric trauma patients is a necessity. The challenge is identification of the hopelessly ill patients. Decisions to limit ICU care should be based on the following principles [84]:

1. Every patient deserves a precise diagnosis.
2. The prognosis often is uncertain.
3. Each decision should be based on a risk-benefit analysis for patients.
4. Patient autonomy is paramount.
5. Due deliberation prior to decision.
6. Communicating with patients, families, and professional colleagues.
7. Framing the discussion within families' cultural context.
8. Achieving consensus before a final decision.

Summary

Geriatric trauma is an important challenge facing trauma surgeons and trauma systems. This problem will assume increasing importance over the next several decades as the population of the United States ages. Training programs should prepare the next generation of surgeons to recognize the unique patterns of injury and meet the physiologic, rehabilitation, and ethical challenges of injury to senior citizens.

References

[1] He W, Sengupta M, Velkoff VA, et al. 65 + in the United States: 2005. Washington, DC: US Government Printing Office; 2005.

[2] MacKenzie EJ, Morris JA Jr, Smith GS, et al. Acute hospital costs of trauma in the United States: implications for regionalized systems of care. J Trauma 1990;30:1096–101 [discussion: 1101–3].

[3] Morris JA Jr, MacKenzie EJ, Damiano AM, et al. Mortality in trauma patients: the interaction between host factors and severity. J Trauma 1990;30:1476–82.

[4] Finelli FC, Jonsson J, Champion HR, et al. A case control study for major trauma in geriatric patients. J Trauma 1989;29:541–8.

[5] Grossman M, Scaff DW, Miller D, et al. Functional outcomes in octogenarian trauma. J Trauma 2003;55:26–32.

[6] Mandavia D, Newton K. Geriatric trauma. Emerg Med Clin North Am 1998;16:257–74.

[7] Roudsari BS, Ebel BE, Corso PS, et al. The acute medical care costs of fall-related injuries among the US older adults. Injury 2005;36:1316–22.

[8] Kong LB, Lekawa M, Navarro RA, et al. Pedestrian-motor vehicle trauma: an analysis of injury profiles by age. J Am Coll Surg 1996;182:17–23.

[9] Shabot MM, Johnson CL. Outcome from critical care in the "oldest old" trauma patients. J Trauma 1995;39:254–9 [discussion: 259–60].

[10] Knudson MM, Lieberman J, Morris JA Jr, et al. Mortality factors in geriatric blunt trauma patients. Arch Surg 1994;129:448–53.

[11] Taylor MD, Tracy JK, Meyer W, et al. Trauma in the elderly: intensive care unit resource use and outcome. J Trauma 2002;53:407–14.

[12] Perdue PW, Watts DD, Kaufmann CR, et al. Differences in mortality between elderly and younger adult trauma patients: geriatric status increases risk of delayed death. J Trauma 1998;45:805–10.

[13] Morris JA Jr, MacKenzie EJ, Edelstein SL. The effect of preexisting conditions on mortality in trauma patients. JAMA 1990;263:1942–6.

[14] Grossman MD, Miller D, Scaff DW, et al. When is an elder old? Effect of preexisting conditions on mortality in geriatric trauma. J Trauma 2002;52:242–6.

[15] Milzman DP, Boulanger BR, Rodriguez A, et al. Pre-existing disease in trauma patients: a predictor of fate independent of age and injury severity score. J Trauma 1992;32:236–43 [discussion: 243–4].

[16] Zimmer-Gembeck MJ, Southard PA, Hedges JR, et al. Triage in an established trauma system. J Trauma 1995;39:922–8.

[17] Ma MH, MacKenzie EJ, Alcorta R, et al. Compliance with prehospital triage protocols for major trauma patients. J Trauma 1999;46:168–75.

[18] Meldon SW, Reilly M, Drew BL, et al. Trauma in the very elderly: a community-based study of outcomes at trauma and nontrauma centers. J Trauma 2002;52:79–84.

[19] Demetriades D, Sava J, Alo K, et al. Old age as a criterion for trauma team activation. J Trauma 2001;51:754–6 [discussion: 756–7].

[20] Demetriades D, Karaiskakis M, Velmahos G, et al. Effect on outcome of early intensive management of geriatric trauma patients. Br J Surg 2002;89:1319–22.

[21] Jacobs DG, Plaisier BR, Barie PS, et al. Practice management guidelines for geriatric trauma: the EAST Practice Management Guidelines Work Group. J Trauma 2003;54: 391–416.

[22] Epstein CD, Peerless J, Martin J, et al. Oxygen transport and organ dysfunction in the older trauma patient. Heart Lung 2002;31:315–26.

[23] Schulman AM, Claridge JA, Young JS. Young versus old: factors affecting mortality after blunt traumatic injury. Am Surg 2002;68:942–7 [discussion: 947–8].

[24] Fishkind D, Paris BE, Aronow WS. Use of digoxin, diuretics, beta blockers, angiotensin-converting enzyme inhibitors, and calcium channel blockers in older patients in an academic hospital-based geriatrics practice. J Am Geriatr Soc 1997;45:809–12.

[25] Hart RG, Boop BS, Anderson DC. Oral anticoagulants and intracranial hemorrhage. Facts and hypotheses. Stroke 1995;26:1471–7.

[26] Mina AA, Bair HA, Howells GA, et al. Complications of preinjury warfarin use in the trauma patient. J Trauma 2003;54:842–7.

[27] Cohen DB, Rinker C, Wilberger JE. Traumatic brain injury in anticoagulated patients. J Trauma 2006;60:553–7.

[28] Wojcik R, Cipolle MD, Seislove E, et al. Preinjury warfarin does not impact outcome in trauma patients. J Trauma 2001;51:1147–51 [discussion: 1151–2].

[29] Ivascu FA, Howells GA, Junn FS, et al. Rapid warfarin reversal in anticoagulated patients with traumatic intracranial hemorrhage reduces hemorrhage progression and mortality. J Trauma 2005;59:1131–7 [discussion: 1137–9].

[30] Dutton RP, McCunn M, Hyder M, et al. Factor VIIa for correction of traumatic coagulopathy. J Trauma 2004;57:709–18 [discussion: 718–9].

[31] Martinowitz U, Michaelson M. Guidelines for the use of recombinant activated factor VII (rFVIIa) in uncontrolled bleeding: a report by the Israeli Multidisciplinary rFVIIa Task Force. J Thromb Haemost 2005;3:640–8.

[32] Lin J, Hanigan WC, Tarantino M, et al. The use of recombinant activated factor VII to reverse warfarin-induced anticoagulation in patients with hemorrhages in the central nervous system: preliminary findings. J Neurosurg 2003;98:737–40.

[33] Spektor S, Agus S, Merkin V, et al. Low-dose aspirin prophylaxis and risk of intracranial hemorrhage in patients older than 60 years of age with mild or moderate head injury: a prospective study. J Neurosurg 2003;99:661–5.

[34] Mina AA, Knipfer JF, Park DY, et al. Intracranial complications of preinjury anticoagulation in trauma patients with head injury. J Trauma 2002;53:668–72.

[35] Ohm C, Mina A, Howells G, et al. Effects of antiplatelet agents on outcomes for elderly patients with traumatic intracranial hemorrhage. J Trauma 2005;58:518–22.

[36] Li J, Brown J, Levine M. Mild head injury, anticoagulants, and risk of intracranial injury. Lancet 2001;357:771–2.

[37] Vollmer DG, Torner JC, Jane JA, et al. Age and outcome following traumatic coma: why do older patients fare worse? J Neurosurg 1991;75:S37–49.

[38] Hukkelhoven CW, Steyerberg EW, Rampen AJ, et al. Patient age and outcome following severe traumatic brain injury: an analysis of 5600 patients. J Neurosurg 2003;99:666–73.

[39] Howard MA 3rd, Gross AS, Dacey RG Jr, et al. Acute subdural hematomas: an age-dependent clinical entity. J Neurosurg 1989;71:858–63.

[40] Kotwica Z, Jakubowski JK. Acute head injuries in the elderly. An analysis of 136 consecutive patients. Acta Neurochir (Wien) 1992;118:98–102.

[41] Kilaru S, Garb J, Emhoff T, et al. Long-term functional status and mortality of elderly patients with severe closed head injuries. J Trauma 1996;41:957–63.

[42] Knudson MM, Maull KI. Nonoperative management of solid organ injuries. Past, present, and future. Surg Clin North Am 1999;79:1357–71.

[43] Barone JE, Burns G, Svehlak SA, et al. Management of blunt splenic trauma in patients older than 55 years. Southern Connecticut Regional Trauma Quality Assurance Committee. J Trauma 1999;46:87–90.

[44] Cocanour CS, Moore FA, Ware DN, et al. Age should not be a consideration for nonoperative management of blunt splenic injury. J Trauma 2000;48:606–10 [discussion: 610–2].

[45] Falimirski ME, Provost D. Nonsurgical management of solid abdominal organ injury in patients over 55 years of age. Am Surg 2000;66:631–5.

[46] Krause KR, Howells GA, Bair HA, et al. Nonoperative management of blunt splenic injury in adults 55 years and older: a twenty-year experience. Am Surg 2000;66:636–40.

[47] Myers JG, Dent DL, Stewart RM, et al. Blunt splenic injuries: dedicated trauma surgeons can achieve a high rate of nonoperative success in patients of all ages. J Trauma 2000;48: 801–5 [discussion: 805–6].

[48] Harbrecht BG, Peitzman AB, Rivera L, et al. Contribution of age and gender to outcome of blunt splenic injury in adults: multicenter study of the eastern association for the surgery of trauma. J Trauma 2001;51:887–95.

[49] Cummings SR, Melton LJ. Epidemiology and outcomes of osteoporotic fractures. Lancet 2002;359:1761–7.

[50] Martin RE, Teberian G. Multiple trauma and the elderly patient. Emerg Med Clin North Am 1990;8:411–20.

[51] Henry SM, Pollak AN, Jones AL, et al. Pelvic fracture in geriatric patients: a distinct clinical entity. J Trauma 2002;53:15–20.

[52] O'Brien DP, Luchette FA, Pereira SJ, et al. Pelvic fracture in the elderly is associated with increased mortality. Surgery 2002;132:710–4 [discussion: 714–5].

[53] Schwartsman R, Brinker MR, Beaver R, et al. Patient self-assessment of tibial plateau fractures in 40 older adults. Am J Orthop 1998;27:512–9.

[54] Koval KJ, Meek R, Schemitsch E, et al. An AOA critical issue. Geriatric trauma: young ideas. J Bone Joint Surg Am 2003;85-A:1380–8.

[55] Zuckerman JD, Sakales SR, Fabian DR, et al. Hip fractures in geriatric patients. Results of an interdisciplinary hospital care program. Clin Orthop Relat Res 1992;27:213–25.

[56] Sexson SB, Lehner JT. Factors affecting hip fracture mortality. J Orthop Trauma 1987;1: 298–305.

[57] Pellicane JV, Byrne K, DeMaria EJ. Preventable complications and death from multiple organ failure among geriatric trauma victims. J Trauma 1992;33:440–4.

[58] Smith DP, Enderson BL, Maull KI. Trauma in the elderly: determinants of outcome. South Med J 1990;83:171–7.

[59] Bochicchio GV, Joshi M, Knorr KM, et al. Impact of nosocomial infections in trauma: does age make a difference? J Trauma 2001;50:612–7 [discussion: 617–9].

[60] Schultz RJ, Whitfield GF, LaMura JJ, et al. The role of physiologic monitoring in patients with fractures of the hip. J Trauma 1985;25:309–16.

[61] Connors AF Jr, Speroff T, Dawson NV, et al. The effectiveness of right heart catheterization in the initial care of critically ill patients. SUPPORT Investigators. JAMA 1996;276:889–97.

[62] Sandham JD, Hull RD, Brant RF, et al. A randomized, controlled trial of the use of pulmonary-artery catheters in high-risk surgical patients. N Engl J Med 2003;348:5–14.

[63] Manasia AR, Nagaraj HM, Kodali RB, et al. Feasibility and potential clinical utility of goal-directed transthoracic echocardiography performed by noncardiologist intensivists using a small hand-carried device (SonoHeart) in critically ill patients. J Cardiothorac Vasc Anesth 2005;19:155–9.

[64] Jensen MB, Sloth E, Larsen KM, et al. Transthoracic echocardiography for cardiopulmonary monitoring in intensive care. Eur J Anaesthesiol 2004;21:700–7.

[65] Khoury AF, Afridi I, Quinones MA, et al. Transesophageal echocardiography in critically ill patients: feasibility, safety, and impact on management. Am Heart J 1994;127:1363–71.

[66] Richmond TS, Kauder D, Strumpf N, et al. Characteristics and outcomes of serious traumatic injury in older adults. J Am Geriatr Soc 2002;50:215–22.

[67] van Aalst JA, Morris JA Jr, Yates HK, et al. Severely injured geriatric patients return to independent living: a study of factors influencing function and independence. J Trauma 1991; 31:1096–101 [discussion: 1101–092].

[68] Battistella FD, Din AM, Perez L. Trauma patients 75 years and older: long-term follow-up results justify aggressive management. J Trauma 1998;44:618–23 [discussion: 623].

[69] Emanuel LL, Barry MJ, Stoeckle JD, et al. Advance directives for medical care—a case for greater use. N Engl J Med 1991;324:889–95.

[70] Shmerling RH, Bedell SE, Lilienfeld A, et al. Discussing cardiopulmonary resuscitation: a study of elderly outpatients. J Gen Intern Med 1988;3:317–21.

[71] Smedira NG, Evans BH, Grais LS, et al. Withholding and withdrawal of life support from the critically ill. N Engl J Med 1990;322:309–15.

[72] Beecher HK. A definition of irreversible coma. Report of the Ad Hoc Committee of the Harvard Medical School to Examine the Definition of Brain Death. JAMA 1968;205: 337–40.

[73] Morenski JD, Oro JJ, Tobias JD, et al. Determination of death by neurological criteria. J Intensive Care Med 2003;18:211–21.

[74] Youngner SJ. Who defines futility? JAMA 1988;260:2094–5.

[75] Tomlinson T, Brody H. Futility and the ethics of resuscitation. JAMA 1990;264:1276–80.

[76] Levy MM. Caring for the caregiver. Crit Care Clin 2004;20:541–7 [xi.].

[77] Lavery GG. Optimum sedation and analgesia in critical illness: we need to keep trying. Crit Care 2004;8:433–4.

[78] Fakhry SM, Kercher KW, Rutledge R. Survival, quality of life, and charges in critically III surgical patients requiring prolonged ICU stays. J Trauma 1996;41:999–1007.

[79] Sluys K, Haggmark T, Iselius L. Outcome and quality of life 5 years after major trauma. J Trauma 2005;59:223–32.

[80] Pande I, Scott DL, O'Neill TW, et al. Quality of life, morbidity, and mortality after low trauma hip fracture in men. Ann Rheum Dis 2006;65:87–92.

[81] Stricker KH, Cavegn R, Takala J, et al. Does ICU length of stay influence quality of life? Acta Anaesthesiol Scand 2005;49:975–83.
[82] Abrams FR. The doctor with two heads. The patient versus the costs. N Engl J Med 1993; 328:975–6.
[83] Cassell J, Buchman TG, Streat S, Stewart RM. Surgeons, intensivists, and the covenant of care: administrative models and values affecting care at the end of life—updated. Crit Care Med 2003;31:1551–7 [discussion: 1557–9].
[84] Schecter WP. Withdrawing and withholding life support in geriatric surgical patients. Ethical considerations. Surg Clin North Am 1994;74:245–59.

ELSEVIER
SAUNDERS

SURGICAL
CLINICS OF
NORTH AMERICA

Surg Clin N Am 87 (2007) 247–267

Environmental Cold-Induced Injury

Gregory J. Jurkovich, MD[a,b,*]

[a]*University of Washington, Seattle, WA, USA*
[b]*Harborview Medical Center, 325 Ninth Avenue, Box 359796, Seattle, WA 98104, USA*

Hypothermia

In the United States, there are more than 650 deaths per year from hypothermia. The Centers for Disease Control and Prevention reports that between 1979 and 2002, a total of 16,555 deaths in the United States (an average of 689 per year; range: 417–1021) were attributed to exposure to excessive natural cold (Fig. 1) [1], an annual death rate of 0.2 per 100,000 population. Most hypothermia-related deaths (66%) occurred in men, but the overall death rate was the same for both men and women. The hypothermia-related death rate was highest in states with characteristically milder climates that experience rapid temperature changes (eg, North Carolina [0.4] and South Carolina [0.4]), and in western states that have high elevations and considerable changes in nighttime temperatures (eg, Arizona [0.3]). States with the highest overall death rates for hypothermia are Alaska, New Mexico, North Dakota, and Montana.

Human physiology requires a constant body temperature, normally 37°C sublingually, 38°C in the rectum, 32°C at the skin, and 38.5°C deep in the liver. Even minor deviation from normal leads to important symptoms and disability [2]. The thermoregulatory drive is such a powerful one that it takes precedence over many other homeostatic functions. The human body can dissipate heat readily by evaporating body water, but it is far less able to cope with cold conditions. As a result, hypothermia can occur in various clinical settings, and from a number of causes (Table 1).

Primary, unintentional hypothermia is a decrease in core temperature from overwhelming environmental cold stress. It occurs most often after cold-water immersion or prolonged environmental exposure. Secondary, unintentional hypothermia occurs in patients with abnormal heat production or thermoregulation who become cold despite only mild cold stress

---
* Harborview Medical Center, 325 Ninth Avenue, Box 359796, Seattle, WA 98104, USA.
  E-mail address: jerryj@u.washington.edu

0039-6109/07/$ - see front matter © 2006 Elsevier Inc. All rights reserved.
doi:10.1016/j.suc.2006.10.003   *surgical.theclinics.com*

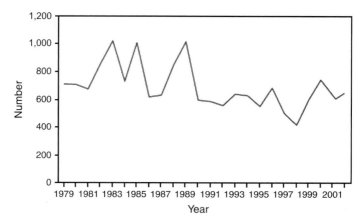

Fig. 1. Number of hypothermia-related deaths, by year: United States, 1979–2002. (*From* Hypothermia-related deaths–United States, 2003–2004. MMWR Morb Mortal Wkly Rep 2005;54(7):173–5.)

[1,3]. The most significant risk factors are advanced age, mental impairment, and substance abuse, although hypothyroidism, hypoadrenalism, trauma, and hypoglycemia are other risk factors. Chronic hypothermia develops in patients with impaired heat generation (ie, the elderly and infirm) who live in nonheated apartments, are under continual cold stress, and after a time are found to have a low temperature, as if they have autoregulated to a new set temperature. A multicenter review of 428 cases of unintentional hypothermia reported an overall mortality rate of 17%, although other reports document mortality rates as high as 80%, primarily when caused by infection and underlying illness [4].

The physiologic response to hypothermia is one of transitional changes, with few exact temperature-dependent responses. To allow for the normal

Table 1
Clinical definitions and causes of hypothermia

Type	Setting
Accidental	Recreational environmental exposure
Therapeutic	Cardiopulmonary bypass, circulatory arrest surgery, organ preservation
Drug-induced	Alcohol, barbiturates, phenothiazines, morphine, anesthetics
Central nervous system dysfunction	Spinal cord injury, hypopituitarism, cerebrovascular accidents
Hypothalamic dysfunction	Wernicke's encephalopathy, anorexia nervosa, head trauma, pinealoma, other tumors
Metabolic	Hypoglycemia, hypothyroidism, hypoadrenalism, malnutrition
Dermal dysfunction	Burns, erythrodermas
Trauma	After major injury

circadian temperature variation of up to 1°C, hypothermia is considered to be present if the core temperature drops below 35°C (95°F). Hypothermia is classified most commonly as mild (32° to 35°C), moderate (28° to 32°C), or severe (<28°C), because these temperature zones relate to varying degrees of physiologic alternations (Table 2) [2]. Broadly speaking, the transition from a "mild zone" of hypothermia (in which physiologic adaptations to heat loss are working) to a more severe hypothermia (in which shivering is abolished, metabolism decreases, and heat loss is accepted passively) occurs between 33° and 30°C. The initial effects of hypothermia mimic those of intense sympathetic stimulation, with tremulousness, profound vasoconstriction, tremendous increases in oxygen consumption, and acceleration of heart rate and minute ventilation.

The cardiovascular response to hypothermia begins with tachycardia, followed by progressive bradycardia at approximately 34°C, and results in a 50% heart rate decrease at 28°C. Cardiac output initially increases with the tachycardia, then progressively decreases, with a concomitant fall in blood pressure. The conduction system is particularly sensitive to hypothermia: the PR, then the QRS, and finally the QT interval become progressively prolonged [5]. As temperature falls below 30°C, atrial fibrillation, bradycardia, and ventricular dysrhythmia become common, with asystole occurring at temperatures below 25°C [6].

Oxygen consumption per unit time (VO_2) increases dramatically with any fall in body temperature. A core temperature decrease of as little as 0.3°C is associated with a 7% increase in VO_2, and temperature reductions between 0.3° and 1.2°C have been reported to result in a 92% increase in VO_2, with proportional increases in minute ventilation [7]. Hypothermic post-op patients increase oxygen consumption by 35% and CO_2 production by 65% after resolution of anesthesia, when the thermostatic drive reappears [8], which often results in shivering in an effort to increase temperature. But this is inefficient because shivering produces heat near the surface of the body, causing most of it to be lost to the environment, with less than 45% being retained by the patient [9]. The resultant increase in oxygen use may result in anaerobic metabolism, acidosis, and significant cardiopulmonary stress, further worsening the abnormal physiology of hypothermia, and potentially increasing surgical wound infections with even mild intraoperative hypothermia [10,11].

Respiratory drive is also increased during the early stages of hypothermia, but progressive respiratory depression occurs below 33°C, resulting

Table 2
Ranges of severity of hypothermia: trauma versus accidental hypothermia.

Hypothermia of trauma		Accidental hypothermia	
Mild:	36°C to 34°C	Mild:	32°C to 35°C
Moderate:	34°C to 32°C	Moderate:	28°C to 32°C
Severe:	<32°C (<90°F)	Severe:	<28°C (<82°F)

in a decrease in minute ventilation. This decrease usually is not a significant problem until temperatures below 29°C are reached. Occasionally, hypothermia results in the production of a large amount of mucus (cold bronchorrhea). Because ciliary action and the cough reflex are also depressed, this predisposes to atelectasis and aspiration. Noncardiogenic pulmonary edema is also reported occasionally, primarily in elderly patients, and especially after prolonged periods of hypothermia [12,13].

The neurologic response to hypothermia is heralded by progressive loss of lucidity and deep tendon reflexes, and, eventually, by flaccid muscular tone. Patients are often amnestic below 32°C, and between 31° and 27°C, they usually lose consciousness.

Although the reduced blood pressure and cardiac output of hypothermia decrease the glomerular filtration rate, urinary output is often maintained because of an impairment in renal tubular Na^+ reabsorption (cold diuresis) [14–16]. Vasoconstriction also results in an initial increase in relative central blood volume that prompts a diuresis. Ileus, bowel wall edema, depressed hepatic drug detoxification, punctate gastric erosions (Wischnevsky's ulcers), hyperamylasemia, and, rarely, hemorrhagic pancreatitis are all hallmarks of the intestinal response to hypothermia. Hyperglycemia is also a relatively common finding because hypothermia inhibits insulin release and insulin uptake by membrane receptors at temperatures below 30°C [17]. Exogenous insulin administration should be avoided because it may result in rebound hypoglycemia during rewarming. Serum electrolyte changes are unpredictable, but serum potassium is often slightly increased in hypothermic patients because of renal tubular dysfunction, acidosis, and the breakdown of liver glycogen. Hypothermia also appears to suppress endothelial cell adhesion molecule function, which may partially explain increased infectious complications in hypothermic patients [18]. Only 1.9°C core hypothermia triples the incidence of surgical wound infection following colon resection and increases the duration of hospitalization by 20% [11]. Further details of specific organ system responses to hypothermia are beyond the scope of this article, but the interested reader is referred to several excellent in-depth monographs [2,19–21].

Hypothermia in trauma

Mild hypothermia is very common after traumatic injury, and can be considered a form of secondary, unintentional hypothermia. After shock or injury, oxygen supplies are often limited, and heat loss occurs owing to cold emergency department and operating room environments, cold fluid resuscitation, and open thoracic and abdominal cavities. This situation is aggravated further by anesthetic and neuromuscular blocking agents that prevent the heat-producing shivering response. In one study, 57% of trauma patients admitted to a level I trauma center were hypothermic at some time, with the most significant temperature loss occurring in the emergency department [22]. Another study reported that the average initial temperature for 94 intubated major trauma victims was 35°C, with no seasonal variation [23]. Sixty-six percent of all patients in this study were hypothermic on admission: 43% were 34° to 36°C, and 23% had temperatures below 34°C. Likewise, Jurkovich and colleagues reported that 42% of 71 adult trauma victims with an injury severity score of 25 or higher had core temperatures below 34°C, and in 13% the core temperature fell below 32°C [24].

Hypothermia in the trauma patient is an ominous sign. Although the mortality rate for moderate levels (28° to 32°C) of primary, unintentional hypothermia is approximately 20% [4], moderate levels of hypothermia in trauma and critically ill patients are associated with a much higher mortality rate. The mortality rate of a trauma patient whose core temperature falls below 32°C is nearly 100%. Both mortality rate and the incidence of hypothermia increase with higher injury severity score, massive fluid resuscitation, and the presence of shock, but controlling for these variables still demonstrates that the mortality rate of the hypothermic trauma patient is greater than that of the warm trauma patient [2,25]. Rutherford and colleagues [26] have reported that 9.4% of surgical intensive care unit patients had a core body temperature less than 35°C; the mortality rate of the hypothermic trauma patients was 53%. Compared with other patient populations, the mortality rate associated with hypothermia in the trauma victim is so high that the definition of mild, moderate, and severe hypothermia in the trauma patient warrants special classification. The following zones of severity for injury hypothermia are therefore more applicable [2]:

Mild hypothermia: 36° to 34°C (<96.8°–93.2°F)
Moderate hypothermia: 34° to 32°C (<93.2°–89.6°F)
Severe hypothermia: less than 32°C (<89.6°F)

Evidence further supporting the harmful effect of hypothermia in the trauma patient is provided by a prospective, randomized trial of rapid rewarming versus conventional rewarming of 57 multiple trauma patients [27]. In this study, trauma patients who were rewarmed rapidly with continuous arteriovenous rewarming (CAVR) from less than 34.5°C to greater than 36°C required less resuscitation fluid volume and had a lower early mortality rate than those rewarmed more slowly. Failure to rewarm in either group was uniformly fatal. The survival rate at 3 days after injury was 82% in the rapid rewarm group, versus 62% in those conventionally managed. Approximately 50% of the patients in both groups had a severe head injury, defined as a head Abbreviated Injury Severity score of 3 or greater. In this well-controlled study, maintenance of hypothermia not only failed to confer an advantage, but was detrimental to early survival.

The detrimental effect of hypothermia in the human trauma victim is contrasted by a large body of animal experimental evidence that suggests that hypothermia has a protective role in shock, organ transplantation, cardiac arrest, and, possibly, brain injury. This extensive body of literature is reviewed elsewhere [2], but, in general, animals subjected to combined hypo-thermia and shock (hemorrhage, burn, blunt trauma) usually survive longer than similarly injured but actively warmed animals. In 1941, Blalock and Mason [28] were among the first in modern times to recognize the ability of hypothermia to prolong survival times after shock, but they emphasized that the overall survival rate was unchanged, an observation reaffirmed in 2003 [29]. However, increases in both survival times and survival rates have been shown in a number of animal models of induced hypothermia after hemorrhagic shock [30,31]. The protective effects of hypothermia in preventing ischemia–reperfusion injury have been described in a number of models, including muscle, intestine, and rabbit ear [32–34].

Hypothermia has also been suggested to protect the traumatically injured brain. The use of therapeutic hypothermia in a patient with traumatic brain injury was first reported in 1943, and then sporadically over the ensuing two decades [35,36]. More recently, a randomized, multicenter, controlled trial of core body hypothermia in trauma patients with severe closed head injury (Glasgow Coma Scale [GCS] scores of 3 to 7) was conducted [37]. Select trauma patients with severe head injury were cooled intentionally within 6 hours of injury to 32° to 33°C for 48 hours after injury, and then rewarmed. The outcome was poor (defined as severe disability, a vegetative state, or death) in 57% of the patients in both groups. Mortality was 28% in the hypothermia group and 27% in the normothermia group ($P = .79$). The patients in the hypothermia group had more hospital days with complica-tions than the patients in the normothermia group. The investigators con-cluded that treatment with hypothermia is not effective in improving outcomes in patients with severe brain injury. Other investigators have also reported higher rates of pneumonia and diabetes insipidus in a small study of induced hypothermia in severely head-injured patients (GCS score <8), with no effect on neurologic outcome [38].

Cooling of the uninjured victim of sudden cardiac arrhythmia has also been receiving considerable attention recently. A trial published in 1997 from Victoria, Australia, reported on the outcome of 22 adults with acute cardiac events who remained unconscious following successful cardiopul-monary resuscitation [39]. These patients were surface cooled in the emer-gency department to 33°C and maintained for 12 hours in the medical intensive care unit. This group had improved GCS outcome scores and a mortality of 45%, versus the historical control mortality of 77%. A similar trial from Vienna, Austria, was published in 2000, in which during 3 years, 27 similar patients from several centers were cooled intentionally to 33°C for 24 hours [40]. These investigators demonstrated the difficulty of getting patients to this target temperature, although it was not as dramatic in out-come. Cooling was initiated an average of 62 minutes after emergency department arrival, and target temperature was reached in 4.75 hours (range 1–7 hours). This same group published further on their multicenter Euro-pean trial, this time a prospective, randomized study of intentional cooling versus standard normothermia in victims of ventricular fibrillation. The intentionally cooled group (n = 136) had a more favorable neurologic outcome (55% versus 39%) and lower mortality (41% versus 55%), although the incidence of bleeding, pneumonia, and sepsis was higher in the hypothermic group. As a result of this growing body of evidence, the International Liaison Committee on Resuscitation published an advisory statement in 2003 on the role of hypothermia following cardiac arrest [41]. This group recommended intentional cooling of the patient to 32° to 34°C for unconscious adults with spontaneous circulation after an out-of-hospital ventricular fibrillation–induced cardiac arrest.

Given this evidence of the protective effect of hypothermia in some clinical situations of shock, why is hypothermia so bad in the trauma patient? The systems most affected by hypothermia in the victim of injury are those involved in clotting. Although hemodilution with volume expanders deficient in clotting factors and platelets is usually the primary cause of nonsurgical bleeding, cold platelets are known to undergo morphologic changes that affect adherence, including loss of shape, cytoplasmic swelling, and dissolution of cytoplasmic microtubules necessary for normal motility [42]. Valeri and associates [43] induced systemic hypothermia to 32°C in baboons, but kept one forearm warm using heating lamps and a warming blanket. Simultaneous bleeding time measurements in the warm and cold arm were 2.4 and 5.8 minutes, respectively. This effect, which was reversible with rewarming, appeared to be mediated by cold-induced slowing of the enzymatic reaction rate of thromboxane synthetase, which resulted in decreased production of thromboxane A_2, a potent vasoconstrictor necessary for normal platelet aggregation [44]. At mildly reduced temperatures (33°–36°C), there is a defect in platelet adhesion, and not reduced enzyme activity or platelet activation. However, at temperatures below 33°C, both reduced platelet function and enzyme activity likely contribute to the coagulopathy, perhaps helping to explain why 32°C is such a critical temperature in the coagulopathic injured patient [45].

Similar to those of blood gases, clinical tests of coagulation are temperature standardized to 37°C. Fibrometers contain a thermal block that heats the plasma and reagents to 37°C before initiating the assay. Thus, tests of coagulation reflect clotting factor deficiencies, but are corrected for any potential effect of hypothermia on clotting factor function. A detailed study of the kinetic effects of hypothermia on clotting factor function has been undertaken by Reed and colleagues [46], who performed clotting tests (prothrombin time [PT], partial thromboplastin time [PTT], and thrombin time) on reference human plasma containing normal clotting factor levels at temperatures ranging from 25° to 37°C. The results showed a significant slowing of all coagulation tests at temperatures below 35°C that was proportional to the degree of hypothermia. The prolongation of clot formation occurred at clinically relevant levels of hypothermia, and was equivalent to that seen in normothermic patients who have significant clotting factor depletion. For example, assays conducted at 35°, 33°, and 31°C prolonged the PTT to the same extent as would occur in a euthermic patient with reductions in factor IX levels to 66%, 32%, and 7% of normal, respectively.

Clotting factor supplementation is not the answer to a hypothermia-induced coagulopathy; rewarming is. However, in many seriously injured patients, clotting factor depletion exists in conjunction with hypothermia. A potentiating effect of hypothermia on coagulation dysfunction occurs in the plasma of patients who have deficient clotting factor levels, although there does not appear to be synergy between the two conditions [47]. Hypothermic, coagulopathic trauma patients still benefit from coagulation profile testing. If prolongation of PT and PTT are evident in plasma warmed to 37°C, clotting factor replacement is indicated. If PT and PTT are near normal, rewarming alone reverses the clinically apparent coagulopathy.

The current status of the role of hypothermia in the patient in shock remains somewhat controversial. It is apparent that the physiologic consequence of severe trauma is a drop in core body temperature. However, it remains unresolved whether this represents a "protective" response to shock, or is the result of diminished heat production caused by failing metabolism, and should be reversed and avoided. The bulk of clinical evidence indicates that hypothermia in the trauma patient is predictive of a poor outcome. Yet many animal studies demonstrate that hypothermia increases survival time following shock; they suggest that the body be allowed to autoregulate its temperature and that attempts at rewarming the cool, hemorrhagic shock patient are misguided.

Hypothermia does diminish metabolic demands and oxygen consumption, but the price appears to be malfunction of body enzyme and physiologic systems necessary to recover from injury. On balance, the occurrence of hypothermia in the multiply injured trauma victim should be considered detrimental to survival, especially as the temperature approaches 32°C. The only prospective, randomized study of the effect of rapid, early rewarming of hypothermic trauma patients demonstrated improved survival and with less fluid and blood resuscitation in patients rapidly rewarmed with CAVR (see later discussion), compared with standard rewarming techniques [27]. On balance, however, the detrimental effects of hypothermia in the multitrauma patient appear to outweigh any theoretical advantage of cooling.

Rewarming the hypothermic patient

Because palpating pulses or measuring blood pressure in cold, stiff, hypothermic patients is difficult, the presence of an organized cardiac electrical rhythm (not fibrillation) should be taken as a sign of life. Cardiopulmonary resuscitation with chest compression is contraindicated in this situation, despite the absence of a palpable pulse. The rhythm that is present is usually adequate to provide sufficient circulation in patients who have severely reduced metabolism, and it is likely that vigorous chest compressions will convert this perfusing rhythm to fibrillation. Rewarming is indicated, with close monitoring of rhythm, pulse, and blood pressure. If cardiac arrest should occur, extracorporeal cardiopulmonary bypass for perfusion and rewarming is indicated, but takes a prepared team [48]. One report noted excellent long-term functional outcomes in 15 of 32 young patients successfully rewarmed in this manner [49]. All patients were intubated and ventilated and had received ongoing cardiac massage during transportation, and all 15 survivors had documented circulatory arrest (ventricular fibrillation or asystole) and fixed, dilated pupils. The mean interval from discovery of the patient to rewarming with cardiopulmonary bypass was 141 ± 50 minutes; the mean temperature was 21.8° ± 2.5°C. A report from Finland documents a 61% (14 of 23) survival to hospital discharge for adults undergoing cardiopulmonary bypass after a mean of 70 minutes cardiopulmonary resuscitation following hypothermic arrest primarily from cold water immersion or exposure [50].

Pupillary dilatation and loss of cerebral autoregulation occur at temperatures below 26°C, and electroencephalography becomes silent at 19° to 20°C [51]. These findings, combined with an unobtainable pulse and apparent rigor mortis, may cause the patient to appear dead. It is important to remember that patients have been revived from core temperatures as low as 14°C [89], and hence, the saying "no one is dead until warm and dead." An exception to this admonition is the patient who has sustained an anoxic event while still normothermic and has a serum potassium level greater than 10 mmol/L [50,52]. The cold trauma patient also represents a particular challenge, but the absence of vital signs in a blunt trauma patient with a core body temperature of less than 32°C is probably lethal, and rewarming would be futile.

Usually, rewarming techniques are classified as passive external rewarming, active external rewarming, or active core rewarming [53]. Passive external rewarming simply implies allowing spontaneous rewarming to occur with the patient removed from a hypothermic environment, and usually is used only for the mildly hypothermic patient. Active external rewarming techniques include surrounding the patient with warm blankets or heating pads, infrared heating lights, and immersion in warm water. Active core rewarming includes heated intravenous fluids; heated peritoneal or thoracic lavage; heated gastric, bladder, or colonic lavage; heated and water-saturated inhaled air; and extracorporeal circulatory rewarming. Currently, blood rewarming is limited to a maximum temperature of 42°C by the American Association of Blood Banks, but rewarming to 49°C with inline microwave blood rewarmers has been reported as safe, as has intravenous fluid rewarming to 65°C [54,55].

The rate of heat transfer to the hypothermic patient is greatest using active core rewarming, particularly extracorporeal circulation rewarming, which may be a critical factor in surgical patients for whom rapid restoration of clotting and cardiac function is necessary. Numerous investigators have described the technique of rewarming the hypothermic victim by extracorporeal circulation, primarily based on a few personal experiences. This technique has appeal in cases of primary, unintentional hypothermia, where maintenance of circulation, correction of hypoxia, and replenishment of intravascular volume may play a role as large as correcting the temperature change itself. The need for systemic anticoagulation has, however, generally limited the usefulness of full cardiopulmonary bypass rewarming in the trauma patient.

A simplified technique of extracorporeal active core rewarming is CAVR [56]. This technique makes use of the patient's own blood pressure to drive an extracorporeal circuit through an efficient, but small counter-current heat exchange device. Systemic anticoagulation is not necessary because the tubing is heparin-bonded and trauma patients are relatively anticoagulated. Its relative ease of use may make this device widely applicable in rewarming severely hypothermic patients with an intact circulation. This device has been used in a prospective, randomized trial of rewarming trauma patients, demonstrating its efficacy [27].

The use of body cavity lavage with warm solutions is a simple, less invasive method of accomplishing active core rewarming. However, rewarming rates with body cavity lavage vary greatly, based on initial core temperature, dialysate temperature, infusion rate, and dwell time. Several studies support the notion that active core rewarming by peritoneal lavage is preferable to active external rewarming [57]. Moss and colleagues [3] examined three techniques of rewarming hypothermic and cardiac-arrested dogs, concluding that both peritoneal lavage (55°C dialysate) and partial extracorporeal circulation were faster than active external rewarming with a heating blanket. A frequently stated disadvantage of external rewarming is that the peripheral tissues are rewarmed in advance of the still cool "core," resulting in peripheral vasodilation. In the presence of inadequate volume resuscitation, this may result in vascular collapse ("rewarming shock") and a subsequent fall in central temperature ("afterdrop") as the cold peripheral blood returns to the core. Whether this is the mechanism of the core afterdrop is debatable, because a core afterdrop has been noted to occur in animal models even during complete circulatory arrest. Volume contraction due to vasoconstriction, cold diuresis, and cellular swelling, coupled with inadequate fluid resuscitation, may be a more appropriate explanation for circulatory collapse during rewarming.

The thermodynamic principles of heat transfer to the hypothermic patient are reviewed in greater detail elsewhere, but some knowledge of rewarming rates and the quantity of heat transferred by various techniques is instructional [53,58]. Ventilating a patient with a core temperature of 32°C with water-saturated air at 41°C results in a maximum heat transfer rate of 9 kcal/h. For comparison, basal metabolic heat generation produces approximately 70 kcal/h, and shivering produces up to 250 kcal/h. Given the specific heat of the body (0.083 kcal/kg/°C), 58 kcal is required to raise the temperature of a 70-kg patient by 1°C. Thus, more than 6 hours would be required to warm a 32°C patient using 41°C humidified inspired air.

Heat transfer rates using body cavity lavage can be calculated similarly, based on the specific heat of water (1 kcal/kg/°C). If 1 L of 44°C water infused into a body cavity dwells long enough to exit at 40°C, 4 kcal of heat will have been transferred to the patient. Thus, more than 14 L of fluid is needed to increase core temperature by 1°C. However, warming becomes less efficient as the patient rewarms because a longer dwell time is required to reduce the temperature of the infusate to 40°C.

Warming by cardiopulmonary bypass or CAVR is the most efficient method of core heating. With flow rates of 15 to 30 L/h, it is possible to deliver 120 to 240 kcal/h if the reinfused blood is heated to 40°C, a rate of heat transfer more than 10 times that of the other methods. In any case, the urgency with which rewarming must be accomplished depends on how adversely the hypothermia is affecting the patient. With the exception of extracorporeal circulatory methods, most rewarming techniques serve primarily to prevent loss of endogenously generated heat, and are ineffective in circumstances during which rapid rewarming is indicated. Early and discrete attention to the mechanisms of heat loss in the first place is preferable to prevent the metabolic and hemorrhagic complications associated with hypothermia in surgical patients.

Cold injury and frostbite

Cold injuries of exposed surfaces are the result of either direct tissue freezing (frostbite) or more chronic cold just above freezing (chilblain or pernio; trench foot). Cold injury has been a major cause of morbidity during war experiences, resulting in more than 7 million lost soldier fighting days by Allied forces in World War II [59].

Chilblain and pernio are descriptive terms for local cold injury characterized by pruritic, red-purple papules, macules, plaques, or nodules on the skin, usually the face, the anterior surface of the tibia, or the dorsum of the hands and feet. The lesions are often associated with edema or blistering and are caused by a chronic vasculitis of the dermis [60]; this entity does not appear to be related to hereditary protein C or S deficiency [61]. This pathologic process is provoked by repeated exposure to cold, but not freezing, temperatures. Treatment consists of sheltering the patient, elevating the affected part on sheepskin, and allowing gradual rewarming at room temperature. Rubbing and massage are contraindicated because they can cause further damage and secondary infection.

Trench foot or cold immersion foot (or hand) is a nonfreezing injury of the hands or feet that is caused by chronic exposure to wet conditions and temperatures just above freezing, as might occur with sailors, fishermen, or soldiers [62]. It appears to involve an alternating arterial vasospasm and vasodilatation, with the affected tissue first cold and anesthetic, and then hyperemic after 24 to 48 hours of exposure. With the hyperemia come an intense, painful burning and dysesthesia, and tissue damage characterized by edema, blistering, redness, ecchymosis, and ulceration. Complications of local infection or cellulitis, lymphangitis, and gangrene may occur. A posthyperemic phase occurs 2 to 6 weeks later, and is characterized by tissue cyanosis with increased sensitivity to cold. Treatment is best started during or before the reactive hyperemia state, and consists of immediate removal of the extremity from the cold, wet environment with exposure of the feet (or hands) to warm, dry air. Elevation to minimize edema, protection of pressure spots, and local and systemic measures to combat infection are indicated. Massage, soaking of the feet, or rapid rewarming are not indicated. Demyelination of nerves, muscle atrophy, fallen arches, and osteoporosis may all present long-term complications, and a tendency toward marked vasospasm during subsequent exposure to cold develops in some patients [63].

Frostnip is the mildest form of cold injury. It is characterized by initial pain and pallor, with subsequent numbness of the affected body part. Skiers and other winter outdoor enthusiasts are most likely to experience this cold injury to the nose, ears, or tips of digits. The injury is reversible, and warming of the cold tissue results in return of sensation and function with no tissue loss.

Frostbite is a common and more severe form of cold injury. Frostbite damage is caused by direct ice crystal formation at the cellular level, with cellular dehydration and microvascular occlusion. Frostbite is traditionally classified into grades I-IV of injury severity, but because the appearance of the lesion changes frequently during the course of treatment, and because the initial treatment regimen is applicable for all degrees of insult, some authorities simply classify frostbite as either superficial or deep [64]. Although the initial symptoms may be mild and overlooked by the patient, severe pain, burning, edema, and even necrosis and gangrene may appear with rewarming. With severe injury, there is a progressive decrease in range of motion, and edema becomes prominent. The injury may progress to numbness and, eventually, to loss of all sensation in the affected tissue. Usually, the progression of severity is characterized as:

First degree: tissue freezing with hyperemia and edema, but without blistering

Second degree: tissue freezing with hyperemia, edema, and characteristic large, clear blisters

Third degree: tissue freezing with death of subcutaneous tissues and skin, resulting in hemorrhagic vesicles that are, in general, smaller than second-degree blisters

Fourth degree: tissue necrosis, gangrene, and eventual full-thickness tissue loss; the affected body part nearly always initially appears hard, cold, white, and anesthetic, regardless of the depth of injury

Evidence suggests that frostbite injury has two components: the initial freeze injury and a reperfusion injury that occurs during rewarming. The initial response to tissue cooling is vasoconstriction and arteriovenous shunting, intermittently relieved (every 5 to 7 minutes) by vasodilation, the so-called "hunting response" [65]. With prolonged exposure, this response fails, and pain sensation is lost between 7°C and 9°C. The temperature of the freezing tissue approximates ambient temperature until –2°C, when extracellular ice crystals form, and, as these crystals enlarge, the osmotic pressure of the interstitium increases, resulting in movement of intracellular water into the interstitium. Cells begin to shrink and become hyperosmolar, disrupting cellular enzyme function. If freezing is rapid (> 10°C/min), intracellular ice crystal formation occurs, resulting in immediate cell death [59]. Intravascularly, endothelial cell disruption and red cell sludging result in cessation of circulation.

During rewarming, red cell, platelet, and leukocyte aggregation is known to occur, and this results in patchy thrombosis of the microcirculation. These accumulated blood elements are thought to release, among other products, the toxic oxygen free radicals and the arachidonic acid metabolites PGF_{2a} and thromboxane A_2, which further aggravate vasoconstriction and platelet and leukocyte aggregation [66,67]. However, the exact mechanism of tissue destruction and death after freeze injury remains poorly defined. Vascular injury may be primarily in the form of endothelial cell damage and subsequent interstitial edema, but not vessel thrombosis, which may be the initial event in the rewarming injury [68,69]. A substantial component of severe cold injury may be neutrophil mediated, as suggested by the observation that a monoclonal antibody to neutrophil–endothelial and neutrophil–neutrophil adherence can markedly ameliorate the pathologic process of a severe cold injury [68]. In this rabbit model, animals treated with anti-CD11/CD18 adhesion molecule after cold injury (30 minutes at –15°C) but before rewarming (39°C water bath) had significantly less tissue loss and edema. The implication of these observations is that much of the injury of severe frostbite occurs during rewarming or reperfusion. Clinical application of these experimental observations remains untested.

Treatment of frostbite

Initial care of the victim of cold injury should focus on removing the patient from the hostile environment and protecting the injured body part from further damage. Rubbing or exercising the affected tissue does not augment blood flow and risks further cold injury or mechanical trauma. Because repeated bouts of freezing and thawing worsen the injury, it is preferable for the patient who has frostbite of the hands or feet to seek definitive shelter and care immediately, rather than rewarm the tissue in the field if there is a risk of refreezing. The emergency room treatment of a frostbite victim should first focus on the basic ABCs (airway, breathing, and circulation) of trauma resuscitation, and systemic hypothermia should be identified and corrected. Most patients are dehydrated, and resuscitation with warm fluids is an important part of early management. Fractures are often accompanied by frostbite in mountaineers, and although manipulation may be required to treat vascular compromise, open reduction is hazardous, and application of traction should be delayed until after post-thawing edema has been assessed.

Rapid rewarming is the goal. Gradual, spontaneous rewarming is inadequate, particularly for deeper injuries, and rubbing the injured part in ice or snow often delays warming and results in marked tissue loss [70]. Rapid rewarming should be achieved by immersing the tissue in a large water bath of 40° to 42°C (104°–108°F). The water should feel warm, but not hot, to the normal hand. The bath should be large enough to prevent rapid loss of heat and the water temperature should be maintained. Dry heat is not advocated because it is difficult to regulate, and the result of using excessive heat is often disastrous. The rewarming process should take approximately 30 to 45 minutes for digits, with the affected area appearing flushed when rewarming is complete and good circulation has been reestablished. Narcotics are required because the rewarming process can be quite painful.

The skin should be cleansed gently but meticulously, air dried, and the affected area elevated to minimize edema. A tetanus toxoid booster should be administered as indicated by immunization history. Sterile cotton should be placed between toes or fingers to prevent skin maceration, and extreme care taken to prevent infection and avoid even the slightest abrasion (Fig. 2). The affected tissue should be protected by a tent or cradle, and pressure spots must be prevented. In one review, infection developed in 13% of urban frostbite victims, but one half of these infections were present at the time of admission [71]. Most clinicians reserve antibiotics for identified infections [72].

Numerous agents have been tried to prevent thrombosis and vascular wall injury, and to ameliorate further tissue damage during the rewarming

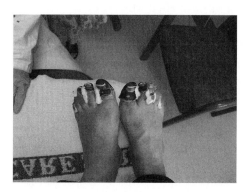

Fig. 2. Sterile cotten between toes to prevent skin maceration.

phase. Until recently, all have proven ineffective. However, two new studies provide evidence that early thrombolytic therapy may prevent or minimize tissue loss. Twomey and colleagues [73] presented an open-label trial confirming the safety of intravenous or intra-arterial tissue plasminogen activator (tPA) in frostbite patients. Bruen and colleagues [74], from the University of Utah, next reported on 32 patients with acute frostbite treated between 1995 and 2006. Six of these patients had early digital angiography and treatment with tPA for abnormal perfusion. In the patients in whom treatment was begun within 24 hours of injury, the amputation rate of involved digits was 10%, compared with a 40% amputation rate of involved digits managed without tPA.

These successful reports contrast with others in which investigators have tried numerous adjuvants to restore blood supply to frostbitten areas. Experience with intra-arterial vasodilating drugs such as reserpine and tolazoline, or heparin alone, have also been unrewarding. Bouwman and colleagues [75] demonstrated in a controlled, clinical study that immediate (mean, 3 hours) ipsilateral intra-arterial reserpine infusion coupled with early (mean, 3 days) ipsilateral operative sympathectomy failed to alter the natural history of acute frostbite injury, compared with the contralateral limb. The intense vasoconstrictive effect of cold injury has lead some to conceptualize an increased sympathetic tone. Sympathetic blockade, and even surgical sympathectomy, continues to be advocated by some investigators, under the theory that it releases the vasospasm that precipitates thrombosis in the affected tissue [76]. No prospective, randomized trials are available, and the results of the isolated reports are difficult to interpret. Although sympathectomy appears to mollify the pain, hyperhidrosis, and vasospasm of cold injuries, it may increase vascular shunting away from the frostbite area, and adversely affect healing. In one series, a more proximal demarcation of injury in sympathectomized limbs was noted than in nonsympathectomized ones, despite apparently equal bilateral injury [77].

After rewarming, the treatment goals are to prevent further injury while awaiting the demarcation of irreversible tissue destruction. Generally, hospitalization is recommended, with the affected tissue gently cleansed once or twice a day in warm (38°C) whirlpool baths, with or without an antiseptic such as chlorhexidine or an iodophor in the bath. Uninfected blebs should be left intact because they provide a sterile biologic dressing for 7 to 10 days and protect underlying epithelialization. After resolution of edema, digits should be exercised during the whirlpool bath, and physical therapy begun. Tobacco, nicotine, and other vasoconstrictive agents must be withheld. Weight bearing is prohibited until complete resolution of edema.

The use of aloe vera (a thromboxane inhibitor), nonsteroidal anti-inflammatory agents (eg, ibuprofen), or aspirin has some theoretic appeal, based on the findings of arachidonic acid metabolites in the blisters of frostbite victims. Heggers and colleagues [78] report on a nonrandomized trial in which 56 patients treated with these agents, plus prophylactic penicillin, had less tissue loss, a lower amputation rate, and a shorter hospital stay than 98 patients treated with warm saline, silver sulfadiazine, or Sulfamylon dressings (Bertek Pharmaceuticals, Sugar Land, Texas). An animal study demonstrated improved tissue viability if systemic pentoxifylline and topical aloe vera cream were used to treat frostbite [79].

The difficulty of determining the depth of tissue destruction in cold injury has led to a conservative approach to the care of frostbite injuries [72,80,81]. As a general rule, amputation and surgical debridement are delayed for 2 to 3 months, unless infection with sepsis intervenes. The natural history of a full-thickness frostbite injury is the gradual demarcation of the injured area, with dry gangrene or mummification clearly delineating nonviable tissue (Fig. 3). Often, the permanent tissue loss is much less than originally suspected. In an Alaskan series, only 10.5% of patients required amputation, usually involving only phalanges or portions of phalanges [62]. The need for emergency surgery is unusual, but vigilance should be maintained during the rewarming phase for the development of a compartment syndrome requiring fasciotomy. Open amputations are indicated in patients who have persistent infection and sepsis that is refractory to debridement and antibiotics. Mills and colleagues [82] convincingly demonstrated that of all the factors in the treatment of frostbite that may influence outcome, premature surgical intervention by any means, in any amount, was by far the greatest contributor to poor results.

The use of technetium 99m methylene diphosphonate bone scanning has shown some promise in the early detection of eventual bone and soft-tissue

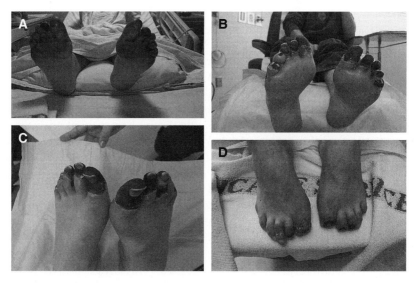

Fig. 3. (*A*) Frostbite injury. (*B*) Frostbite injury. (*C*) Clear delineation of nonviable tissue. (*D*) Postoperative, same patient.

viability [83], as has the use of MRI [84]. Technetium 99m "triple-phase" scanning (1 minute, 2 hours, 7 hours) performed 48 hours after admission has been used to assess early tissue perfusion and viability, in an attempt to define the extent of fatally damaged tissues and to allow for early debridement and wound closure [85,86]. However, the usefulness of this diagnostic modality continues to evolve, with one recent study suggesting that moderate to severe frostbite lesion can be identified by Tc 99 scans to be "hibernating" (viable) tissue, which can show improvement up to 6 months after injury [87].

Frostbitten tissues seldom recover completely. Some degree of cold insensitivity invariably remains. Hyperhidrosis (in up to 72% of patients), neuropathy, decreased nail and hair growth, and a persistent Raynaud's phenomenon in the affected part are frequent sequelae to cold injury [88]. The affected tissue remains at risk for reinjury and should be protected carefully during any cold exposure. Chilblain (or chronic pernio) is a specific form of dermopathy secondary to cold-induced skin vasculitis. Treatment with antiadrenergics (prazosin hydrochloride, 1 to 2 mg/day) or calcium channel blockers (nifedipine, 30 to 60 mg/day) and careful protection from further exposure is often helpful [60,88]. However, few therapies afford significant relief to the chronic symptoms after tissue freeze injury, although b- and a-adrenergic blocking agents, calcium channel blockers, topical and systemic steroids, and a host of home remedies have been tried with occasional individual success.

References

[1] Hypothermia-related deaths–United States, 2003–2004. MMWR Morb Mortal Wkly Rep 2005;54(7):173–5.
[2] Jurkovich G. Hypothermia in the trauma patient. Adv Trauma 1989;4:111–40.
[3] Moss J. Accidental severe hypothermia. Surg Gynecol Obstet 1986;162:501–13.
[4] Danzl D, Pozos R, Auerbach P, et al. Multicenter hypothermia survey. Ann Emerg Med 1987;16:1042–55.
[5] Trevino A, Razi B, Beller B. The characteristic electrocardiogram of accidental hypothermia. Arch Intern Med 1971;127:470–3.
[6] Aslam AF, Aslam AK, Vasavada BC, et al. Hypothermia: evaluation, electrocardiographic manifestations, and management. Am J Med 2006;119(4):297–301.
[7] Roe C, Goldberg M, Blair C, et al. The influence of body temperature on early postoperative oxygen consumption. Surgery 1966;60:85–92.
[8] Zwischenberger J, Kirsh M, Dechert R, et al. Suppression of shivering decreases oxygen consumption and improves hemodynamic stability during postoperative rewarming. Ann Thorac Surg 1987;43:428–31.
[9] Iampietro P, Vaughan J, Goldman R, et al. Heat production from shivering. J Appl Physiol 1960;15:632–4.
[10] Doufas AG. Consequences of inadvertent perioperative hypothermia. Best Pract Res Clin Anaesthesiol 2003;17(4):535–49.
[11] Kurz A, Sessler DI, Lenhardt R. Perioperative normothermia to reduce the incidence of surgical-wound infection and shorten hospitalization. Study of Wound Infection and Temperature Group. N Engl J Med 1996;334(19):1209–15.

[12] Cohen D, Cline J, Lepinski S, et al. Resuscitation of the hypothermic patient. Am J Emerg Med 1988;6:475–8.

[13] Ledingham I, Mone J. Treatment of accidental hypothermia: a prospective clinical study. BMJ 1980;1:1102–5.

[14] Broman M, Kallskog O, Nygren K, et al. The role of antidiuretic hormone in cold-induced diuresis in the anaesthetized rat. Acta Physiol Scand 1998;162(4):475–80.

[15] Granberg PO. Human physiology under cold exposure. Arctic Med Res 1991;50(Suppl 6):23–7.

[16] Sabharwal R, Johns EJ, Egginton S. The influence of acute hypothermia on renal function of anaesthetized euthermic and acclimatized rats. Exp Physiol 2004;89(4):455–63.

[17] Helman A, Gilbert M, Pfister-Lemaire N, et al. Glucagon and insulin secretion and their biological activities in hypothermic rats. Endocrinology 1984;115(5):1722–8.

[18] Haddix T, Pohlman T, Noel R, et al. Hypothermia inhibits human E-selectin transcription. J Surg Res 1996;64(2):176–82.

[19] Hildebrand F, Giannoudis PV, van Griensven M, et al. Pathophysiologic changes and effects of hypothermia on outcome in elective surgery and trauma patients. Am J Surg 2004;187(3): 363–71.

[20] Gentilello L. Practical approaches to hypothermia. Advances in Trauma and Critical Care 1994;39–79.

[21] Paton B. Accidental hypothermia. Pharmacol Ther 1983;22:331–7.

[22] Gregory J, Townsend M, Cloutier C, et al. Timing and incidence of hypothermia (T < 36C) in operated trauma patients. Presented at the 50th Annual Meeting of the AAST. Tucson (AZ), September 22, 1990.

[23] Luna G, Maier R, Pavlin E, et al. Incidence and effect of hypothermia in seriously injured patients. J Trauma 1987;27(9):1014–8.

[24] Jurkovich G, Greiser W, Luterman A, et al. Hypothermia in trauma victims: an ominous predictor of survival. J Trauma 1987;27:1019–24.

[25] Psarras P, Ivatury R, Rohman M, et al. Hypothermia in trauma: incidence and prognostic significance. Presented at East Ass Surg Trauma. Longboat Key (FL); January 1988.

[26] Rutherford EJ, Fusco MA, Nunn CR, et al. Hypothermia in critically ill trauma patients. Injury 1998;29(8):605–8.

[27] Gentilello LM, Jurkovich GJ, Stark MS, et al. Is hypothermia in the victim of major trauma protective or harmful? A randomized, prospective study. Ann Surg 1997;226(4):439–47 [discussion: 47–9].

[28] Blalock A, Mason M. A comparison of the effects of heat and those of cold in the prevention and treatment of shock. Arch Surg 1945;42:1054–9.

[29] Wu X, Stezoski J, Safar P, et al. After spontaneous hypothermia during hemorrhagic shock, continuing mild hypothermia (34 degrees C) improves early but not late survival in rats. J Trauma 2003;55(2):308–16.

[30] Alam HB, Bowyer MW, Koustova E, et al. Learning and memory is preserved after induced asanguineous hyperkalemic hypothermic arrest in a swine model of traumatic exsanguination. Surgery 2002;132(2):278–88.

[31] Sori A, El-Assuooty A, Rush B, et al. The effect of temperature on survival in hemorrhagic shock. Am Surg 1987;53:706–10.

[32] Cornejo CJ, Kierney PC, Vedder NB, et al. Mild hypothermia during reperfusion reduces injury following ischemia of the rabbit ear. Shock 1998;9(2):116–20.

[33] Jurkovich G, Pitt R, Curreri P, et al. Hypothermia prevents increased capillary permeability following ischemia-reperfusion injury. J Surg Res 1988;44:514–21.

[34] Wright J, Kerr J, Valeri C, et al. Regional hypothermia protects against ischemia-reperfusion injury in isolated canine gracilis muscle. J Trauma 1988;28:1027–31.

[35] Fay T. Observations on generalized refrigeration in cases of severe cerebral trauma. Assoc Res Nerv Ment Dis Proc 1943;24:611–9.

[36] Milde LN. Clinical use of mild hypothermia for brain protection: a dream revisited. J Neurosurg Anesthesiol 1992;4(3):211–5.

[37] Clifton GL, Miller ER, Choi SC, et al. Lack of effect of induction of hypothermia after acute brain injury. N Engl J Med 2001;344(8):556–63.

[38] Shiozaki T, Kato A, Taneda M, et al. Little benefit from mild hypothermia therapy for severely head injured patients with low intracranial pressure. J Neurosurg 1999;91(2): 185–91.

[39] Bernard SA, Jones BM, Horne MK. Clinical trial of induced hypothermia in comatose survivors of out-of- hospital cardiac arrest. Ann Emerg Med 1997;30(2):146–53.

[40] Zeiner A, Holzer M, Sterz F, et al. Mild resuscitative hypothermia to improve neurological outcome after cardiac arrest. A clinical feasibility trial. Hypothermia After Cardiac Arrest (HACA) Study Group. Stroke 2000;31(1):86–94.

[41] Nolan JP, Morley PT, Vanden Hoek TL, et al. Therapeutic hypothermia after cardiac arrest: an advisory statement by the advanced life support task force of the International Liaison Committee on Resuscitation. Circulation 2003;108(1):118–21.

[42] Kattlove H, Alexander B. The effect of cold on platelets: 1. Cold-induced platelet aggregation. Blood 1971;38:39–47.

[43] Valeri C, Feingold H, Cassidy G, et al. Hypothermia induced reversible platelet dysfunction. Ann Surg 1987;205:175–81.

[44] Patt A, McCroskey B, Moore E. Hypothermia-induced coagulopathies in trauma. Surg Clin N Am 1988;68:775–89.

[45] Wolberg AS, Meng ZH, Monroe DM 3rd, et al. A systematic evaluation of the effect of temperature on coagulation enzyme activity and platelet function. J Trauma 2004;56(6):1221–8.

[46] Reed R, Bracey A, Hudson J, et al. Hypothermia and blood coagulation: dissociation between enzyme activity and clotting factor levels. Circ Shock 1990;32:141–52.

[47] Gubler K, Gentilello L, Hassantash S, et al. The impact of hypothermia on dilutional coagulopathy. J Trauma 1994;36:847–51.

[48] Hauty MG, Esrig BC, Hill JG, et al. Prognostic factors in severe accidental hypothermia: experience from the Mt. Hood tragedy. J Trauma 1987;27(10):1107–12.

[49] Walpoth B, Walpoth-Aslan B, Mattle H, et al. Outcome of survivors of accidental deep hypothermia and circulatory arrest treated with extracorporeal blood warming. N Engl J Med 1997;337:1500–5.

[50] Silfvast T, Pettila V. Outcome from severe accidental hypothermia in Southern Finland– a 10-year review. Resuscitation 2003;59(3):285–90.

[51] Orlowski J, Erenberg G, Lueders H, et al. Hypothermia and barbiturate coma for refractory status epilepticus. Crit Care Med 1984;12:367–72.

[52] Schaller M, Fischer A, Perret C. Hyperkalemia: a prognostic factor during acute severe hypothermia. JAMA 1990;264(14):1842–5.

[53] Gentilello L, Moujaes S. Treatment of hypothermia in trauma victims: thermodynamic considerations. J Intensive Care Med 1995;10:5–13.

[54] Herron D, Grabowy R, Connolly R, et al. The limits of bloodwarming: maximally heating blood with an inline microwave bloodwarmer. J Trauma 1997;43(2):219–28.

[55] Sheaff C, Fildes J, Keogh P, et al. Safety of 65 C intravenous fluid for the treatment of hypothermia. Am J Surg 1996;172:52–5.

[56] Gentilello L, Cobean R, Offner P, et al. Continuous arteriovenous rewarming: rapid reversal of hypothermia in critically ill patients. J Trauma 1992;32(3):316–27.

[57] Patton J, Doolittle W. Core rewarming by peritoneal dialysis following induced hypothermia in the dog. J Appl Physiol 1972;33:800–4.

[58] Gentilello L, Jurkovich G, Moujaes S. Hypothermia and injury: thermodynamic principles of prevention and treatment. In: Levine B, editor. Perspectives in surgery. St. Louis: Quality Medical Publishers; 1991. p. 25–56.

[59] Britt LD, Dascombe WH, Rodriguez A. New horizons in management of hypothermia and frostbite injury. Surg Clin N Am 1991;71(2):345–70.

[60] Jacob J, Weisman M, Rosenblatt S, et al. Chronic pernio. A historical perspective of cold-induced vascular disease. Arch Intern Med 1986;146:1589–92.

[61] Benchikhi H, Roujeau JC, Levent M, et al. Chilblains and Raynaud phenomenon are usually not a sign of hereditary protein C and S deficiencies. Acta Derm Venereol 1998; 78(5):351–2.

[62] Auerbach P. Disorders due to physical and environmental agents. In: Mills J, Ho MT, Salber PR, et al, editors. Current emergency diagnosis and treatment. Los Altos (CA): Lange Medical Publications; 1985.

[63] Francis T, Golden FSC. Non-freezing cold injury: the pathogenesis. J R Nav Med Serv 1985; 71:3–8.

[64] Mills WJ Jr. Frostbite and hypothermia–current concepts [1973 classical article]. Alaska Med 1993;35(1):28.

[65] Dana H, Rex I, Samitz M. The hunting reaction. Arch Dermatol 1969;99:441.

[66] Murphy JV, Banwell PE, Roberts AH, et al. Frostbite: pathogenesis and treatment. J Trauma 2000;48(1):171–8.

[67] Ozyazgan I, Tercan M, Melli M, et al. Eicosanoids and inflammatory cells in frostbitten tissue: prostacyclin, thromboxane, polymorphonuclear leukocytes, and mast cells. Plast Reconstr Surg 1998;101(7):1881–6.

[68] Mileski W, Raymond J, Winn R, et al. Inhibition of leukocyte adherence and aggregation for treatment of severe cold injury in rabbits. J Appl Physiol 1993;74(3):1432–6.

[69] Zook N, Hussmann J, Brown R, et al. Microcirculatory studies of frostbite injury. Ann Plast Surg 1998;40(3):246–53 [discussion: 54–5].

[70] MillsFrostbite WJ Jr. A discussion of the problem and a review of the Alaskan experience [1973 classical article]. Alaska Med 1993;35(1):29–40.

[71] Urschel J. Frostbite: predisposing factors and predictors of poor outcome. J Trauma 1990; 30(3):340–3.

[72] Petrone P, Kuncir EJ, Asensio JA. Surgical management and strategies in the treatment of hypothermia and cold injury. Emerg Med Clin North Am 2003;21(4):1165–78.

[73] Twomey JA, Peltier GL, Zera RT. An open-label study to evaluate the safety and efficacy of tissue plasminogen activator in treatment of severe frostbite. J Trauma 2005;59(6):1350–4 [discussion: 4–5].

[74] Bruen KJ, Ballard J, Morris SE, et al. Thrombolytic therapy reduces the incidence of amputation following acute frostbite. Presented at Western Surgical Association. Los Cabos (Mexico), November 12, 2006.

[75] Bouwman D, Morrison S, Lucas C, et al. Early sympathetic blockade for frostbite - Is it of value? J Trauma 1980;20:744–9.

[76] Rakower S, Shahgoli S, Wong SL. Doppler ultrasound and digital plethysmography to determine the need for sympathetic blockade after frostbite. J Trauma 1978;18(10):713–8.

[77] Mills WJ Jr, Whaley R. Frostbite: experience with rapid rewarming and ultrasonic therapy: part I and II [1960 classical article]. Alaska Med 1993;35(1):6–18.

[78] Heggers J, Robson M, Weingarten M, et al. Experimental and clinical observations on frostbite. Ann Emerg Med 1987;16(9):1056–62.

[79] Miller MB, Koltai PJ. Treatment of experimental frostbite with pentoxifylline and aloe vera cream. Arch Otolaryngol Head Neck Surg 1995;121(6):678–80.

[80] Mills W Jr. Comment and recapitulation. Alaskan Medicine 1993;35(1):69–87.

[81] Edlich RF, Chang DE, Birk KA, et al. Cold injuries. Compr Ther 1989;15(9):13–21.

[82] Mills WJ Jr. Summary of treatment of the cold injured patient: hypothermia [1980 classical article]. Alaska Med 1993;35(1):50–3.

[83] Mehta RC, Wilson MA. Frostbite injury: prediction of tissue viability with triple-phase bone scanning. Radiology 1989;170:511–4.

[84] Barker JR, Haws MJ, Brown RE, et al. Magnetic resonance imaging of severe frostbite injuries. Ann Plast Surg 1997;38(3):275–9.

[85] Cauchy E, Marsigny B, Allamel G, et al. The value of technetium 99 scintigraphy in the prognosis of amputation in severe frostbite injuries of the extremities: a retrospective study of 92 severe frostbite injuries. J Hand Surg [Am] 2000;25(5):969–78.

[86] Greenwald D, Cooper B, Gottlieb L. An algorithm for early aggressive treatment of frostbite with limb salvage directed by triple-phase scanning. Plast Reconstr Surg 1998;102(4): 1069–74.

[87] Bhatnagar A, Sarker BB, Sawroop K, et al. Diagnosis, characterisation and evaluation of treatment response of frostbite using pertechnetate scintigraphy: a prospective study. Eur J Nucl Med Mol Imaging 2002;29(2):170–5.

[88] Rustin M, Newton J, Smith N, et al. The treatment of chilblains with nifedipine: the results of a pilot study, a double-blind placebo-controlled randomized study and a long-term open trial. Br J Dermatol 1989;120:267–75.

[89] Dobson JA, Burgess JJ. Resuscitation of severe hypothermia by extracorporeal rewarming in a child. J Trauma 1996;40:483–5.

ELSEVIER
SAUNDERS

SURGICAL
CLINICS OF
NORTH AMERICA

Surg Clin N Am 87 (2007) 269–278

Index

Note: Page numbers of article titles are in **boldface** type.

A

Abdominal aortic aneurysm repair, and abdominal compartment syndrome, 79

Abdominal compartment syndrome, etiology of, 77–79

Abdominal injuries, trauma care for in children. *See* Trauma care, in children.
in elderly, 235–236

Abdominal wall reconstruction, in damage control laparotomy, 86–88, 92

Active core rewarming, for hypothermia, 255–256

Acute care centers, in trauma systems, 28

Advance directives, in trauma care, 239

Aeromedical transport, in military surgery, 178

Airway burn injuries. *See* Burns, inhalation injuries.

Airway management
in prehospital care. *See* Prehospital care.
in trauma care
for traumatic brain injury, 135
in children, 210–211

Amputation, for frostbite, 262

Anemia, in burn patients, 193–194

Antibiotics
in burn care, 187–188
in military surgery, 166
and multi–drug-resistant infections, 166

Anticoagulation, and trauma care, in elderly, 232–234

Anticonvulsants, prophylactic, for traumatic brain injury, 141

Anti–drunk driving efforts, in injury prevention, 5–6

Antioxidant therapy, in fluid resuscitation, in burn care, 190–191

Antiplatelet agents, for cardiovascular disease, 233–234

Artificial blood, in fluid resuscitation, 65–66

Artificial colloids, in fluid resuscitation, 65

Aspirin, for cardiovascular disease, 233–234

B

Baxter formula, in fluid resuscitation, in burn care, 189–190

Beta-blockers
and trauma care, in elderly, 232
for rupture of thoracic aorta, 111

Biologic dressings, in burn care, 187

Body cavity lavage, for hypothermia, 256

Bogota bag, in damage control laparotomy, 81

Bone scintigraphy, to determine tissue viability, in frostbite, 262–263

Brain herniation, trauma care for, 123

Brain injury
penetrating, trauma care for, 152–153
traumatic. *See* Traumatic brain injury.

Burns, trauma care for, **185–206**
access to, 197–199
antibiotics in, 187–188
dermal substitutes in, 188–189
disaster planning in, 199–200
dressings in, 186–187
biologic, 187
electrical injuries, 195–196
eschar excision in, 185–187
fluid resuscitation in, 189–191
and edema, 190
antioxidant therapy in, 190–191
Parkland formula for, 189–190
plasma exchange in, 191
for anemia, 193–194

Burns (*continued*)
    inhalation injuries, 191–193
        carbon monoxide poisoning with,
            191–192
        tracheostomy for, 192–193
        ventilation for, 192
    modulation of post-burn
        hypermetabolism in, 194–195
    noncontact laser Doppler imaging
        in, 186
    reconstructive surgery in, 196–197
    referral criteria for, 198
    rehabilitation in, 196
    research on, 200
    skin grafts in, 188–189
    thromboembolic disease prophylaxis
        in, 193–194

Burr holes, for increased intracranial
    pressure, 148–149

C

Carbon monoxide poisoning, with
    inhalation burn injuries, 191–192

Cardiac arrhythmia, therapeutic
    hypothermia for, 252–253

Cardiac injuries, trauma care for, 102–104

Cardiopulmonary bypass, for hypothermia,
    257

Cardiovascular response, to hypothermia,
    249

Cellular injury, markers of, fluid
    resuscitation and, 59–60

Central nervous system injuries. *See also*
    Traumatic brain injury.
    trauma care for, **119–156**
        brain herniation, 123
        cerebral blood flow in, 122, 123,
            125, 126
        cerebral edema, 133
        cerebral microdialysis in, 126
        computed tomography in,
            128–133
        depressed skull fractures,
            151–152
        epidural hematomas, 150
        Glasgow Coma Scale in,
            127–128, 150–151
        hematomas, 130–131
        increased cerebral perfusion
            pressure in, 123–126
        increased intracranial pressure in,
            122–126
        intracerebral contusions, 131–132
        intraparenchymal lesions, 151
        jugular venous saturation in, 126

        motor system in, 128
        patient assessment in, 127
        penetrating brain injuries,
            152–153
        posterior fossa lesions, 151
        primary brain injury, 120–121
        pupillary reactions in, 128
        secondary brain injury, 121–122
            hypotension with, 121
            hypoxia with, 121
            pyrexia with, 121–122
        subarachnoid hemorrhage, 133
        subdural hematomas, 150–151
        targeted therapies in, 126–127

Cerebral blood flow, in central nervous
    system injuries, 122, 123, 125, 126

Cerebral edema, computed tomography
    of, 133

Cerebral microdialysis, in central nervous
    system injuries, 126

Cerebral perfusion pressure, increased, in
    central nervous system injuries, 123–126

Cerebrospinal fluid drainage, for increased
    intracranial pressure, 143

Cerebrospinal fluid leaks, traumatic brain
    injury and, 149–150

Chilblain, trauma care for, 257, 263

Child abuse, trauma care for, 222

Chitosan dressings, in military surgery,
    162–163

Circulation management
    in prehospital care. *See* Prehospital
        care.
    in traumatic brain injury, 137

Clam shell incision, in thoracotomy,
    101–102

Clopidogrel, for cardiovascular disease,
    233–234

Coagulation system, hypothermia and,
    253–254

Cold injuries, trauma care for, **247–267**
    chilblain, 257, 263
    frostbite, 258–263
        amputation for, 262
        initial freeze injury in, 259
        preventing tissue damage in,
            260–261
        progression of severity of, 258
        rapid rewarming for, 260
        reperfusion injury in, 259
        restoration of blood supply in,
            261

sympathectomy for, 261
technetium-99m bone scanning of, 262–263
thrombolytic therapy for, 261
frostnip, 258
hypothermia, 247–257
active core rewarming for, 255–256
and coagulation system, 253–254
and lack of vital signs, 255
body cavity lavage for, 256
cardiopulmonary bypass for, 257
cardiovascular response to, 249
continuous arteriovenous rewarming for, 256, 257
heat transfer rates in, 256–257
in combat casualties, 167–168
incidence of, 247
mortality rate in, 251
neurologic response to, 250
oxygen consumption in, 249
physiologic response to, 248–249
physiology of, 247
respiratory drive in, 249–250
rewarming for, 251, 254–257
rewarming rates for, 256–257
risk factors for, 248
therapeutic, 147, 252–253
pernio, 257, 263
trench foot, 257–258

Colloids, in fluid resuscitation, 65

Coma, pentobarbital, for increased intracranial pressure, 145, 147

Combat casualties. See Military surgery.

Communication systems, in trauma systems, 26

Compartment syndrome
abdominal, etiology of, 77–79
damage control laparotomy and. See Damage control laparotomy.
prevention of, in combat casualties, 174

Component separation technique, in damage control laparotomy, 88–92

Computed tomography
in trauma care, in children, 213
of brain, for increased intracranial pressure, 139
of central nervous system injuries, 128–133

Continuous arteriovenous rewarming, for hypothermia, 256, 257

Continuous peripheral nerve block, in military surgery, 165

Craniectomy, decompressive, for increased intracranial pressure, 147, 148

Crystalloids, in fluid resuscitation, 64–65

D

Damage control laparotomy, in trauma care, 73–93
and compartment syndromes, 74–79
abdominal, 77–79
etiology of, 75–76
ischemia reperfusion and, 76
secondary, 79
open abdomen techniques in, 80–92
abdominal wall reconstruction in, 86–88, 92
biomaterials in, 92
Bogota bag in, 81
component separation in, 88–92
intestinal fistulae in, 85–86
muscle flaps in, 88
planned ventral hernia in, 84
propylene mesh in, 82–83
prosthetic insertion in, 81–84
skin grafts in, 85–86
suturing of prosthetic material in, 82
vacuum pack technique, 83–84
principles of, 73–74

Deaths, preventable, in trauma systems, 30–31

Decompressive craniectomy, for increased intracranial pressure, 147, 148

Deep venous thrombosis, prevention of, in burn patients, 193–194

Delayed thoracotomy, for thoracic trauma, 112–113

Depressed skull fractures, trauma care for, 151–152

Dermal substitutes, in burn care, 188–189

E

Echocardiography, in trauma care, in elderly, 239

Edema
cerebral, computed tomography of, 133
in burn patients, fluid resuscitation and, 190

Electrical injuries, trauma care for, 195–196

Emergency department thoracotomy, for thoracic trauma, 95–97

Endobronchial intubation, for tracheobronchial injuries, 109

Endotracheal intubation
in prehospital airway management, 39
in trauma care
for traumatic brain injury, 135
in children, 211

Epidural hematomas
computed tomography of, 130–131
trauma care for, 150

Eschar excision, in burn care, 185–187

Esophageal injuries, trauma care for, 110–111

Essential Trauma Care Project. See Trauma care.

Exploratory thoracotomy, for thoracic trauma, 102

Extremity fractures, trauma care for, in elderly, 236–238

F

Factor VIIa, to reverse anticoagulation, 233

Fallen lung sign, in tracheobronchial injuries, 108

Fasciotomy, in military surgery, 174

Fentanyl, in military surgery, 165

Fistulae, intestinal, in damage control laparotomy, 85–86

Fluid resuscitation
in burn care. See Burns.
in military surgery, 55–56, 63–64, 167
in prehospital care, 56–57
in trauma care, **55–72**
and gene regulation, 60
and immune activation, 58–59
and inflammation, 57–58
and markers of cellular injury, 59–60
and neutrophil excitation, 58–59
and white cell function, 59
artificial blood in, 65–66
artificial colloids in, 65
fresh whole blood in, 65
hypertonic saline in, 59, 61–65
clinical experience with, 61–63
immune dysfunction and, 57
in children, 212
isotonic crystalloids in, 64
lactated Ringer's solution in, 58–61
patient selection for, 66–67

pharmacologic, 60–61, 66
plasma in, 65
timing of, 66–67

Focused abdominal sonography for trauma
in children, 212–213
in military surgery, 171

Fractures
depressed skull, trauma care for, 151–152
pelvic, trauma care for
in children, 217
in elderly, 236–238

Fresh frozen plasma
in military surgery, 175, 176
to reverse anticoagulation, 233

Fresh whole blood, in fluid resuscitation, 65

Frostbite. See Cold injuries.

Frostnip, trauma care for, 258

G

Gene regulation, fluid resuscitation and, 60

Glasgow Coma Scale, in trauma care
for central nervous system injuries, 127–128, 150–151
for combat casualties, 168
for traumatic brain injury, 128
in elderly, 235

Graduated drivers licensing, in injury prevention, 4–5

Grafts, skin
in burn care, 188–189
in damage control laparotomy, 85–86

Great vessel injuries. See Thoracic trauma.

Guidelines for Essential Trauma Care, development process for, 10–13

H

Head injuries, trauma care for, in elderly, 234–235

Health care proxies, in trauma care, 239

Hematomas
cerebral, computed tomography of, 130–131
trauma care for, 150–151
in elderly, 234–235

HemCon dressings, in military surgery, 162–163

Hemodynamic monitoring, in trauma care, in elderly, 238–239

Hemoglobin-based blood substitute oxygen carriers, in prehospital circulation management, 45

Hemolink, in prehospital circulation management, 45

Hemopericardium, and emergency department thoracotomy, 97

Hemopure, in prehospital circulation management, 45

Hemostatic dressings, in military surgery, 161–163

Hemothorax, incompletely drained, delayed thoracotomy for, 112–113

Heparin-induced thrombocytopenia, in burn patients, 193–194

Hepatic injuries, trauma care for, in children, 220

Hernia, planned ventral, in damage control laparotomy, 84

Hextend, in military surgery, 167

Histone deacetylase inhibitors, in fluid resuscitation, 61

Hyperbaric oxygen therapy, for carbon monoxide poisoning, 191–192

Hypermetabolism, modulation of, in burn patients, 194–195

Hyperosmolar therapy, for increased intracranial pressure, 143, 145

Hypertonic resuscitation, in prehospital circulation management, 43–45

Hypertonic saline, in fluid resuscitation, 59, 61–65
    clinical experience with, 61–63

Hypertonic saline with dextran, in prehospital circulation management, 43–45

Hyperventilation
    for increased intracranial pressure, 143, 147
    for traumatic brain injury, 135
    in prehospital care, 41

Hypotension
    permissive, in military surgery, 168–169
    secondary brain injury and, 121

Hypothermia. *See* Cold injuries.

Hypoxia, secondary brain injury and, 121

I

Immersion foot, trauma care for, 257–258

Immune activation, fluid resuscitation and, 58–59

Immune dysfunction, trauma and, 57

Infections, nosocomial, in elderly, intensive care and, 238

Inhalation injuries. *See* Burns.

Injury prevention, global perspective on, 1–7
    advances in, 6–7
    anti-drunk driving efforts in, 5–6
    graduated drivers licensing in, 4–5
    Haddon's matrix in, 3–4
    surveillance in, 3

Intestinal fistulae, in damage control laparotomy, 85–86

Intra-abdominal pressure, increased, in abdominal compartment syndrome, 78–79

Intracerebral contusions, computed tomography of, 131–132

Intracranial pressure
    increased
        in abdominal compartment syndrome, 77–78
        in central nervous system injuries, 122–126
        in traumatic brain injury, 139–141, 143, 145, 147
    monitoring of, 149

Intraosseous access
    in military surgery, 164–165
    in prehospital circulation management, 43

Intraparenchymal lesions, trauma care for, 151

Intravenous access, in trauma care, in children, 211–212

Intravenous fluids, in prehospital circulation management, 42–43

Isotonic crystalloids, in fluid resuscitation, 64

J

Jugular venous desaturation, in central nervous system injuries, 126

L

Lactated Ringer's solution
in fluid resuscitation, 58–60, 64
in prehospital circulation
management, 43

Laparotomy, damage control. *See* Damage
control laparotomy.

Laser Doppler imaging, in burn care, 186

Left thoracotomy, for thoracic trauma, 101

Life support, in elderly, withdrawing and
withholding, 240–241

Lobar injuries, trauma care for, 107

M

Maltreatment, trauma care for, in children,
222

Median sternotomy, for thoracic trauma,
100

Medical direction, in trauma systems, 26

Microdialysis, cerebral, in central nervous
system injuries, 126

Military surgery, **157–184**
aeromedical transport in, 178
antibiotics in, 166
and multi–drug-resistant
infections, 166
hemostatic dressings in, 161–163
Hextend in, 167
hospital concepts in, 170–178
damage control for truncal
injuries, 171–172
damage control for vascular
injuries, 172–173
fasciotomy, 174
shunts, 172–173
transfusions, 174–178
triage and evaluation of
casualties, 170–171
hypothermia prevention in, 167–168
improved helmets and body armor in,
158–159
intraosseous access in, 164–165
needle thoracostomy in, 163–164
pain medications in, 165
prehospital concepts in, 168–170
casualty evacuation, 169–170
permissive hypotension, 168–169
triage guidelines, 168
tourniquets in, 159–161
training in, 179–180

Monro-Kellie doctrine, of management, for
increased intracranial pressure, 122,
123

Morphine, in military surgery, 165

Motor system assessment, in central
nervous system injuries, 128

Multi–drug-resistant infections, in military
surgery, 166

N

Needle thoracostomy, in military surgery,
163–164

Nerve block, continuous peripheral, in
military surgery, 165

Neurologic response, to hypothermia, 250

Neuromuscular blocking agents
for increased intracranial pressure, 143
in prehospital airway management, 39

Neutrophil function, fluid resuscitation and,
58–59

Noncontact laser Doppler imaging, in burn
care, 186

Normal saline, in prehospital circulation
management, 43

Nosocomial infections, in elderly, intensive
care and, 238

O

Orthopedic injuries, trauma care for, in
children, 217–218

Oxandrolone, to modulate
hypermetabolism, in burn patients,
194–195

Oxygen consumption, in hypothermia, 249

P

Pain management, in military surgery, 165

Pancreatic injuries, trauma care for, in
children, 222

Parkland formula, in fluid resuscitation, in
burn care, 189–190

Pelvic fractures, trauma care for
in children, 217
in elderly, 236–238

Penetrating brain injuries, trauma care for,
152–153

Pentobarbital coma, for increased
intracranial pressure, 145, 147

Pericardial tamponade, trauma care for, 103

Perihilar injuries, trauma care for, 107–108

Permissive hypotension, in military surgery, 168–169

Pernio, trauma care for, 257, 263

Plain films, in trauma care, in children, 212–213, 216

Plasma
in fluid resuscitation, 65
in military surgery, 175, 176

Plasma exchange, in fluid resuscitation, in burn care, 191

Pneumothorax, tension, in combat casualties, needle thoracostomy for, 163–164

Polyheme, in prehospital circulation management, 45

Polypropylene mesh, in damage control laparotomy, 82–83

Posterior fossa lesions, trauma care for, 151

Posterolateral thoracotomy, for thoracic trauma, 100–101

Prehospital care, 26, **37–53**
airway management in, 38–41
endotracheal intubation in, 39
for traumatic brain injury, 39–31
neuromuscular blocking agents in, 39
rapid sequence induction in, 39–41
circulation management in, 42–45
choice of fluid for, 43
for traumatic brain injury, 43–45
hypertonic resuscitation in, 43–45
intraosseous access in, 43
intravenous fluids in, 42–43
fluid resuscitation in, 56–57
for disability/spinal injury, 45–46
historical aspects of, 37
in children, 210–211
in combat casualties. *See* Military surgery.
triage system in, 46–48
withholding or terminating treatment in, 47–48
ventilation in, 41–42

Pulmonary artery catheter, in hemodynamic monitoring, in elderly, 238–239

Pulmonary contusions, trauma care for, in children, 218

Pulmonary embolism, prevention of, in burn patients, 193–194

Pulmonary injuries. *See* Thoracic trauma.

Pupillary reactions, in central nervous system injuries, 128

Pyrexia
with secondary brain injury, 121–122
with traumatic brain injury, 143

Q

QuikClot dressings, in military surgery, 162

R

Rapid sequence induction, in prehospital airway management, 39–41

Reconstructive surgery, in burn care, 196–197

Red blood cell transfusions, in military surgery, 174, 175, 176

Rehabilitation centers, in trauma systems, 29

Renal injuries, trauma care for, in children, 221–222

Reperfusion injury
and compartment syndromes, 76
in frostbite, 259

Respiratory drive, in hypothermia, 249–250

Right thoracotomy, for thoracic trauma, 101

S

Shunts, in military surgery, 172–173

Skin grafts
in burn care, 188–189
in damage control laparotomy, 85–86

Skull fractures, depressed, trauma care for, 151–152

Sodium bicarbonate, prophylactic, for secondary compartment syndrome, 79

Spinal cord injuries, trauma care for, in children, 215–217

Spinal immobilization devices, in prehospital care, 45–46

Spinal injuries
prehospital care for, 45–46
trauma care for, in children, 215–217

Splenic injuries, trauma care for
in children, 220–221
in elderly, 235–236

Steroids, for spinal injuries, in children, 217

Subarachnoid hemorrhage, computed
    tomography of, 133
Subdural hematomas
    computed tomography of, 131
    trauma care for, 150–151
Subxiphoid pericardial window, in trauma
    care, 103
Sundt shunts, in military surgery, 173
Sympathectomy, for frostbite, 261

T

Technetium-99m bone scintigraphy, to
    determine tissue viability, in frostbite,
    262–263
Tension pneumothorax, in combat casualties,
    needle thoracostomy for, 163–164
Testosterone analogs, to modulate
    hypermetabolism, in burn patients,
    194–195
Thermal Angel, in hypothermia prevention,
    in combat casualties, 167
Thermal injuries. *See* Burns.
Thoracic aorta, rupture of. *See* Thoracic
    trauma.
Thoracic trauma, **95–118**
    cardiac injuries, 102–104
    delayed thoracotomy for, 112–113
    emergency department thoracotomy
        for, 95–97
        hemopericardium and, 97
    esophageal injuries, 110–111
    exploratory thoracotomy for, 102
    great vessel injuries, 104–106
        choice of incision for, 105
        stab wounds, 105
    in children, 218–219
    pulmonary injuries, 106–108
        deep lobar, 107
        perihilar, 107–108
    rupture of thoracic aorta, 111–112
        beta blockade for, 111
        plain films of, 111
    tracheobronchial injuries, 108–110
        endotracheal intubation for, 109
        fallen lung sign in, 108
    urgent thoracotomy for, 97–102
        clam shell incision in, 101–102
        incision selection for, 98, 100–102
        indications for, 97–98
        left thoracotomy in, 101
        median sternotomy in, 100
        posterolateral thoracotomy in,
            100–101

right thoracotomy in, 101
Thoracostomy, needle, in military surgery,
    163–164
Thoracotomy, for thoracic trauma.
    See Thoracic trauma.
Thrombocytopenia, heparin-induced, in
    burn patients, 193–194
Thromboembolic disease, prevention of, in
    burn patients, 193–194
Thrombolytic therapy, for frostbite, 261
Tourniquets, in military surgery, 159–161
Tracheobronchial injuries. *See* Thoracic
    trauma.
Tracheostomy, for inhalation burn injuries,
    192–193
Transfusions
    for anemia, in burn patients, 193
    for traumatic brain injury, 141
    in military surgery, 174–178
Trauma care
    damage control laparotomy in.
        See Damage control laparotomy.
    fluid resuscitation in. *See* Fluid
        resuscitation.
    for burns. *See* Burns.
    for central nervous system injuries. *See*
        Central nervous system injuries.
    for cold injuries. *See* Cold injuries.
    for thoracic trauma. *See* Thoracic
        trauma.
    global perspective on, 1–2, 7–16
        Essential Trauma Care Project
            in, 8–16
            foundations of, 8–9
            future steps in, 15–16
            *Guidelines for Essential
                Trauma Care* in, 10–13
            international public health
                in, 9
            rights of the injured in, 11
            trauma system development
                in, 9
        progress in implementing
            essential trauma care, 13–14
            in Ghana, 14
            in India, 14
            in Mexico, 15
            in Sri Lanka, 15
            in Vietnam, 15
    in children, **207–228**
        agricultural accidents and, 209
        airway management in, 210–211
        alcohol-related accidents and,
            210

all-terrain vehicle accidents and,
    208–209
firearm accidents and, 210
for abdominal injuries, 219–222
    kidneys, 221–222
    liver, 220
    pancreas, 222
    spleen, 220–221
for maltreatment, 222
for orthopedic injuries, 217–218
for spinal and spinal cord
    injuries, 215–217
for thoracic injuries, 218–219
for traumatic brain injury,
    214–215
initial evaluation in, 211–214
    airway, 211
    computed tomography, 213
    fluid resuscitation, 212
    focused abdominal
        sonography for
        trauma, 212–213
    imaging, 212–213
    intravenous access, 211–212
injury prevention in, 208–210
    automobile restraints in,
        209–210
prehospital care in, 210–211
recovery phase in, 222–223
in elderly, **229–245**
    advance directives and health
        care proxies in, 239
    anticoagulation and, 232–234
    beta-blockers and, 232
    case report of, 229
    definition of geriatric trauma, 230
    epidemiology of aging in,
        229–230
    for abdominal injuries, 235–236
    for head injuries, 234–235
    for pelvic and extremity
        fractures, 236–238
    intensive care in, 238–239
        and nosocomial infections,
            238
        echocardiography in, 239
        hemodynamic monitoring
            in, 238–239
    life support in, withdrawing and
        withholding, 240–241
    long-term functional outcome in,
        239
    mechanisms of injury, 230
    physiologic reserve and, 232
    predictors of morbidity and
        mortality, 230–231
        age, 230–231
        comorbidities, 231
        severity of injury, 231

triage in, age as criterion for,
    231–232
in military. *See* Military surgery.

Trauma systems, **21–35**
    acute care facilities, 28
    communication systems in, 26
    components of, 24–25
    criteria for, 24
    definition of, 21
    development of, 9, 24
    evaluation of, 29
    historical aspects of, 21–24
    human resources in, 25
    Level I centers in, 27–28
    Level II centers in, 28
    Level III centers in, 28
    Level IV centers in, 28
    medical direction in, 26
    performance of, analysis of, 31–32
    prehospital care in. *See* Prehospital
        care.
    preventable deaths in, 30–31
    problems in, 32
    public information and education in,
        25
    quality improvement in, 29–30
    rehabilitation centers in, 29
    report card on, 32–33
    specialty centers in, 28
    standardized definition of errors in,
        30–31
    triage and transport in, 26–27

Traumatic brain injury. *See also* Central
    nervous system injuries.
    and hypotension, 121
    trauma care for, 119, 121, 128, 129,
        134–150
        airway management in, 135
        before intensive care unit,
            139–140
        cerebrospinal fluid drainage in,
            143
        circulation management in, 137
        decompressive craniectomy in,
            147, 148
        evidence-based, 134–135
        for cerebrospinal fluid rhinorrhea
            and otorrhea, 149–150
        for intracranial hypertension,
            141, 143, 145
        for pyrexia, 143
        Glasgow Coma Scale in, 128
        hyperosmolar therapy in, 143,
            145
        hyperventilation in, 143, 147
        hypothermia in, 147
        in children, 214–215
        in intensive care unit, 140–141

Traumatic (*continued*)
    intracranial pressure monitoring
        in, 139–141, 143, 145, 147, 149
    neurologic status in, 137
    neuromuscular blocking agents
        in, 143
    patient observation in, 150
    pentobarbital coma in, 145, 147
    prehospital airway management
        for, 39–41
    prehospital circulation
        management for, 43–45
    prophylactic anticonvulsants in,
        141
    second-tier therapy in, 145, 147
    therapeutic hypothermia in, 252
    transfusions in, 141
    trephination in, 148–149

Trench foot, trauma care for, 257–258

Trephination, for increased intracranial
    pressure, 148–149

Triage
    in combat casualties, 168, 170–171
    in prehospital care, 46–48
        withholding or terminating
            treatment in, 47–48
    in trauma care, 26–27
        age as criterion in, 231–232

Truncal injuries, damage control for, in
    military surgery, 171–172

U

Urgent thoracotomy, for thoracic trauma.
    See Thoracic trauma.

V

Vacuum pack technique, in damage control
    laparotomy, 83–84

Vascular injuries, damage control for, in
    military surgery, 172–173

Ventilation
    for inhalation burn injuries, 192
    for traumatic brain injury, 135
    in prehospital care, 41–42

Ventral hernia, planned, in damage control
    laparotomy, 84

W

Warfarin, and trauma care, in elderly,
    232–234

White blood cell function, fluid
    resuscitation and, 59

Whole blood, in fluid resuscitation, 65

Z

Zeolite dressings, in military surgery, 162

Moving?

Make sure your subscription moves with you!

To notify us of your new address, find your **Clinics Account Number** (located on your mailing label above your name), and contact customer service at:

E-mail: elspcs@elsevier.com

800-654-2452 (subscribers in the U.S. & Canada)
407-345-4000 (subscribers outside of the U.S. & Canada)

Fax number: 407-363-9661

Elsevier Periodicals Customer Service
6277 Sea Harbor Drive
Orlando, FL 32887-4800

*To ensure uninterrupted delivery of your subscription, please notify us at least 4 weeks in advance of move.

ELSEVIER